Testing Baby

Critical Issues in Health and Medicine

Edited by Rima D. Apple, University of Wisconsin–Madison,
and Janet Golden, Rutgers University, Camden

Growing criticism of the U.S. health care system is coming from consumers, politicians, the media, activists, and healthcare professionals. Critical Issues in Health and Medicine is a collection of books that explores these contemporary dilemmas from a variety of perspectives, among them political, legal, historical, sociological, and comparative, and with attention to crucial dimensions such as race, gender, ethnicity, sexuality, and culture.

For a list of titles in the series, see the last page of the book.

Testing Baby

The Transformation of Newborn Screening, Parenting, and Policy Making

Rachel Grob

Rutgers University Press

New Brunswick, New Jersey, and London

Library of Congress Cataloging-in-Publication Data

Grob, Rachel, 1966–
    Testing baby : the transformation of newborn screening, parenting, and policymaking /
Rachel Grob.
        p. ; cm.—(Critical issues in health and medicine)
    Includes bibliographical references and index.
    ISBN 978–0-8135–5135–7 (hardcover : alk. paper)—ISBN 978–0-8135–5136–4
(pbk. : alk. paper)
    1. Newborn infants—Diseases—Diagnosis. 2. Medical screening. I. Title.
II. Series: Critical issues in health and medicine.
    [DNLM: 1. Infant, Newborn—United States. 2. Neonatal Screening—United States.
3. Health Policy—United States. 4. Parents—United States. WS 420]
    RJ255.5.G76 2011
    362.198′9201—dc22

                                                        2010049959

A British Cataloging-in-Publication record for this book is available from the British Library.

Visit our Web site: http://rutgerspress.rutgers.edu

Manufactured in the United States of America

This book is dedicated to my children, Jonah and Talia,
who inspire me every day.

Contents

Acknowledgments

What draws me most compellingly to the discipline of sociology is its fundamental claim that context matters. This seems such a self-evident observation, yet I continue to marvel at how profound an insight it really is. And never has the structural power of my own life context been demonstrated to me more concretely than during the process of researching and writing this book. I could never have completed it without the advice, support, and encouragement of the family members, friends, teachers, interviewees, and colleagues who have formed my own personal context.

The parents who volunteered to be interviewed for my study gave generously of their time. They also shared intimate feelings, thoughts, and ideas. I am grateful to all of them, and I wish them and their children all the very best. I also thank the newborn screening administrators who allowed my colleagues and me to interview them.

Barbara Katz Rothman has been magnificent in every way. Practical advisor, partner in our Robert Wood Johnson Investigator Award, fellow mother, friend, role model as public sociologist—Barbara is all of this and more. Jack Levinson was been with me through every stage of my intellectual life, and our now decades-long dialogue continues to shape my thinking and to give me great pleasure. Thanks are due also to Martine Hackett.

I am hugely grateful to Diane Paul and Ellen Clayton, who both read the entire manuscript and offered insightful feedback.

My friends and colleagues at Sarah Lawrence College have provided me with support of many kinds. Marsha Hurst (now at Columbia), Caroline Lieber, Linwood Lewis, Sarah Wilcox, Laura Weil, Constance Peterson, Laura Long, Rebecca Johnson, and others have spent many hours with me talking through a wide range of conceptual, practical, ideological, and technical issues directly or indirectly related to *Testing Baby*. Human Genetics students Vicki Lyus, Meenakshi Mahi, and Karina Achrich provided skillful and patient research assistance of many kinds for my early research, and students Vicki Lyus, Shawna Irish, and Kathleen Erskine all did a terrific job transcribing interviews. Nicole Zolofra and Tracey Thomas (at Yale University) also assisted with the manuscript in various ways. Barbara Robb provided expert assistance with the newborn-screening program administrator interviews and several other aspects of this research, and also assisted greatly with preparing the manuscript for publication: very special thanks and acknowledgment to her for all of this. Human Genetics students Jessica Giordano, Alison Janson, and Emily Place were skilled research assistants for the media analysis discussed in chapter 5, and my thinking benefited from discussions with them. The Child Development Institute's Faculty Group (Abigail Canfield, Lorayne Carbon, Jan Drucker, Cheryl French, Barbara Schecter, and Sara Wilford) provided an intellectual home for me at Sarah Lawrence, and I am grateful to all my colleagues there. I want also to thank the Dean's Office for funding to assist with manuscript preparation.

This work was funded primarily by a grant from the Robert Wood Johnson Foundation's Investigator Awards program in health policy research. I thank the foundation and the national program office for their investment in my project, and for nourishing the community of investigators I have now been privileged to join. Conversations with Beatrix Hoffman, Nancy Tomes, Eugene DeClerque, Betsy Armstrong, Joe Finns, Lori Andrews, and others have improved *Testing Baby* in many ways. Mark Peterson is generous with advice of all kinds and has become a treasured friend.

My family is unfailingly wonderful, but knowing that they are always here for me does not make me any less appreciative. My dad, Lenny Grob, has been an example all my life of the ideal intellectual—someone who approaches each endeavor with passion and rigor but who never forgets that his work must ultimately be in the service of generosity, inclusiveness, and kindness. Many thanks also to Lenny (Papa) and dear Susan (Spooz) for spending time with my children during some crucial times when I needed to write. My husband Andy's mother, Lucy Noyes, gave me the incredible gift of time to write at her lovely house in Mexico. Thanks to her and Dick Hopkins.

My mother, Naomi Grob, deserves a paragraph all her own. Since this is one of the only paragraphs in *Testing Baby* that will not benefit from her skillful editing, I cannot dare hope it will convey more than a fraction of my gratitude to and love for her—but here goes. Naomi truly joined me inside this book. She carefully read the entire thing once it was drafted; talked with me about it in depth (or sometimes just listened); told me how interesting, moving, and important it was; and helped hone the prose in innumerable ways. The editing work we did together was nothing short of joyful; I treasure already the memory of every late-night session.

Andy has been steadfast, patient, and generous—as ever—throughout this process. He never failed to encourage me; to tell me it was fine for me to go write despite the dishes in the sink or laundry in the basket; to talk with me about my latest interview, idea, or epiphany. The intellectual friendship we began more than twenty years ago in the Science in Society Program reading room at Wesleyan continues to bear very precious fruit, held as it is within the larger, multidimensional, always-growing framework of our lives together. I know well that the collective energy we had to focus on *Testing Baby* has meant putting on hold other adventures and other priorities. That Andy could make this sacrifice without begrudging it one iota is a true act of love, and also a true testament to his generosity and goodness.

The last words here are for Mark Schlesinger. I acknowledge in the text itself his most tangible contributions to *Testing Baby*, as a partner in some of the research presented in chapter 5. Here, I want to express something different. Over the last four years, Mark and I have been in continuous discussion (most often in person, but other times by e-mail or phone) about issues that matter deeply to both of us: how policy making can be made more participatory; how research can be simultaneously rigorous and imaginative; how engaged scholarship can best be nurtured in ourselves, our students, and our community. Mark's conviction that the work I have done for *Testing Baby matters*, his confidence in my ability to write about it with the nuance it deserves, and his eagerness to talk through with me so many evolving thoughts have meant more to me than I can easily express. His faith—bestowed so lightly, yet so completely—has been nothing short of transformative.

Testing Baby

Chapter 1

Saving Babies, Changing Lives

Within forty-eight hours after birth, the heel of every baby in the United States has been pricked and the blood sent to a laboratory. There it will be tested for the many disorders the baby's birth state has mandated for universal screening. Almost always without parental consent, and often without parental knowledge or understanding, the newborn's blood is analyzed for molecular clues to her future. Many of these tests do what the highly regarded newborn-screening public health program was originally intended to do: provide information that, if acted on quickly, can be used to protect the infant's health or even to save her life. Others have much more complex or indeterminate consequences. Some identify variants that may in fact never cause manifest signs or symptoms. Others find mutations that will result in serious or fatal disease for which there is as yet no cure. And in almost all cases, these tests provide information about what at the time of screening are abstractions: genetic traits that have not yet been expressed and will not result in recognizable effects for weeks, months, years, or—for those who are most fortunate—ever.

Mandatory, population-wide screening for noninfectious disease is unprecedented in U.S. public health. Until the mid 1960s, it did not exist. Yet by a decade later, every state had begun newborn screening. Why? Largely because advocates compellingly argued that immediate identification of phenylketonuria (PKU)—a serious, early-onset, treatable genetic condition—was the only way to prevent death or permanent disability for affected babies. Newborn screening (NBS) programs continue today, and they do indeed save lives. But they have expanded to cover not just one but up to eighty-plus genetic disorders, many of which are neither classifiable nor treatable in straightforward ways, and with this expansion have come increasingly to *change lives.* This book is about those changes.

By design, population screening seeks evidence of disease processes before the onset of symptoms. Every member of the group is tested, regardless of whether symptoms of any kind have been shown or specific identifiable risks carried. Most of us have participated in screening programs of one sort or another in the context of primary health care: our blood pressure is routinely taken, for example, and our cholesterol levels measured. Yet as NBS programs grew exponentially at the beginning of the new century, with more and more parents inevitably receiving abnormal results with less and less clear implications for their child's health, I wondered about the impact of this particular kind of universal screening on families, on identity, and on the role of genetic information in health care and in society at large.

I have given birth myself, so I know both from experience and from what I have heard and read how momentous, complicated, and overwhelming those first weeks after birth can be. What is the effect of genetic diagnosis, I wanted to know, when it comes before parents have gotten to know their infant? How might this news shape parenting roles and perceptions of the baby differently from diagnoses that come after the onset of symptoms? How is newborn screening altering the experience, for affected families, of medically defined disease as distinct from the social experience of lived illness? I also wondered how relationships between families and health care providers would unfold in the wake of an abnormal screen. Professional expertise is already a powerful influence on many parents as they navigate their new responsibilities and identities after childbirth. How might the role of expertise be altered for families with an NBS diagnosis, who get the news so close to birth and who have not, in most cases, been meaningfully engaged in decisions to conduct the screening procedure in the first place?

I could tell right away that these were good questions when I began asking them of parents whose children were diagnosed with cystic fibrosis. Parents wanted to talk—in detail—about their experiences with diagnostic processes. They told me their rich, complicated, and often heartbreaking stories with very little prompting, pouring out narrative accounts full of just the kinds of nuanced testimony that qualitative researchers hope to have the privilege of hearing.

If you had asked me back then what sort of book might emerge from my inquiry, I would have imagined a volume devoted solely to answering legal scholar Ellen Clayton's trenchant yet long-ignored plea that researchers find out how NBS programs actually "feel to those they touch" (Clayton 1992b, 94). But before long, I came to understand that my questions about how newborn screening influences people's lives were impossible to separate from a corollary inquiry: how have parents' experiences, actions, and perspectives influenced NBS itself—both its actual practices and public perceptions about it? In pursuit of answers to this latter set of questions, I began to explore why it is that certain narratives about screening have become dominant in policy discourse while others have remained almost completely unexplored—and how it is that a cacophony of opinions about NBS has made it difficult to stand back and learn about experiences with it. These questions led me to undertake, in partnership with my colleague Mark Schlesinger and with expert assistance from Barbara Robb, another set of primary interviews—this time with those who direct state NBS programs. Mark Schlesinger and I also conducted, with assistance from graduate students Jessica Giordano, Alison Janson, and Emily Place, a content analysis of NBS's media coverage in the United States and in the Commonwealth countries.

Recently, newborn screening has expanded so rapidly, in fact so exponentially, that physician Rodney Howell likened it some years ago to a house on fire (Grob, forthcoming; Kolata 2005). A number of important factors have driven this rise, including technological innovation, political opportunity, interstate rivalries, and competitive pressure on state programs from private laboratories. It has also been substantially influenced by parent advocates who argue with great heart and forceful emotion that their own child was, or could have been, saved by NBS. These stories of tragedy suffered or averted are compelling beyond easy description. The devastation of suddenly losing a child—what pain could be greater for those who endure it, or loom larger in the imaginations of those who contemplate it? Only one thing, perhaps: learning afterward that the loss was needless because it could have been easily prevented.

Families whose children have died or been permanently disabled because the state in which they lived did not yet screen for a specific treatable disorder are in precisely this worst-case situation. To their enormous credit, many of them have gone public about these excruciating experiences in the hope that so doing might spare other families the same fate. As one couple-turned-NBS-advocates put it: "Although our lives will never be the same because losing Ben was so unnecessary and unacceptable, we are proud of Ben's impact on the future of children's health in our state."[1] "This should not have happened," says another parent, "[and] it shouldn't happen again to somebody else's child" (Waldholz 2004).

These narratives are hugely powerful. Powerful enough to bring tears to our eyes, and make us clutch tightly the living children we treasure. Powerful enough to convince some state health departments to expand their NBS panels without further ado (see chapter 5). And powerful enough, too, that they have often come to represent, in public discourse, the totality of parental experiences with NBS.

In a national context where newborn screening is best known for its initial aspiration to save lives and its laudable track record of doing so, and where the most insistent voices talking about screening are those of bereaved, grateful, or desperate parents, there is a reason why we don't understand much about how it also changes lives. After families with affected kids tell their "horrible stories," observed a public health official I interviewed for this book, there is "virtually nobody willing to speak" about any other aspect of the newborn screening experience.

Parents I interviewed for *Testing Baby* did speak, however—and I tried to listen very carefully. In extended qualitative interviews about their experiences having children, getting diagnoses, and coping with knowledge of genetic disorders, parents had a lot to say—some of it familiar, but much of it redolent with insights not given voice anywhere that I know of in the public domain. I do not offer their stories here to negate the importance of NBS's lifesaving and health-improving functions, or to attempt any sort of calculus of pain meant to delegitimize NBS's contributions to children's health—no. I offer these stories because like all forms of genetic testing—and indeed all kinds of health care— NBS is a complex social intervention, as well as a medical one. If we neglect to acknowledge that this is so, or we pretend it isn't for fear of undermining political commitment to the benefits screening offers, we lose the opportunity to understand the multidimensional consequences NBS has for families in the present, and to more fully anticipate where yet further expansion of the program may take us.

The experiences with NBS recounted in the next three chapters of this book reveal much about how—as sociologist Barbara Katz Rothman said of prenatal testing when it first came to the fore—"technological changes can force us to confront questions we never before faced, to see ourselves and each other in new ways" (1986, 3). Although some of the parents' stories highlight how newborn screening (like prenatal testing before it) creates problems as well as solutions, these chapters are not intended as a referendum on current NBS practice. Rather, they are an exploration of underexamined aspects of the current technological shift in childhood genetic diagnostics, and a mechanism for giving voice to a broader range of parental narratives about the consequences of this shift than is common in either the popular or the scientific literature.

The last two chapters of *Testing Baby* introduce other perspectives on NBS, and explicitly take up more value-laden questions—again not about the costs and benefits of newborn screening, but about the way discourse on this life-changing issue has been framed in the past and might best be usefully reframed as screening shifts away from its original lifesaving paradigm and as genetic technologies make it possible to test our babies in more and more ways right at birth.

Newborn Screening: A Historical Overview

Newborn screening procedures, defined here broadly as biochemical testing of an infant's blood to detect disorders, began in the mid 1960s when Dr. Robert Guthrie developed a test for phenylketonuria (PKU), a metabolic disease causing severe mental retardation but controllable with a phenylalanine-restricted diet introduced soon after birth (AAP 2000; Therrell 2001). The screen Guthrie created—which detects elevated phenylalanine levels by analyzing bacterial growth in a dried blood spot under specific chemical conditions—could be conducted shortly after birth using just a few drops of blood taken from the newborn's heel. Guthrie, who himself had a family member with PKU, worked tirelessly to make the test mandatory for newborns, taking his impassioned plea for NBS "directly to parents, politicians, and the press" (Paul 2008, 10). Children's advocacy groups, such as the Association for Retarded Citizens and the March of Dimes Birth Defects Foundation, were also outspoken advocates for universal screening. Within a few years, Guthrie and his allies had overcome the challenges of what he called—with considerable relish—a "hard sell" to gain acceptance for universal application of his assay (Guthrie 1996, S5). By the early 1970s, almost every state had passed a law to establish compulsory PKU screening at birth, making the heel stick a routine part of well-baby care in hospitals. With relatively little public attention or debate (Clayton 1992a), but with significant impetus from parent advocates (Paul 2008), newborn screening pioneered new terrain for U.S. medicine and public health: state-mandated diagnosis of noninfectious disease. Newborn screening systems were also developed in conjunction with the laboratory procedure itself, to provide notification to parents of abnormal results, follow-up, education of parents and clinicians, tracking, and a range of other services (see chapter 2).

Since the early 1970s, then, nearly every newborn in the United States—more than four million each year—has undergone screening. Since almost all the conditions detected by screening are considered genetic disorders, NBS has long been and remains far and away the single most widely utilized form of genetic testing in the United States (AAP 2000; Hiller, Landenburger, and Natowicz 1997; Paul 1999).[2] But until roughly the turn of the twenty-first century, the number of conditions states tested for with collected blood spots remained very small (Alexander and Hanson 2006). Decisions about what to include besides PKU have always been made—as they still are—at the state level. However, in an effort to provide guidance to states and to make the policy process more consistent and evidence-based, the World Health Organization, the National Academy of Sciences, the Institute of Medicine, the American Academy of Pediatrics, and various national task forces have developed iterative sets of recommended principles or guidelines since as early as 1968, often at the request of Congress (AAP 2000; ACMG 2005; Clayton 1992b; Downie and Wildeman 2001; Therrell 2001; U.S. GAO 2003; Watson 2006). Over time, these bodies have become more specific in their analyses and have taken into account the impact of ongoing technological changes in both screening capacity and treatment. But the core aspirations for screening, and the central criteria used to determine if a given condition was suitable for this public mandate, changed relatively little over newborn screening's first thirty-five years.

First, principles for decision making about candidate NBS conditions held that the screen must be clearly beneficial for the affected infant. James Wilson and Gunner Jungner, writing for the World Health Organization in 1968, were emphatic on this point with respect to screening tests in general, and their words have been quoted often in the forty years since they were published. "Of all the criteria that a screening test should fulfill," they write,

> the ability to treat the condition adequately, when discovered, is perhaps the most important. In adhering to the principle of avoiding harm to the patient at all costs (the *primum non nocere* of Hippocrates), treatment must be the first aim. For declared disease there is, of course, the ethical obligation to provide an accepted treatment whether or not this is of scientifically proved value; but, when new territory is being explored by the earlier detection of disease, it is clearly vital to determine by experimental surveys whether a better prognosis is given by treating the conditions found at an earlier stage than was previously the practice. (1968, 27–28)

Although Wilson and Jungner were writing about adult screening rather than NBS, most subsequent advisory panels have affirmed and reaffirmed this core principle (Andrews et al. 1994). NBS advisory panels also embraced a number of other principles set out in that seminal World Health Organization report: that conditions should be tested for only if they are relatively prevalent, if technology can identify the disorder with sufficient accuracy, if the costs incurred by identifying cases (for both diagnosis and treatment) is "balanced" by economic benefits of screening, if early detection and treatment are necessary to prevent substantial harm, if onset of symptoms is early, if the natural history of the condition is adequately understood, and if facilities for diagnosis and treatment are available (Therrell 2001). Wilson and Jungner's original principles also specified—though this particular aspiration received far less attention in subsequent reports or policy making—that "the test should be acceptable to the population to which it is offered," taking into serious account such considerations as the nature of the risk involved and how health education has "prepared the ground" for testing (Wilson and Jungner 1968, 31).

Through the end of the twentieth century, states did gradually expand screening to include additional conditions using the same spot of heel blood taken to test for PKU. But they added just a few more, and only those considered to satisfy the Wilson and Jungner criteria reasonably well—albeit usually not without substantial contestation, both before and after their adoption for NBS (Grosse et al. 2006; Paul 1997, 2008; Watson 2006). Congenital hypothyroidism was added in the late 1970s, followed by several metabolic disorders. And then came sickle cell disease, which states began screening for in the late 1980s, after research suggested that early treatment with penicillin could significantly improve affected children's health (Kolata 1987).

The New Newborn Screening

So why did NBS begin to grow so dramatically around the turn of the century? And what led programs to begin (or continue) shifting away from traditional NBS—which tested for (ostensibly) early-onset, reasonably predictable, treatable disorders—and toward what I will call here the "new NBS," which includes tests for disorders that clearly do not fit these criteria?[3] Many factors contributed, as I discuss with greater depth elsewhere. But here I will touch on just two of the three that I believe matter most: changing technology and changing conceptions of NBS's purpose. (The third, intensified parent advocacy, I explore more fully in chapter 5.)

So, first, technology. Until the 1990s, each new condition added to NBS panels necessitated a separate test. This meant that each also necessitated additional labor, additional cost, and its own share of the tiny collected blood spot. Enter a new technology, tandem mass spectrometry (MS/MS), and all this changed. MS/MS works by fragmenting and quantifying ions based on their mass/charge ratio—and it is able to accomplish many such separations all at once, in contrast to the one-at-a-time chromatography techniques of the past. As a result, MS/MS "permits very rapid, sensitive and . . . accurate measurement of many different types of metabolites with minimal sample preparation and without prior chromatographic separation" (ACMG/ASHG 2000, 267).

The advent of this new technology meant that suddenly a spot of newborn blood could in one fell swoop be analyzed quickly, and at very low cost, for metabolites associated with as many as fifty distinct gene mutations.

The families of conditions newly detectable by MS/MS included disorders of the metabolism, hemoglobin disorders, and disorders of the endocrine system. Early NBS conditions such as PKU and sickle cell disease are included among these. However, the new technology also made it possible to easily identify metabolites that "may not be associated with serious—or indeed any—clinical symptoms as well as conditions of low penetrance or where no effective treatment exists" (Paul 2008, 10). And as use of MS/MS technology spread (from thirteen states in 2002 to forty-nine states by 2007), so too did the number of conditions that states included in their mandatory screening panels.[4]

Meanwhile, another technological capacity with broad implications for NBS also advanced significantly: DNA analysis (also known as molecular genetic diagnosis). This form of testing, as the name implies, looks for DNA mutations directly instead of identifying proteins, metabolites, or other evidence of changes in body function that suggest an underlying genetic abnormality. When applied in the context of NBS, DNA testing is beginning to change things significantly. First, when molecular analysis is routinely done directly on the infant's blood spot, clinicians sometimes cease to view NBS as a screening process and instead treat DNA results as a presumptive diagnosis. As I explore in chapter 2, this is a substantial shift for a program that was designed to trigger a system of notification and follow-up testing in response to abnormal screening results rather than to deliver diagnoses directly to families.

Second, DNA testing is significant because it directly produces genetic information, and in the context of twenty-first-century U.S. culture this explanatory model automatically tends to be accorded more power than others. As Michael Green and Jeffrey Botkin observe in their analysis of genetic exceptionalism: "Right or wrong, genetic information is believed to reveal who we 'really' are, so information from genetic testing is often seen as more consequential than that from other sources" (2003, 572).

Third, and perhaps most significantly, molecular analysis is solidly on track to transform the future of NBS even more radically than MS/MS has already done. The DNA chip—a next iteration of diagnostic technology already in use in the private sector—will soon make possible additional, exponential expansion of NBS programs.[5] Chip technology is capable of identifying ten thousand alleles—ten thousand conditions (or perhaps just variations from the norm) that might be part of each baby's genetic makeup—and many believe it will soon be adapted for use in testing the blood of every U.S. infant

(ACOG 2003; Alexander and Hanson 2006; Alexander and van Dyck 2006; Bailey, Skinner, and Warren 2005; Lloyd-Puryear and Forsman 2002; Wilcken 2003). Under a scenario of "truly vast expansion"—a future for which a number of commentators confidently believe "the stage has been set"—infants would be "routinely screened at birth for almost all medically significant genetic markers (with a few conditions deliberately excluded), to be treated immediately when possible, and otherwise to be enrolled in registries to await trials of experimental therapies" (President's Council on Bioethics 2008, 55).

This vision for actualizing what Deborah Heath, Rayna Rapp, and Karen-Sue Taussig (2004) have characterized as the "increasingly screenable future" in the newborn period has been enthusiastically embraced by the National Institute of Child Health and Human Development, which is hard at work developing "a multiplex screening technology prototype for newborn screening" (Alexander and Hanson 2006, 302) capable of identifying "every medically significant genetic marker" (President's Council 2008, 54). If implemented, this plan for newborn screening would result in pediatricians (and parents) receiving "a complete map of each young patient's known genetic defects, vulnerabilities, and susceptibilities"—a veritable "newborn profile"—at each child's birth (55).

As MS/MS began to make testing for a vastly increased number of conditions not only technologically feasible but in fact the path of least resistance, and as DNA applications began to be employed for newborns, the paradigm guiding NBS decision making also started to shift. In 2005, the American College of Medical Genetics (ACMG) released its influential NBS report, "Newborn Screening: Toward a Uniform Screening Panel and System." This report had been commissioned by the federal Department of Health and Human Services to analyze the contemporary state of newborn screening (ACMG 2005, 7), and to formulate recommendations about how to standardize "outcomes and guidelines for state newborn screening programs" and thus reduce what were then large interstate variations in the number of conditions on state panels (Watson et al. 2006, S297).

The ACMG considered eighty-four candidate conditions for its "uniform panel." It concluded by recommending inclusion of fifty-four of these. Twenty-nine were categorized by ACMG as part of a "core" constellation that, according to their criteria and methodology, merited screening.[6] ACMG's own description of why it recommended nationwide screening for these twenty-nine suggests significant fidelity to Wilson and Jungner: in ACMG's judgment, each of the twenty-nine is identifiable within the first two days after birth via an appropriately specific and sensitive screening test, and early detection of each is linked

to "demonstrated benefits of early detection, timely intervention, and efficacious treatment" (Moyer et al. 2008, 36). Not everyone agrees. Critics argue that
the report asserts far more certainty about "the incidence of these abnormalities
and their natural history," and thus about the probability of direct benefit to the
child, than is warranted (37). Further, they point out that a European evidence-
based assessment of conditions screenable using MS/MS conducted just one
year before the ACMG report found that only two of the twenty possible metabolic disorders it can identify should be screened because "robust evidence on
the underlying incidence and outcomes for many of the disorders was lacking"
(President's Council on Bioethics 2008, 36–37, including quotation from Pandor
et al. 2004).

ACMG also recommended mandatory screening for twenty-five "secondary" targets that it acknowledged did not meet traditional Wilson and Jungner
criteria, but that either would be identified in the process of differential diagnosis for one of the core conditions, or could just be detected using the MS/MS
technology at its fullest capacity (President's Council on Bioethics 2008,
45; Watson 2006, S298). These conditions lack efficacious treatment, a well-
understood natural history, or both.

Creating what has come to function as a national NBS standard for many
states was thus not the only new ground forged by the ACMG report. Perhaps
even more notable was the way it broke decisively from earlier guidance by
considering "benefits to family and society"—rather than just direct benefits to
the child—as a central criterion for assessing whether a specific screen should
be mandated. When it recommended mandatory screening in every state for
conditions with no demonstrated treatment and/or poorly understood natural
history, the ACMG intentionally opened wide the door to continued expansion
of NBS panels based merely on whether testing for them is possible. The rationale for compulsory testing in the absence of direct benefit to the infant? That
families can "benefit from establishing that there may be a genetic risk to others
in the family" and society can "benefit by a reduction in medical diagnostic
odysseys that are costly to the healthcare system" (ACMG 2005, 493). In addition, and perhaps most significantly, "early information provides opportunity
for better understanding of disease history and characteristics, and for earlier
medical interventions that might be systematically studied to determine the
risks and benefits. Multiplex testing and the identification of conditions falling
outside of the uniform screening panel provides the opportunity for such
conditions to be included in research protocols" (Watson et al. 2006, S17).

Among the ACMG's considerations when assessing candidate NBS conditions, then, was the ability of mandatory population-wide screening to advance

biomedical research, to influence future reproductive decision-making for parents of screened children, and to identify diseases at birth (even if they are not early onset or preventable) so as to avoid a delayed diagnosis in clinical settings once symptoms begin to emerge. And the influence of this sea change in criteria extends well beyond the implementation of ACMG's uniform panel of fifty-four conditions recommended in 2005 and then almost universally adopted across the fifty states. What was codified with publication of that report was also a model methodology—contested (Baily and Murray 2008; Botkin et al. 2006; Moyer et al. 2008; President's Council on Bioethics 2008), yet still powerful—for assessing candidate conditions in the future, when technology is able to identify not just fifty or sixty but hundreds of thousands of genetic variants.[7] The "new paradigm" for NBS that some have called for (Alexander and Hanson 2006; Alexander and van Dyck 2006; Bailey et al. 2006) thus seems to have already arrived. As articulated by Duane Alexander and Peter van Dyck (2006, S351, S352), this means changing "the dogma that it is appropriate to screen only for conditions for which effective treatment already exists." That traditional tenet, they contend, "served a useful purpose in the early years of newborn screening, but it is now being challenged as outmoded because it fails to consider other benefits of diagnosis in the newborn period and dooms us to continued ignorance and unavailability of treatment because affected individuals are not identified until they exhibit symptoms, too late for effective preventive treatments to be tested or applied."[8]

The new NBS means more screening—a lot more. Just between 2004 and 2005, the average number of conditions screened for across the states rose from eight to twenty.[9] By 2009, the March of Dimes was proudly reporting that all fifty states mandated screening for at least twenty-one of the twenty-nine core ACMG conditions.[10] The majority also screen for most of the twenty-five so-called secondary conditions. New York's arrival, by late 2005, at a panel numbering forty-six soon became old news when California announced expansion of its NBS program to more than eighty tests, and Missouri boasted screening for seventy-two, including all five of the controversial lysosomal storage diseases (all very serious, and all with as-yet-unproven treatments). The number of true positive screens now produced by newborn screening each year has roughly tripled, from approximately 2,500 in the mid 1990s to roughly 7,500 by 2008.[11] In ways I describe in more detail later, abnormal NBS results also change the lives of hundreds of thousands of parents who receive unsolicited and unanticipated information about their baby (in the form of false positive results) via the mandatory screen.

Expanded NBS entails not only a vast increase in the number of parents receiving notification of abnormal screens, but also an accelerating change in the very nature of childhood diagnostics. Formerly, testing for a genetic disorder was initiated only after the emergence of symptoms had impelled a search to find the cause of physiological—or, to use the genetic term, "phenotypic"—problems. Genetic diagnosis, in such cases, is made only when a looked-for mutation in gene function coexists with manifest clinical signs in a particular person. Further, the very meaning of genetic disease X, in this diagnostic paradigm, is a combination of collection of symptoms Y and genetic mutation(s) Z.

Now, consider NBS. Here every infant—the entire healthy population—is screened for evidence of genetic disorders. But for each new test, a whole set of questions arises about the actual implications of an abnormal result—or, to again use the technical term, a particular "genotype." This is because although it may be clear that everyone with both symptoms and genetic mutation has genetic disease X, it cannot be known prospectively, in the absence of large-scale longitudinal research, if all people who have that same kind of genetic mutation will in fact develop symptoms. In other words, in the world of genetics, the fact that Y + Z = X in clinically diagnosed cases does not reliably mean that Z (mutation[s]) invariably causes Y (symptoms) and will therefore lead to X (disease) as formerly defined. To complicate things even further, Z might refer to not just one but a variety of mutations associated with a particular gene. Each of these mutations may have a different pattern of phenotypic influence. Each may also be modified by other genetic or environmental factors. When NBS for any new condition begins—and often long afterward—these complex patterns and probabilities are unlikely to be thoroughly understood.

Lack of predictive precision associated with presymptomatic diagnosis has been an issue from NBS's inception. Beginning with PKU, newborn screening's "'paradigm therapeutic case' of postnatal diagnosis and proof of the value of genetic medicine" (Paul 1998, 176, including quote from Kevles 1985, 254), it was not possible to accurately know what the severity of many NBS disorders would be in a particular child—or even to establish presence of the disease as classically defined (Watson 2006). As historian of science Diane Paul has documented in her case study, "PKU screening counts as a success" and has, at relatively low cost, "prevented mental retardation in thousands of infants worldwide" (1997, 138; see also Paul 2000). However, PKU screening is not an unqualified success. In addition to high rates of false-negative and false-positive test results, early PKU screening resulted in inappropriate diagnosis of babies with a relatively benign condition called hyperphenylalaninemia, and in exaggerated claims about "the ease and efficacy of treatment" (Paul 1997).

Uncertainty about the implications of positive screening results and follow-up testing has continued to grow with NBS's inclusion of a larger number of complex conditions, of disorders for which little natural history exists, and of new testing technologies. As ACMG's executive director himself noted: "Conditions being considered for newborn screening are increasingly difficult to define as the genetic basis for many of the conditions often subdivides the condition on the basis of the genes and the mutations within those genes that are involved in causing the condition" (Watson 2006, 231). When screening at birth relies on analytes of one kind or another—those signals that a gene disorder may exist based on enzyme or protein levels—it is not always clear where the cutoff value separating normal from abnormal results should be set. As a result, variation and uncertainty about which infants are considered screen positive and in need of further testing can occur (see chapter 4).

Nobody knows how many asymptomatic and mildly affected children will be identified via NBS over time, since the epidemiological data now being collected for the entire infant population has never before been available. As Virginia Moyer and her colleagues trenchantly observe, it is simply not possible to accurately predict for each condition "how many infants will be identified as having [it], and of those identified, how many will go on to develop noticeable symptoms. . . . Even when the natural history of clinically detected cases of a condition is known, the natural history for *screen-detected* cases is often poorly understood. Many children with screen-detected conditions may never develop clinically important morbidity and mortality, or they may be likelier to have milder cases than those who are detected clinically" (2008, 35).

What is clear, however, is that many of the conditions now screened for have complex and varied forms of phenotypic expression, and that asymptomatic and mildly affected children are being identified along with those expressing classical forms of tested disorders. In some cases, this occurs with the shift to population-level screening for conditions characterized by multiple mutations (some causing severe and others much more mild or undetectable symptoms), that are nonetheless considered to have had a fairly well understood natural history before NBS. Some of the metabolic disorders are examples: with newborn screening for these has come both (1) a higher overall number of cases diagnosed in the infant population than had been predicted based on clinically identified cases (presumably at least in part because the mild and asymptomatic cases in the unscreened general population never came to medical attention), and (2) screen-detected subgroups displaying much higher rates of mild mutations and lower rates of severe ones than the clinically diagnosed population (see, e.g., Waisbren et al. 2003). Cystic fibrosis (Wilcken et al. 2003) and the hemoglobinopathies are additional cases in point. As Scott Grosse and his colleagues document, screening for sickle-cell disease (SCD) is a "public health success" that has reduced mortality during the first three years of life for affected children. However, NBS for SCD and other hemoglobinopathies "results in the detection and reporting of multiple disorders and variants." Some of these "are benign, whereas other disorders are associated with mild outcomes or with severe outcomes that cannot be avoided with early treatment" (2006, 924). In other cases, NBS is initiated for a genetic mutation classified as a disorder and presumed to cause symptoms, but later determined decisively to be just a normal variant—though not necessarily before tens or hundreds of children have been diagnosed and treated (see, e.g., Brosco et al. 2010).[12]

Krabbe disease is another prime exemplar of diagnostic uncertainty—and one which merits a paragraph of its own since it and the family of disorders to which it belongs are arguably NBS's next frontier. The infantile form of Krabbe has always been considered fatal during early childhood, but experimental stem cell transplants in infancy are now reported to have had some success in delaying or preventing mortality (Knapp et al. 2009). Once symptoms emerge, however, it is too late for this treatment, so affected children must be identified at birth if they are to have the transplant opportunity. New York has had three years' experience conducting mandatory screening for Krabbe (as of 2010), and at least two other states are poised to begin. Data from New York illustrate, however, just how much uncertainty continues to surround screening. During the first three years of implementation, 140 infants screened positive and proceeded to diagnostic testing. Of these, thirty-six have been classified as "low risk," thirteen as "moderate risk," and seven as "high risk" for the infantile form of the disease that is the target of screening. Two of the seven high-risk infants have been diagnosed and referred for the transplant procedure: one survived and is being followed, and the other died shortly after the operation. Monitoring has been prescribed for the remaining fifty-four children, but it is not possible to "predict which, if any, of the moderate- and low-risk patients will become symptomatic" (20). The number of infants identified by NBS is "many times higher than the predicted incidence of Krabbe disease," but it is not at all clear what being identified through screening means for these children's lives. Clinicians acknowledge "the dilemma created by the identification of novel variants" but are clear that the level of uncertainty around Krabbe NBS means that "physicians are unable to provide prognostic information to parents of asymptomatic patients at the present time" (ibid.). For families of the fifty-four at-risk babies in New York, this means that the result of mandatory screening— at least for the moment—is that they have been informed their child may or may not develop symptoms indicating fatal disease, and instructed to follow up with medical specialists for routine monitoring. Whether early identification will produce better health outcomes for these children, if they do indeed become ill, remains to be seen.

The fluidity of the boundary that rules out and rules in disease classifications is arguably even more evident with the advent of increased molecular testing (Miller et al. 2005). Use of DNA analysis introduces a "seemingly definitive diagnostic resource" (ibid.) in clinical settings, since it places genetic material itself—rather than a byproduct produced through altered organism function—center stage. Leaders of the so-called genomic revolution have argued forcefully that reclassification of "all human illnesses on the basis of detailed molecular characterization" will result in a new taxonomy of illness "which would replace our present, largely empirical, classification schemes and advance both disease prevention and treatment" (Collins et al. 2003, 841). Indeed, many claim (as reported in the popular media) that DNA testing has brought us to "a unique position in the history of medicine to define human disease precisely, uniquely and unequivocally" (Pollack 2008).

However, despite the sophisticated achievements of bench science in mapping the entire human genome, it turns out that DNA does not present a straightforward or easily cracked code in terms of clinical implications (Khoury et al. 2007). In other words, the capacity that now exists to identify a staggering number of DNA variations rarely translates into an understanding of the implications those variations have for the health of individuals. Even proponents of increased DNA testing for NBS thus note that a "significant disadvantage" of this methodology is that "the correlation between the genetic mutation and the phenotype is not always well known" (Alexander and van Dyck 2006, S351–S352).

Representations and Research: Newborn Screening in the Popular, Scientific, and Social Science Literature

The rapid growth of NBS has been the focus of considerable research, commentary, and media attention—especially in the period leading up to and just after release of the ACMG report, throughout which the venerable March of Dimes carried out a sustained public campaign and media blitz advocating NBS expansion (Howse, Weiss, and Green 2006). "Newborn screening" has yet to become a household term, but it does have a significant public presence that frames parents' encounters with it—as well as researchers' approaches to it—in various ways.

Some stories in the popular media try to present a balanced view of the complex issues raised by expanded newborn screening. For example, Gina Kolata of the *New York Times* reported back in 2005 that "while no one argues with the idea of saving babies, [the ACMG]'s proposed [uniform panel of twenty-nine diseases] is generating fierce debate" because experts dispute both "whether treatments help" and "how often a baby will test positive but never show signs of serious disease." More and more public critiques and lawsuits focus on the use for research, without parental consent, of stored NBS blood spots. This issue has begun to generate significant negative U.S. media attention for the first time in NBS's history.[13] But even these controversies are about privacy concerns after NBS is completed rather than about the ethics or research-related functions of NBS itself.

The vast majority of articles on the web, in the popular press, and in the parenting literature do not capture the complexities of NBS in any substantial depth. Rather, they tell a simplified story that emphasizes the benefits of NBS and downplays its complexities (Grob and Schlesinger 2008). Most often, these pieces use firsthand stories about or by affected families to add emotional emphasis.[14] They begin with a heart-wrenching vignette about a baby whose death could have been prevented by newborn screening, or a heart-warming story about a baby who was saved by it. They then go on to talk about the failure of states to protect the public by expanding their mandatory panels, or about new tests that will make it possible to save yet more lives. This introductory text from an Associated Press piece entitled "Parents Seek Expanded Newborn Screening" is illustrative: "Debra Gara held 9-month-old Cristal in her arms, singing her to sleep, and then dozed off herself. An hour later, she awoke with a start to find her baby ice-cold and not breathing. An autopsy diagnosed a rare metabolic disease, one treatable if Cristal's parents had known—and one of more than 40 genetic and metabolic disorders that can be diagnosed easily at birth."[15]

Headlines of similar articles proclaim, with little content to balance bold claims in the lead lines, that "early screening will save lives," that "few states offer adequate newborn screening," and that "early tests can reduce later problems."[16] Even stories focused on controversial issues related to NBS, such as the storage and use of infants' blood spots, continue to describe the program itself in terms of its original mission, with little or no reference to unintended consequences or to the new NBS. Rob Stein's recent piece in the *Washington Post* provides an example: "Hospitals prick the heels of more than 4 million babies born each year in the United States to collect a few drops of blood under state programs requiring that all newborns be screened for dozens of genetic disorders. The programs enable doctors to save lives and prevent permanent neurological damage by diagnosing and treating the conditions early" (Stein 2009).

Sociologist Peter Conrad has noted that the media's overall coverage of genetics suggests an overly deterministic view of genetic contributions to illness, downplaying complexities such as gene/gene and gene/environment interactions. Coverage also disproportionately focuses on success stories, without counterbalancing examples of "failures" or "disconfirmations." His conclusion that the media therefore reinforce the "idea that genetics can explain more of the world than it can" certainly appears to hold true for press coverage of newborn screening (1997, 149).[17]

The medical and public health literatures also tend toward a favorable view of newborn screening, and toward endorsing screening program expansion (see, e.g., Arn 2007; Goodwin et al. 2002; Wright, Brown, and Davidson-Mundt 1992). It's not hard to see why this is so. PKU screening is widely acknowledged to have prevented mental retardation in thousands of newborns, and this success story is almost universally—and rightly—regarded as a huge win for public health. Pediatricians and other clinicians speak with pride and generosity about the good work that has been accomplished by newborn screening. "Our ability to identify affected newborn infants, when totally asymptomatic," writes one prominent physician, "and institute programs and treatments that prevent serious morbidity and mortality is a great privilege" (Howell 2006b, 1800).

Further, as the first decade of the new millennium comes to a close, NBS is arguably a prime example of the way much-touted genetic research is being "translated" from bench science to tangible improvements in population health (Khoury et al. 2007)—even though NBS's original success with PKU and other metabolic disorders predated the mapping of the human genome and other advances in genetic research. Many predicted benefits of the $2.7 billion Human Genome Project have yet to materialize, such as gene therapy, personalized medicine, and the promised $100 whole-body DNA scan. But newborn-screening programs are different. Here, despite NBS's origins in public health rather than genetics, the promise of genetic medicine has indeed been matched at the bedside, where screening can so dramatically save lives and improve health. As the literature often sums it up, NBS is "a triumph of medicine and public policy in the U.S. over the last 50 years"—a model program that "represents one of the major advances in child health of the past century" and is now growing up in the genomic era of expanded screening (Brosco, Seider, and Dunn 2006, 4; Arn 2007, 559).

At the same time, a number of problematic issues continue to be raised by practitioners, researchers, and analysts who publish in the clinical literature, and—even more commonly—in public policy and bioethics. One recurrent worry is that children who are being promptly diagnosed by newborn screening don't then have adequate access to follow-up services and ongoing treatment, since no guaranteed right to health care complements the mandatory

diagnosis. Another is that states have inadequate capacity for genetic counseling and health education in connection with the screening process, and for
treating the increasingly large number of disorders being identified. Lack of
parental informed consent is repeatedly cited as problematic, and this criticism
grows more intense as the vast expansion of panels makes it increasingly difficult to justify mandated screening on the basis of an exigent need to protect
the child. Inadequate protection of genetic information gathered by newborn
screening is yet another concern, particularly with respect to insurance coverage, future employment, and confidentiality. Critics also raise questions about
the ethics and legality of implementing mandatory testing that then acts as a
back door for giving parents unsought (and potentially unwanted) genetic
information they might or might not have voluntarily consented to obtain in the
form of prenatal testing (Annas 1982; Botkin et al. 2006; Clayton 1992a; CDC
2004; Downie and Wildeman 2001; Hoff and Hoyt 2005; Mehlman and Botkin
1998; Moyer et al. 2008; Nelson et al. 2001; Paul 1999; President's Council on
Bioethics 2008; Therrell 2001; Warren et al. 1982).

The vast majority of research in the field of newborn screening has been
designed to determine whether testing produces tangible benefits for children
in terms of clinical outcomes, and for families by reducing the stress caused
by undiagnosed symptoms. However, researchers have also increasingly sought
to examine some of the unintended consequences for families of this broad-
reaching policy, whose intended consequence is the prevention and avoidance
of disease.

The high rate of false-positive screening results has been one of NBS's
most problematic ancillary effects since the inception of screening. The impact
of this unintended consequence of NBS is an issue more thoroughly researched
than most—although even this "most obvious" potentially harmful byproduct
of screening had been investigated "only a few times" over the thirty years of
NBS's history (Wilcken et al. 2003, 2311; Wilcken 2003, S64) and began receiving more serious attention only over the last decade (Gurian et al. 2006; Hewlett
and Waisbren 2006; Lipstein et al. 2009; Prosser et al. 2008; Tarini, Christakis,
and Welch 2006; Waisbren et al. 2003). False positives are defined as "initial
out-of-range screening results that do not signify a . . . disorder on further evaluation of the child. Generally, these are not laboratory errors, but rather transient findings" (Waisbren et al. 2003, 2565).

The rate of false positives is astoundingly high. The overall average is difficult
to calculate because of differences in technology and laboratory practices among
programs, but the rate has been estimated to be between eight and sixty false
positives for every true positive (Hewlett and Waisbren 2006; Prosser et al. 2008).

One study has determined that nationally, NBS using MS/MS produces tens of thousands of false positives annually (Tarini, Christakis, and Welch 2006)—and statistics compiled by the National Newborn Screening Information System suggest the number now well exceeds 100,000. For some specific conditions, such as congenital adrenal hyperplasia and galactosemia, the rate has been more than two hundred false positives for each confirmed case (Goodwin et al. 2002, 165). Maple syrup urine disease presents another dramatic example, with only 18 of 1,249 abnormal NBS results representing a true positive for the condition (President's Council 2008, 14). For cystic fibrosis, with the screening method most commonly used, only eight of every one hundred infants who screen positive will be diagnosed with the disorder, ten will be identified as unaffected carriers, and the remaining eighty-two will be false positives (Duff and Brownlee 2008, 24). It thus continues to be the case, despite improved technology, that for every infant confirmed to have a genetic disorder, many, many parents will be notified of an abnormal screen and will undergo the worry and suffering of subsequent testing, only to find out that their child is not affected.

Some parents with false positives will be told simply that the result was erroneous, a mistake that indicates nothing whatsoever about their child's health. Other parents will learn as a result of screening that their child (and thus one of them as well) is a carrier of a single mutated gene. According to conventional genetic medicine, this would mean that the child will remain without symptoms, since two copies of the gene are necessary to produce the condition. However, such children will be at risk for passing on the gene—and the disorder, if their partner is also a carrier—to their own offspring.[18] In either case, this effect of NBS programs on families is not consistent with the programs' stated mission to improve infants' health or with the recommendations of a number of prominent expert advisory panels (Andrews et al. 1994).

In discussions, debates, commentaries, and research studies, the stress and expense caused by false-positive screening results are consistently cited as a serious unsolved problem associated with NBS programs. The high rate of false positives has been called "perhaps the single major drawback to newborn screening" (Goodwin et al. 2002, 165). As summarized in Centers for Disease Control workgroup proceedings in the late 1990s: "The greatest harms [associated with screening] may be transient distress or long-term confusion among families who have infants with false-positive results on screening tests" (CDC 1997, 10).

These worries are not idle. Some research demonstrates that, even after follow-up tests indicate to the satisfaction of clinicians that an infant's health is not imperiled, parents receiving false-positive results experience increased anxiety levels, remain more vigilant overall, and take their children to emergency departments for a disproportionate number of visits (Clayton 1992b; Gurian et al. 2006; Lipstein et al. 2009; Tluczek et al. 2005; Waisbren et al. 2003).[19] A Swedish study found that three of four families who got false-positive newborn screen results had strong reactions at the time they received the news, and that nearly 20 percent of them continued to be concerned about their child's health six to twelve months later (Fyro and Bodegard 1987). Research from the United States documents clinically significant emotional distress among parents as a result of positive NBS results for cystic fibrosis (CF) (Tluczek et al. 2005). Other studies of children with positive CF screens have shown that "at least 5% of parents whose infants had false positive results . . . believed their infants might have [the disease] one year later, despite consultation" (Holtzman 1991, 803).

Another set of unintended consequences occurs when newborn screening identifies a child as (merely) a carrier of a mutated gene. This result has complex implications that are perhaps even more difficult for parents to fully comprehend—particularly if, as is so often the case, they don't have adequate access to a genetic counselor or other knowledgeable health professional (Clayton 1992a; Mischler et al. 1998). One study found that 11 percent of parents whose children were identified via newborn screening as carriers for CF believed that the disease would develop later in their child, or were unsure whether this could happen (CDC 2004, 28). Another study concluded that 43 percent of parents whose children were found to be carriers of sickle-cell disease believed their child to have the disease, and 66 percent of this subgroup thought their children required dietary supplements in order to remain healthy (Hampton et al. 1974; Marteau et al. 1992).

The unintended consequences for families of true positive results have received considerably less attention than have those of false positives. Parents whose children's lives were dramatically saved by timely diagnosis of a treatable early-onset disorder are highly vocal and visible, but what of parents who receive an unsought diagnosis that changes their lives in other ways? What other kinds of impact does the diagnosis have—regardless of whether or not it improves the child's physical health?

As I have already suggested, several voices active in the NBS discourse have signaled concern over these questions—MaryAnn Baily and Thomas Murray at the Hastings Center for Bioethics among them. What about parents who "are told that testing confirms that their child has an abnormal laboratory finding associated with serious illness in some children," they ask,

> but as it turns out, their child never becomes symptomatic. Perhaps the child has a mild or subclinical form that was unknown before newborns

were routinely screened for the disorder. . . . Meanwhile, the family reorganizes its life around medical monitoring and planning for something terrible that never happens. Or a family may be told that a child has a genuinely serious disorder for which there is no proven treatment. The family begins a treatment odyssey—searching the Internet, visiting specialists, running up debt, medicalizing the child's life—only to have that life end in early death anyway. Or perhaps treatment options exist, but they are terribly expensive and burdensome—perhaps to the child as well as to the parents—and bring at best a slight, fleeting improvement in the child's condition. (2008, 29)

These sorts of open-ended questions about the diverse consequences of NBS remain much more the exception than the rule in the NBS-related literature, however—and research designed to answer them is in short supply. Much more commonly voiced is concern about the impact of early diagnosis on specific phenomena such as parent/child bonding, parental perceptions of disease, and the child's own emerging identity. One researcher, for example, suggests that "there is concern that early diagnosis of untreatable diseases may disrupt parental bonding to their infant if the disease presence or carrier status is determined" and asks: "How will the knowledge that the child has a gene-linked disorder or is a carrier affect these children's socialization into the customary roles that anticipate future childbearing?" (Penticuff 1996, 787). Others also speculate that early diagnosis can have an impact on "the family's ability to bond with a labeled child and on the child's own developing self image" (Mischler et al. 1998, 44). In a report on the implications of all kinds of genetic testing of children, jointly authored by the American Society of Human Genetics and the American College of Medical Genetics, the authors summarize research demonstrating that "presymptomatic diagnosis in children . . . has the potential to alter the relationships that exist between parents and their offspring and among siblings. . . . A child known to have a deleterious gene may be overindulged, rejected, or treated as a scapegoat" (ASHG/ACMG 1995, 1236). Another concern has been that parents will view a baby with an abnormal screen as what psychologists Morris Green and Albert J. Solnit (1964) first termed a "vulnerable child" and will become overprotective in response.

A few studies have investigated these issues, usually using psychometric techniques designed to quantify the impact of a positive newborn-screening experience. One large-scale study funded through the Human Genome Project's Ethical, Legal, and Social Issues program compared "impact on the family" of newborn-screening versus clinical diagnoses for metabolic disorders, as one relatively minor component of a much larger project whose primary objective was to "assess the impact on families of a false-positive screening result compared with a normal result" (Waisbren et al. 2003, 2564). Based on analysis of parents' scores on the standardized Parenting Stress Index, the authors found that "parents of children who were newborn screened compared with parents of children who were clinically identified expressed lower levels of stress and greater satisfaction with their support network" (2570). They attribute this difference partly to the fact that children of parents in the former group had markedly fewer developmental and health problems. They also note that— as suggested here earlier—results may reflect the fact that newborn-screening programs appear to be identifying children with mild or benign forms of genetic disorders compared to the phenotypic norm in the clinically identified group (2571).

Other studies have also examined the impact of diagnosis via newborn screening—particularly for cystic fibrosis—on parenting practices, parental stress levels, and attitudes toward diagnostic processes (Al-Jader et al. 1990; Boland and Thompson 1990; Tluczek et al. 2005; see summaries in Duff and Brownlee 2008 and Whitehead, Brown, and Layton 2010). As I document in the chapters that follow, these studies generated some intriguing preliminary data. They found that receiving a newborn-screen diagnosis is less stressful for parents than is a prolonged "diagnostic odyssey" (CDC 2004) during which their child is symptomatic and physicians fail to identify the problem correctly. They also discovered that "neonatal screening for CF can have a psychological impact on the parent-child bonding" and that "the experiences [with diagnosis] of mothers of apparently healthy children are qualitatively different" from the experience of those whose children are symptomatic (Al-Jader et al. 1990, 460; Boland and Thompson 1990, 1244).[20]

However, because most of these published studies used standardized testing instruments and a survey research design, they do not address questions about what NBS means to parents in the context of their lives overall, and what it may mean—as it grows ever larger—for the very nature of early childhood, identity, and parenthood. Further, several studies have concluded there are no lasting problems along these dimensions (see Parsons and Bradley 2003). As a result, many NBS researchers and commentators have concluded that there is "scant evidence" that NBS for "untreatable" conditions results in problematic risks (Bailey et al. 2006, 278), and that worries about these issues are unfounded because "there have been no reported increases in mothers' tendencies to overprotect and no evidence of significant disruption to parent-child attachment" (Duff and Brownlee 2008, 28).

Researchers mostly refer to the specific issue of diagnosing healthy children with genotypic disease as a potentially confounding factor in studies designed to assess the impact of screening on children's health outcomes. If some of the children would have been healthy without any intervention, researchers note, it is much more difficult or even impossible to tell how effective early intervention was in improving children's health—yet early intervention will likely be credited for the healthier outcomes (Botkin 2005). Reference to the consequences for families of identifying healthy children with genotypic disease is less common, and is almost always included as an afterthought. Virginie Scotet and her colleagues, for example, who found at least 5 asymptomatic children with CF mutations out of 118 in their study, note that "the uncertainty of the evolution of the disease can be a source of anxiety for some couples, so genetic counseling remains of the utmost importance in the management of these families" (2000, 793). And other commentators write that one of the costs of newborn screening for CF is that it is "a difficult condition to define and early asymptomatic detection may exacerbate these difficulties" (Bonham, Downing, and Dalton 2003, S44). But the experience of parents getting a genetic diagnosis for a healthy child has been considered by most researchers, when at all, as a theoretical side effect of current testing policy rather than as an empirical reality worthy of research in its own right.

Testing at Birth: What Kind of Results Will We Get?

In any given situation, how and what we ask has everything to do, of course, with the answers we get. I came to NBS research clear that I did not intend to address the specific questions about cost and benefit most often posed in the bioethical, policy, public health, and clinical literature. The predominant charge to social science from those close to NBS has been for evaluative studies able to produce outcomes data. It was never my goal, however, to generate (for example) quantifiable empirical evidence about the risks associated with expanded newborn screening nor was I intending to elicit parents' opinions about the relative merits of NBS and other diagnostic procedures.

What I wanted to do instead was look at newborn screening from within the tradition of sociological inquiry that explores how science and technology shape human experience in new ways. NBS offers incredibly rich terrain for such an approach, bridging as it does questions about the influence of medical context on parent/child relationships, questions about how health and disease categories become defined and redefined, and questions about the impact of genetics and genomics on identity.[21] Most importantly, though, I found myself repeatedly drawn back to that query about NBS's texture that Ellen Clayton raised—How do NBS programs "feel to those they touch"?—a question that has since been echoed by others imploring society to pay attention to "the way in which an expanded program of newborn screening touches and transforms the relation between parents and children" (Meilaender 2008, 118) and to how NBS "shapes the way parents employ their resources (of time, energy, money, and medical services)" (Schneider 2008, 122). It struck me as self-evident that as more and more parents get abnormal screening results, disease diagnoses, and genetic information about their child at birth, many things besides their children's physical health would be changing—but how?

When I set out to investigate these issues I knew that I would discover crucial differences between NBS-diagnosed diseases as defined by diagnosticians and treatment specialists, and these same conditions experienced as illness by parents of the young children who are diagnosed (Kleinman 1988). This would be especially true, I thought, for complex disorders that express themselves in diverse ways, such as cystic fibrosis (CF)—the condition on which I focused much of my primary research with parents. CF symptoms can begin at birth, sometime in the first few months or years of life, or not until much later. The disorder can be debilitating or very mild or may in men cause only infertility. In some cases, people have no symptoms whatever. In the face of these complex variations in the disease itself and in parents' experience of it, professionals nevertheless often offer parents highly standardized information and highly standardized treatment protocols. Ironically, they do this in part because the very complexity of the disease makes its course difficult to predict.[22] Diagnostic experiences with CF thus promised a rich arena for investigating the relationship between medically defined disease and the actual experience of CF by parents of genetically diagnosed children.

Sociologist Arthur Frank writes that the "modernist 'sick role' carries the expectation that ill people get well, cease to be patients, and return to their normal obligations" (1995, 9). But in postmodern times, he continues, the line between "sick" and "well" is much more complex. Part of Frank's own prodigious work focuses on the roles and stories of people who are effectively well, or at least able to function on a day-to-day basis, yet "could never be considered cured" (8). He uses the term "remission society" to describe this group of individuals (along with the family members who share their struggles), and he argues that modernist medicine lacks a story appropriate to describe their experiences. I approached my NBS research with the intention of understanding the parents of children diagnosed with CF as a subgroup of Frank's "remission society": a group of people who are profoundly affected by disease, but who do not fit the classic modernist "sick role"—in this case both because they are caregivers rather than persons directly affected, and because the meanings of the diagnosis are so complex, varied, and unpredictable. I embarked on my interviews with the expectation that these parents would have their own narrative accounts of what the diagnosis has meant to them, and that they would be generous enough to share these accounts with me. I was not disappointed.

Newborn Screening through New Eyes:
A Qualitative Sociologist's Perspective

Two distinct yet intertwined strands of primary research form the substance of this book. The first is an examination of expanded screening's qualitative impact on families, drawn from fifty in-depth interviews with parents conducted primarily between 2005 and 2009. The second strand focuses on the particular way citizen participation has been shaped, and parents' experiences have been publicly represented, in this highly publicized, emotionally charged policy arena. Here I draw on varied sources—written work (published, unpublished, and Web-based); information gained and observations made at conferences, meetings, and other public forums; content analysis of media coverage; and formal and informal primary interviews in 2008 and 2009 with a range of actors, including at least one NBS program representative in nearly every state.

I relied heavily on the methodologies of grounded theory in designing and implementing my research, since I share this tradition's commitment to inductive theory building and its belief that much useful social science insight emerges through the iterative process of thinking about what questions to ask, analyzing and interpreting what is learned on the ground, and then rethinking the research questions. Grounded theory is also well suited to an exploration of complex social phenomena such as those I set out to examine: I did not anticipate—nor did I discover—simple relationships between diagnostic systems for genetic disorders and human interactions among affected children, parents, and health care professionals. Although I did hypothesize, as noted earlier, that diagnostic systems matter and are likely to have complicated social effects, I approached the inquiry itself with as few assumptions about the nature of these effects as I could manage. In other words, I set out to "discover . . . , develop . . . , and provisionally verify [theory] through systematic data collection and analysis" (Strauss and Corbin 1990, 23), rather than to posit a specific theory and proceed to prove or disprove it.

Using grounded theory by no means implies, of course, that I came to the inquiry as a blank slate or that I encountered parents' experiences without in turn influencing them. Throughout the research I was keenly aware that by asking particular kinds of questions and sparking certain kinds of dialogue, I became an actor in the construction of what I was studying, as do all who investigate social phenomena. I listened intently to the stories parents, and (later) state NBS program officials, told. While I was doing so, I felt that Catherine Riessman's description of narrative as, ideally, a process that draws the listener deeply into the teller's experience so that "a kind of intersubjective agreement about 'how it was' is reached" applied fully (1990, 1197). But I also structured the conversations in specific ways, both implicitly (for example, by seeking to have parents contact me in the first place) and explicitly (for example, by pointedly inquiring about particular aspects of experience). I was—and remain—"a participant in the co-construction of meanings, not . . . a separate, isolated, neutral, and 'objective' scientific analyst" (Alford 1998, 85). I am also aware that recounting parts of what I heard according to themes, as I have done in this book, rather than retaining each person's narrative as a coherent whole in just the way it was told to me, constitutes an interpretive act on my part.

In addition to interviews with more than one hundred people, research for *Testing Baby* included many informal conversations with parents of children (with and without genetic diagnoses) whom I know through personal or professional connections; and with genetic counselors, physicians, public health workers, and other professionals involved in the design and delivery of newborn-screening services. These discussions were enormously useful: they helped me test out my ideas, shape my study, and formulate germane interview questions for my primary research. Throughout the years that I spent preparing for and conducting interviews, I was also fortunate to have regular contact with a number of researchers, scholars, and practitioners whose work is related to my study; to attend and make presentations at a large number of professional conferences of relevance; to participate in national meetings about the impact and future of NBS; and to visit a state newborn-screening program and tour its laboratory (including the MS/MS equipment it had recently acquired). These opportunities to discuss ideas, double-check data, talk through early interview findings, and continually challenge my own thinking were invaluable.

The interview data presented in chapters 2, 3, and 4 of this book derive from my interviews with fifty parents of children who were diagnosed with genetic disorders. Forty-seven of the parents had a child or children with cystic fibrosis, and the other three had children with ambiguous diagnoses. When appropriate, I integrated perspectives from the latter interviews with the CF interviews; in other instances, I kept them separate. Because I was interested in the qualitative aspects of parents' experience, I used a semi-structured design, flexibly implemented to elicit the parent's own narrative as freely as possible. At the outset I developed an interview guide consisting of questions designed to elicit parents' stories.

Since my intention was to learn in an open-ended way about how genetic diagnosis touches and transforms people's lives, it was critical that I first understand something about the flow of experience and perspective—the lifeworld—that was shaping the family's household and web of relationships. Each interview therefore began with a broad discussion about the context and process of parenthood for the interviewee. I asked how the pregnancy (or, for parents with more than one child, pregnancies) went; what kinds of testing, if any, had been sought or accepted prenatally for each child; how the birthing process felt in each instance; what the homecoming was like; how adjustments to parenting unfolded. We then moved on—usually spontaneously and with little steering from me—to focus explicitly on the diagnostic experience and its impact on parenting, on perceptions of the child, on the household at large and the extended family, and on relationships with professionals.

With the exception of the first few interviews and one or two later ones with notably reticent parents, I found little need to rely on my interview guide. The interactions flowed naturally, and it was easy to find seamless ways of moving from one topic to the next in an order that felt respectful and right within the context of each person's narrative. Often, little or no prompting was necessary on my part; as parents recounted in narrative form what had happened in their lives before, during, and after genetic diagnosis, they were spontaneously providing answers to the questions I had written in my guide.

The parents I spoke with were generally eager to talk about their experiences with diagnostic processes, and to tell stories about their lives as parents of children diagnosed with CF. These parents' generosity in sharing both their time and their personal, often emotional narratives was a great gift. My gratitude for it is not in the least lessened by my clear sense that the interviews were also meaningful to the parents who volunteered for the study. That my research questions coincided so well with what parents wanted to talk about encouraged me throughout the research process, and I consider the very richness of the interviews a finding in itself—a crucial piece of evidence that it matters to at least a substantial subset of parents to have their illness narratives recognized, and that they want to claim their own voices with respect to their diagnostic experiences rather than allow them to be "reduced to 'clinical material'" (Frank 1995, 12) or summarized via statistical analysis. A few parents, by exception, contacted me more out of a desire to register their favorable assessment of newborn screening than out of a desire to tell their stories. Despite the informed-consent process and my best efforts to explain the nature of my work, I am aware that this subgroup of parents might feel that my inclusion here of the complex narratives they ended up recounting is an example of what sociologist

Charles Bosk has called "obtain[ing] data that it is not necessarily in our subjects' best interest to reveal" (2001, 206). An even larger subset of parents I interviewed might feel this is true with respect to parts of this book where I have placed their description of events, perspectives, and experiences in a sociological context they did not specifically articulate (207). I agree with Bosk that such "betrayals" probably inhere in the very nature of qualitative research. However, it pains me greatly to imagine perpetrating them, particularly since a central reason I wanted to write this book was to give voice to the stories parents entrusted to me when we spoke.

I began recruiting parents for *Testing Baby* by sharing my Institutional Review Board–approved flier with genetic counselors and other professionals associated with CF specialty centers and asking them to help me identify parents appropriate for the study. A colleague who is herself a parent of children with disabilities also posted the flier on a national listserv. From early interviews conducted as a result of this outreach, I proceeded with snowball sampling, that is, asking each participant to assist in identifying and recruiting other eligible families. Several parents soon posted copies of my flier on their CF listservs, and a steady stream of people who read about the study online contacted me, volunteering to participate. When I decided to expand the study, I again conducted outreach to specialty-center staff and on listservs and was contacted by new families volunteering to be interviewed.

I conducted all but a few of these interviews by telephone. In many cases, this was a necessity because of geographical distance. However, even most parents who lived close enough for an in-person interview preferred the telephone for their own convenience and, I gathered, because they felt greater freedom to speak plainly than they would have felt face-to-face. Somewhat to my surprise, I found the phone provided a balance of intimacy and privacy that facilitated rich and often highly emotional conversations. People may be reticent to weep or to voice the feelings closest to their hearts in front of a stranger. From the other end of the telephone receiver, I found no such inhibitions at work—though of course I regret losing the opportunity to directly observe more about the lives of those I interviewed. The interviews generally lasted between an hour and two hours. Often, parents offered their most poignant insights toward the close of our time together, after they had talked through their narrative and had some time to reflect on it. A number of mothers also sent me follow-up e-mails with additional thoughts, or with attached photos of their beautiful children.

I drew heavily on the methodologies of grounded theory in my analysis, just as I did in my study design. Each interview was transcribed word for word from the tape, usually very soon after it was conducted. This enabled me to read the transcripts from interviews that had just been completed even as I was scheduling and holding subsequent ones. I continually derived concepts from my recollection of interviews and from interview notes, which I then verified through review and comparison of the written transcripts. As I worked with concepts and gained confidence in their "theory-observation" congruence (Corbin and Strauss 1990, 7), I began grouping these into the more complex categories that I use as subheadings in the chapters that follow. Throughout the book I have used extended quotes from the transcripts—removing some of the "ums" and "you knows"—to illustrate thematic findings and connect the reader as directly as possible to the narratives parents recounted. I have also tried to capture nuances of emotion and tone that I gathered from my interviews in passages where I paraphrase or link together several direct quotes; in these parts of the text, the adjectives and phrases I employ are intended to evoke parents' sentiments rather than my own.

When I began to build on my qualitative research with parents by investigating how parents' experiences and perspectives were represented in the public domain, I again did not set out with a specific hypothesis. I had, however, observed that the kinds of "thick" descriptions I was hearing in my interviews were not represented elsewhere in the published literature, and my inquiry was designed to discover why. I talk more about this aspect of my research at the beginning of chapter 5.

My Choice to Focus on Cystic Fibrosis

The great majority of parent interviews I conducted for this book were with people whose child was diagnosed with cystic fibrosis (CF). CF is an autosomal recessive genetic disease. This means that an individual must have two defective copies of the gene—in this case, the cystic fibrosis transmembrane conductance regulator, or CFTR, gene—in order to fully express the disorder.[23] Mutated CFTR genes can cause problems (sometimes terrible, sometimes more mild) with a specific protein that is critical for the healthy functioning of many organs, including the gastrointestinal tract, pancreas, liver, lungs, sweat glands, and genitourinary tract. As a result, people with CF often have problems digesting food, experience recurrent lung infections, and are infertile. The average life span for people with CF in the United States, as of 2008, is thirty-seven years; in 1969, the average lifespan was only fourteen years.[24] Why? Better treatments, and more techniques for managing the disorder. People with symptomatic CF usually die from respiratory failure as a result of chronic obstructive pulmonary disease.[25] Clinical diagnosis in children is often delayed because many of the initial symptoms of CF, such as wheezing, coughing, and diarrhea, are also signs of other childhood illnesses. As a result, doctors just don't think at first appearance that these might be warning signs of CF (ACMG 2005; CDC 2004; Wilfond 1995).

I decided to organize my research primarily around parents of children with CF for several reasons. For one thing, I assumed that my data would be more internally consistent and that identifiable themes would more likely emerge if I interviewed a group of parents whose children share a diagnosis rather than a group whose children have an array of disorders. Given that decision, I needed to select a condition that was screened for in a sufficient number of states, and that has a high enough prevalence, to allow me to recruit an adequate number of parents for interviews. Here again CF fit my requirements. CF is the most common "life-shortening . . . inherited disorder in the United States" (CDC 2004, 1) after sickle-cell disease, which affects 1 in 346 African Americans and approximately 1 of every 2,250 Americans (Kaye and the Committee on Genetics 2006, E958). Its overall prevalence is 1 of every 3,700 births. The disorder is most common among "non-Hispanic whites," where it occurs in 1 of every 2,500 to 3,500 live births (ibid.; ACMG 2005).[26] Prevalence among "Hispanics" and "non-Hispanic Blacks" is 1 in 4,000 to 10,000 and 1 in 15,000 to 20,000, respectively (CDC 2004, 2). One of every twenty-eight "Caucasians" is a carrier, as is one of every sixty-one African Americans, one of every forty-six "Hispanics," and one of every ninety Asian Americans.[27] Colorado began screening newborns for CF in 1982, and Wisconsin and Wyoming followed suit in 1985 and 1988, respectively. Between 1998 and the middle of 2004, six more states added statewide screening programs, and a number of others opted to make their regional or hospital-based pilot screening programs statewide, bringing the total number of states screening for CF to approximately thirteen by 2004. When the ACMG report was released in 2005, CF was among the twenty-nine conditions recommended as part of the core screening panel— although it is notable that CF's rating within the methodology of that study placed it precisely at the cutoff mark between conditions that warrant universal screening and those that do not. By the end of the decade, all fifty states had added CF to their panels, and screening for CF became mandatory for all U.S. infants.

Perhaps most critical for my choice of CF is that it embodies a number of characteristics essential to the new NBS. It is a complex disorder that manifests in many different ways, ranging from severe symptoms beginning in infancy to no symptoms until adulthood or, indeed, ever. This is because there are so many different variations the gene can have: more than one thousand distinct mutations have been identified, and along with them many different manifes-tations of the disorder.[28] CF's broad spectrum of expression is also explained by the fact that even the most common mutations (e.g., DeltaF508, which is thought to comprise up to two-thirds of all CF mutations worldwide [CDC 2004, 2]) have what is known as "poor genotype/phenotype correlation"—that is, even individuals with the same mutation do not all have the same traits and symptoms. Before newborn screening for CF, one subset of symptomatic infants was reliably identified in the newborn period: those with meconium ileus (MI), an intestinal blockage that plagues approximately 15 percent of all newborns with CF. This condition generally results in a distended abdomen, inability to pass stool, vomiting, or all of these. It nearly always requires surgical interven-tion within a few days of birth. Because it is most likely (though not always) indicative of CF, a diagnosis of MI is regarded by many as a presumptive diag-nosis for CF.

CF's complex variability and high prevalence has made it a prime exem-plar of how "genetic classification [can] bring its own ambiguities," writes journalist Andrew Pollack, paraphrasing health policy professor Fiona Miller. Further, Pollack continues, "newborns are now often screened for cystic fibrosis with the idea that they can be treated early to help avoid complications. But some infants with a mutation in the gene responsible for the disease are unlikely ever to have symptoms. Do they have the disease? 'We don't know what to call these infants,' said Dr. Frank J. Accurso, a professor of pediatrics at the University of Colorado. 'We don't even have a good language for it yet'" (Pollack 2008).

Although the impact of this prognostic uncertainty remains little studied for NBS in general, related research suggests that it is an important issue for parents. Indeed, when parents are surveyed about the appropriate scope of NBS, the prognostic reliability of the screen is a major influence on whether they conclude that NBS is appropriate for any given condition (Whitehead, Brown, and Layton 2010).

State NBS directors whom my colleagues and I interviewed also pinpointed CF as an exemplar of NBS's expanding complexities. The most "ambiguous results that we get are in cystic fibrosis," says the director in one state with longstanding CF testing.

> We've detected a lot, a number of mutations, genotypes—not mutations but genotypes—that are not truly CF causing mutations . . . [and] the pulmonologists and whatever, they get these genotypes and they have no idea what to do with them, you know. These are fine, they look

healthy, they're healthy and so on and so forth . . . so what do we do with these kids, what should we do with these kids? . . . There's been . . . unfortunately a fairly large group of kids fall into that "Well, what do we do with them?" category. . . . As far as ambiguous disorders about what to do, right there's the biggest group, in my view. And as more states, almost every state now has added cystic fibrosis, and I think that we're going to start to see that . . . more and more.

Other directors emphatically concur. Identifying asymptomatic kids who have some sort of CF "variant of unknown significance" is "very much of an issue relative to CF," says one. States are finding "atypical CF" and "mutations that we don't know the clinical significance of"—prime examples of how, "gee, a lot of us might be walking around with kind of benign forms of [genetic disorders], actually."

CF also usefully epitomizes the new NBS because direct DNA analysis (rather than testing for analytes) can be and increasingly often is part of the screening process. As more and more states have elected to employ this diagnostic method, ever-larger numbers of children are being classified based on mutation analysis results. Here then is a disorder that, to cite Fiona Miller once again, perfectly "exemplifies the paradoxical challenges of nosological change, where increasingly accurate diagnostic technology creates increased uncertainty about disease identity and clinical management" (Miller et al. 2005, 2542). At the same time, there is some evidence that a combination of newborn screening and CF testing during pregnancy is causing a drop in the percentage of babies carrying the most common mutation (DeltaF508), and a concomitant increase in the proportion of infants with more rare and less well understood variations (Hale, Parad, and Corneau 2008).[29] What counts as CF is thus changing with technology and diagnostic protocols, while at the same time resulting medico-social practices are literally beginning to reconstruct the very nature of the disorder itself, genetics and all.

Until roughly 2005, CF screening was highly controversial in the United States. The debate about whether CF is a disorder appropriate for newborn screening has centered mostly on treatment efficacy, although other factors— such as the (assumed) benefit to families of learning about a CF diagnosis before conceiving subsequent children, the efficacy of screening technology, and the adverse impact of false-positive results—have also been considered. There is no cure for CF, and no clear way to prevent symptoms from developing altogether. However, a number of palliative treatments are available to address the complicated array of digestive and pulmonary symptoms CF can cause. These include medications to control infections, manual chest percussions or mechanical vests used to clear mucus out of the lungs, and replacement enzymes to improve digestion and nutritional status (ACMG 2005; Elborn, Hodson, and Bertram 2009). The central question in the CF newborn-screening debate for many years was, Do the available medical interventions make a demonstrable difference in children's health if started at birth?

The process of answering that question is one aspect of CF newborn screening that sharply differentiates it not only from the new NBS, but also from NBS in general. For CF, two large-scale, longitudinal, randomized clinical trials (RCTs) have been implemented. These studies randomly assigned neonates to either a screened or a control group, and then followed all infants with CF (diagnosed either by newborn screen, or—in the control group—later, with the onset of symptoms) over time to assess health outcomes. A number of cohort and registry studies have also been published. These use retrospective data to see if there were significant differences in childhood health between newborn-screened and clinically identified children (but such studies do not randomly assign children to one group or the other, and therefore do not ascertain how much of the difference in outcomes between the two groups is reliably attributable to screening). The quantity of data thus collected, combined with the rigor of the RCT methodology, makes CF one of the most broadly and rigorously researched conditions on many state NBS panels today. As physician/ethicist Jeffrey Botkin noted several years ago in the context of critiquing NBS's generally weak research base compared with evidence on CF: "Although the magnitude and nature of the benefits of CF NBS remain controversial, the Wisconsin trial has been critical in providing data for policy development" (Botkin 2005, 868).

While I was researching and working on this book, hot controversy over the efficacy of early intervention for CF cooled significantly, and the tide of professional opinion turned in favor of screening.[30] Evidence seems to point convincingly to improved nutritional status, growth, and life expectancy for children identified at birth compared with those identified clinically (Grosse et al. 2006; Sims et al. 2007), thus putting newborn screening for CF in the category of conditions for which there are direct health benefits for many affected children. The efficacy of pulmonary treatments remains contested, as do standards of care for treating diagnosed children who do not have pulmonary symptoms (Elborn, Hodson, and Bertram 2009; Prasad, Main, and Dodd 2008).

The Use of Comparative Design in *Testing Baby*

It was the rapid expansion of newborn-screening programs, and the concomitant changes I hypothesized must be occurring in parents' experiences with genetic diagnosis, that originally excited my interest in NBS research. To understand how newborn screening may be changing the way parents perceive, experience, and respond to their children's genetic disorders, however, it was important to interview not only parents who received a diagnosis for their child through newborn screening, but also their counterparts who learned of their child's disease after the emergence of clinical symptoms. This comparative design—that is, conducting interviews with parents of children with the same condition who arrived at diagnosis through different routes—was very helpful in illuminating the impact of newborn screening and in my attempt to isolate its effects. Indeed, the differences in experience were often striking.

Another compelling reason to interview parents whose children were diagnosed later is that while this diagnostic experience was once the rule, it will soon become an exception. I was aware throughout the interviewing process that these parents' accounts may prove very valuable in future, since nationwide NBS for CF, in combination with increased carrier screening during pregnancy, are bound to make clinical identification of CF an increasingly rare phenomenon.

That I interviewed parents with different diagnostic experiences should not be taken to imply, however, that I employed a strict comparative design. For one thing, I did not set out to interview equal numbers of parents from each group; the primary focus of this work is on NBS, and the majority of the interviews were with parents who had experienced this diagnostic process. For another, I found during the research process that there were actually many more subgroups and defining categories than I had initially anticipated. For example, some experiences—though by no means all of them—were shared among all parents who received what I call in my text an "early diagnosis," regardless of whether their child was diagnosed by prenatal testing, by newborn screening, or by telltale symptoms immediately after birth. Other experiences—though again only a subset—were common to those with asymptomatic children or, again, to those with actively ill children, regardless of the age of the affected child or of how the diagnosis occurred. Despite this complex pattern of subgroups, however, the elements of comparative design as I initially conceived them continued to be useful with respect to extrapolating the potential impact of newborn-screening policy on parents' lives.

Elements of comparative design were also helpful because they kept before me throughout my research what remains constant for all parents regardless of diagnostic routes—that is, the pain of learning that something is or could be devastatingly wrong with their child. I discovered through these interviews many ways in which parents' experience of CF is socially constructed by diagnostic processes, and I believe that how we as a society organize these experiences makes a profound difference. At the same time, I was humbled by constant reminders that there is no good way to get hard news, and that when one's child is actively symptomatic this terrible fact becomes the dominant reality no matter what the route of diagnosis. In the day-to-day life of parents whose children are ill, being forced to bear witness as CF "wreaks havoc" on their children's bodies (to quote one mother) is the most profoundly structuring experience they confront. It is this that creates the deepest grief for parents, and it is one of the things that makes them weep as they tell me their stories. They would give their own lives to free their child from CF if they could, but the reality is that for many parents nothing—not the complex medical interventions available today, not strict adherence to prescribed preventive care, and not the most perfect of diagnostic processes we could design—can fulfill this fervent wish for their child's good health and long life.

The Parents I Interviewed

Of the fifty parents I interviewed for *Testing Baby*, thirty-three received at least one newborn-screening diagnosis; seven received at least one prenatal diagnosis; four received a diagnosis within a few days or weeks of birth when symptoms prompted testing; and eleven received a later diagnosis (between ages two months and seven years) for a symptomatic child or children. Most children were between the ages of one and seven at the time of my interview with their parent, but there were some outliers on both ends of that spectrum. About half the children in my study who were diagnosed by NBS are reported by their parents as having remained entirely asymptomatic since birth; for a subset of these children, parents report that health care providers have concurred that the case is "mild," "borderline," or even "to be declassified as CF." Of the three parents whose children have or had ambiguous diagnoses, two remain profoundly uncertain about whether their child will ever develop symptoms.

I intentionally designed *Testing Baby* as a study of parents' experiences rather than of mothers' experiences. This is largely because my review of the literature led me to agree with the authors of one study that "the experience of fathers has been generally neglected in parent-child research" (Morgan, Robinson, and Aldridge 2002, 222). It is also because of the way my own experience has colored and contextualized my research. The father of my two children has been such a completely equal partner in the parenting process, and my own father has played such a central role in raising and nurturing both me and my children, that the idea of excluding fathers from the outset felt wrong—even though I am well aware (as a parent, as a sociologist, as a feminist) that in general mothers do a hugely disproportionate amount of caregiving work of every kind. Despite my explicit call for parents rather than mothers to volunteer for the study, and despite efforts to recruit more men at about the halfway point, I ended up interviewing forty-three mothers and only seven fathers. I have nonetheless chosen to retain the term "parents" as a descriptor for the group I spoke to at large, and to revert to the word "mothers" when discussing phenomena that were specific only to the women in my sample.

All but one of the parents I interviewed identified themselves as "white" or "Caucasian" when I asked them to describe their ethnic identity. This is not surprising given that CF is a disease most common among non-Hispanic white people, but this ethnic homogeneity impoverished my sample in many regrettable ways. Based on stated occupation, I deduced that parents I interviewed were a more or less equal mix of working and middle class.

Because parents who participated in the study had volunteered to do so, I ended up interviewing people who were motivated—for whatever reason—to join. This may have resulted in an overrepresentation of parents who had dramatic experiences of one sort or another—either very satisfactory or very unsatisfactory—and were therefore eager to tell their story. It may also have resulted in an overrepresentation of highly conscientious parents, as reflected by the fact that they found out about the study through a network of contacts in the CF world they had already built for themselves. However, I believe that these issues of who was represented in my study are not highly problematic, since my intent was to find dense, intensive, and—to use the sociological term—"thick" descriptions from a variety of parents rather than to define a statistically valid norm.

What Follows

In the next chapter, I describe various ways parents learn that their child has CF, and how these different diagnostic pathways shape family experiences of and responses to the disorder. Chapter 2 thus raises broad issues about the power of NBS to shape identity and structure social relationships. In chapters 3 and 4, I go on to examine these issues with more specificity in two domains. Chapter 3 focuses on how NBS is influencing the way parents encounter and care for their children: changes in the bonding process, increased vigilance, new definitions of parental success and failure, hope for increased control over health outcomes alongside the ongoing adverse experience of the disease's inevitability. In chapter 4, I turn to the impact of NBS on relationships between parents and professionals. Early diagnosis via state-mandated testing sets the stage for particular assertions of power, demonstrations of expertise, and approaches to uncertainty in the medical domain, and also at home. Here, I explore how these dramas unfold from the point of view of parents.

Chapters 2, 3, and 4 immerse you in the private lives of families getting diagnoses, caring for their children, and navigating health services. In chapter 5, I examine why the lives just described have remained private, while another set of stories about diagnosis has gone public—significantly influencing policy and structuring assumptions about NBS in the process.

The specific issues addressed in the first five chapters of *Testing Baby* provide a platform for exploring larger questions: about how the discourse of risk and the availability of technology influence our lives; about the challenge and promise of participatory democracy, where policy is informed by lay as well as expert perspectives; about how advocates' interests can both conflict and intersect with the interests of other stakeholders in policy debates; and about the role of qualitative social science research in constructing a more nuanced voice for lay actors in health policy debates. In chapter 6, I connect these broader issues to an analysis of NBS's sociological consequences and public policy implications both at present and in the "increasingly screenable future" (Heath, Rapp, and Taussig 2004) that technology is rapidly bringing our way. I also suggest a framework for encouraging more deliberative, inclusive policy processes that would rectify the omission of the crucial kinds of parental perspectives this book presents without promoting predetermined or prescriptive policy outcomes.

Chapter 2

Diagnostic Odysseys, Old and New

How Newborn Screening Transforms Parents' Encounters with Disease

No research is needed to demonstrate that for parents, news that their child has been diagnosed with a serious genetic disease is devastating to receive. Regardless of how and when the diagnosis comes, it brings with it a range of painful responses: shock, grief, anger, numbness, fear, and very often the feeling that—as a number of parents put it—"our little world just crashed." Worry about the future, questions about what the diagnosis means, and a sense that life is irretrievably altered—these experiences are a somber province shared by all parents receiving their child's cystic fibrosis diagnosis.

Other aspects of parents' experience with genetic diagnosis, however, vary significantly, not just because of individual differences in emotional makeup and ways of coping under stress, but also according to when, how, and why the diagnosis is made. With the rapid expansion of newborn screening, the context in which parents most often receive diagnostic information about their children—and thus too the context of early parenting—is being definitively transformed. This chapter begins to answer the question, How might expanded newborn screening be changing the experience, the significance, and the impact of childhood CF diagnosis? It explores diagnostic processes for CF, drawing on parents' narratives about the NBS process—as well as on comparisons between parents' experiences when diagnosis is at birth and when diagnosis comes after symptoms emerge.

The particular diagnostic pathway parents travel to arrive at CF influences their experience of the destination. I examine here various aspects of first encounters with CF, including their impact on parents' postbirth period; on their sense of the affected child; and on their relationships with family and

community. This chapter also lays important groundwork for deeper exploration of NBS's implications for parenting (chapter 3) and for relationships
with health care professionals (chapter 4).

CF is the second-most common genetic disorder affecting the U.S. population (sickle-cell anemia is the most common), and the most common for people
of Northern European descent. As noted in chapter 1, one in 3,700 newborns in
the general population has the genotype (CDC 2004). Approximately thirty
thousand people in the United States were living with the disease in 2010.[1]
While these statistics are well known to clinicians, most people outside
medical circles still have little awareness of CF. Down syndrome is a genetic
disorder that has gradually made its way into the public consciousness, and
certainly the inherited factor at play in breast cancer rapidly became common
knowledge after the BRCA gene was identified in the 1990s, despite the
fact that it actually contributes to the disease in only 5 to 7 percent of cases
(Rothman 1998). But at the end of the first decade of the twenty-first century,
CF has not yet become part of the popular lexicon of genetic risk and disease.
It is not something parents actively worry about during pregnancy, nor is it
something they are likely to think of as the culprit if their child develops one or
more early symptoms of the disease—especially since these symptoms can also
indicate many other childhood illnesses.

NBS for CF is now mandatory in all fifty states, yet most parents still know
little or nothing about the condition before their own child is tested. No parent
I interviewed had any specific concern about her child's risk for the disease
ahead of time, with the exception of six mothers who had had routine carrier
screening during pregnancy but had chosen not to find out if the fetus was
affected. In this context of little or no knowledge from elsewhere, the diagnostic process itself—the rolling out of procedures designed to determine if the
disease is in fact present—looms very large for families with affected children.

From Sober Confirmation to Devastating Surprise:
The Influence of Context on Parents' First Encounters with CF

Diagnosis of a genetic disorder can mean the long-sought answer to the question, What is wrong with my child? It can mean unsuspected, unsolicited
revelation of invisible chromosomal abnormalities within the body of a healthy,
or seemingly healthy, newborn. It can mean the relief of finally having a label
and some appropriate medical treatment; the confirmation of a half-conscious
suspicion; the death of blissful ignorance; the advent of needless worry. In each
case, what preceded the diagnosis, and what brought parent and child to the
point of getting it, profoundly influence its impact.

Pediatricians often do not recognize clinical manifestations of genetic disorders, including cystic fibrosis, in babies and young children. Because CF is not always rapidly identified as a possible cause for symptoms, many families with later diagnoses have been caring for and worrying about a sick child for months or years before being able to name and address the underlying disease. Many have felt helpless in the face of their child's repeated illnesses, apparent failure to thrive, digestive problems, or other symptoms. And all too often, parents have had their observations, suggestions, and concerns dismissed by health care professionals (see chapter 4).

The frightening, maddening process that occurs when diagnosis comes significantly later than the emergence of persistent, serious symptoms has been dubbed the "diagnostic odyssey," and its harmful impact is well documented in the newborn-screening literature. Research highlights a number of possible damaging effects on parents, including anxiety; loss of trust in health care providers; conviction that their child's well-being was adversely affected in the short or long term; and "a growing sense of fear that their child's deteriorating health [is] the result of their own incompetence" (Boland and Thompson 1990, 1243; CDC 2004; Clayton 1992a; Mérelle et al. 2003; Skinner, Sparkman, and Bailey 2003; Waisbren et al. 2003). In my own research, almost two-thirds of those with later diagnoses experienced some or all of these adverse effects. Annie describes her experience with a mixture of poignancy and vitriol that captures many dimensions of the suffering she and her family endured en route to a diagnosis of CF: "I am angry about [the delayed diagnosis] to this day, like in my, in myself, that nobody would listen to me. Doing all these things to him, [other tests and treatments] that were totally unnecessary. I mean, I've carried that anger inside of me for a long time because I was like—I knew from the day he was born. You know how frustrating that is? So flipping frustrating. Because I knew from the day he was born and for seven years, and I was intimidated by doctors, you know, and it was like, Okay, the doctor said no [to testing for CF], so we're not gonna do it." Another mother, whose symptomatic one-year-old was correctly diagnosed only after her healthy second baby tested positive on his newborn screen, describes the process she underwent with her older boy as "the blind leading the blind," noting: "It takes a newborn before someone figures out what is wrong with my fifteen-month-old. . . . You trust your doctor," she continues, "and they are telling me the first time it is RSV [respiratory syncytial virus], the second time they are so baffled they don't know what is wrong with him that they do a spinal tap, and they *still* can't figure out what is wrong with him."

The process of arriving at CF testing is heart-wrenchingly difficult for many with later diagnoses. But in the context of active illness, the desire to know what is wrong—beginning with having a disease label and a coherent explanation for the problem—is fierce. Parents of older symptomatic children are generally well aware that testing for CF is being done to establish or to rule out the disorder. These parents may have varying levels of familiarity with CF at the time of the test, but it would only be by extreme exception that the procedure itself would be performed without their knowledge or consent, as is the case with newborn screening. This is partly because the test takes place in the context of a health care environment where active symptoms are being addressed and a search for diagnostic information has been explicitly undertaken. It is also because in this case the patient is a child—not a fetus, not a newborn in the liminal hospital environment where professionals retain significant control, but a tangible, individuated child who is symptomatic and whose parents are seeking information about what is wrong. These children are in the custody of their parents, and it is their parents who bring them to health care providers to ask for assistance.

When testing is prompted by the emergence of symptoms that could signal CF, clinicians skip screening processes altogether and move directly to a confirmatory test (Moskowitz et al. 2005, 2–3). This may happen at any age, but as of 2004 the median age of CF diagnosis on the basis of symptoms and signs other than meconium ileus was 14.5 months (CDC 2004, 4).[2] Parents may have been observing their child's symptoms for quite some time when testing occurs, or symptoms may have emerged relatively recently; symptoms may already be severe, or they may still be mild.

Most often what is performed for CF diagnosis is a sweat test, a "simple and painless procedure [that] measures the amount of salt in the sweat." Results of this test are available to parents within hours, and CF is diagnosed if the salt level is above an established cutoff.[3] Alternatively, or if sweat testing is inconclusive (as it not uncommonly is), the child's blood might be sent off to a laboratory for DNA mutation analysis. If two mutations are identified as present in the cystic fibrosis transmembrane conductance regulator (CFTR) gene, then a CF diagnosis is established (Moskowitz et al. 2005, 1–3).

When children are already sick, parents' sadness and fear about the actual CF diagnosis is mixed with tremendous relief. Here is Annie again, recalling her son's eventual diagnosis: "When we got it I was totally relieved. Even though he had cystic fibrosis and I knew what it was and I knew the outcome of it, it was a relief, because I knew he was gonna be treated correctly. I knew . . . that I wasn't crazy, that I wasn't looking for something to be wrong with him, you know?" For these parents, the reality of their child's suffering has already unavoidably asserted itself, and the idea of a healthy, "perfect" child has already receded—sometimes long since. What matters now is to find out what the problem is and take action to make things better for the child, so parents can at long last have "all our questions" answered and "watch all the pieces fall in place." In Jody's words: "We knew that there was something wrong, so tell us what it is and we'll go forward. [After the diagnosis] we had a name. At least we had something to deal with—it's better than nothing. We had some under-standing of what it was." And, perhaps, some medical treatment—at last—that might alleviate suffering and prolong life.

Catherine's baby was only seven months old when the diagnosis came. But her child had been gravely ill, and she had been trying to convince others that there was a serious problem for quite some time. A "mixture of horror and relief" was her response to confirmation that CF was the cause. At least, she goes on, it wasn't some exotic, unknown condition. "I had envisioned flying around the world looking for specialists trying to figure out what was wrong with this child. But it was a relief to know that there was help, you know, at hand and that they knew about the disease and it could be—I don't want to say treated, but you know what I mean."

These parents with symptomatic, undiagnosed children affirm sociologist Douglas Maynard's conclusion that it can be "worse to live in an ill-defined or ambiguous everyday world . . . than in one where something has changed for the worse but can be named and mutually recognized through interaction" (1996, 121). But for parents whose infants receive an abnormal newborn screen and subsequent diagnosis, news of CF is not generally a confirmation of estab-lished suspicions. Rather, it arrives unbidden and unexpected, a devastating surprise.

Every baby's heel is pricked while the newborn is still in the hospital after birth, and the blood is then sent to a state health department or regional or con-tract laboratory to be screened for whichever genetic conditions are included in the newborn-screening panel mandated by law in that state. This is not an indi-vidualized clinical procedure like the sweat test. Instead, it's a mandated and universal public health screening—an intervention designed by the state for all babies and delivered to them without substantial parental involvement and almost always without parental consent.

In the case of CF, the newborn-screening procedure itself is complex and multistaged. In all thirty-six states that mandated newborn screening for CF in December 2007, the first step in that process was a test that measures immunoreactive trypsinogen (IRT), a possible indicator of CF, in the blood taken from the infant's heel in the hospital. If the IRT levels placed the infant in the abnormal range for the state in which the child was born, a second test was run (the range varies from state to state). In some states (in 2007, twenty-two of the thirty-six with CF screening programs), the second test was a DNA analysis of the same blood sample obtained in the hospital. DNA analysis may look for only the most common CF mutation (DeltaF508), or for multiple mutations.[4] If one or more mutations were identified, the baby's doctor, the clinic or hospital of birth, or the most proximate CF specialty center was notified of the positive screen.[5] The infant's parents were then contacted—usually by telephone—and told to bring the infant in for the sweat test.

In the fourteen remaining states that tested for CF in 2007, an elevated IRT prompted direct notification of the baby's health care provider, and then of the parents, again almost always by telephone. In this case, parents were told to bring the baby in for a second heel prick at the age of about two weeks so another IRT test could be run. At this age, "values are more specific for CF because IRT values decrease with age in infants without CF" (CDC 2004, 6). If the IRT was still above whatever value the state had set as a cutoff for this second screen, the child was referred for confirmatory sweat testing (CDC 2004).[6]

Arriving at a CF diagnosis via newborn screening, then, is a complex process involving multiple steps that evolves differently for parents in different states. In some cases, for example, a positive screen means just one elevated IRT, which can be merely an artifact of when the sample was collected (i.e., immediately after birth, when levels for many healthy babies remain elevated). In others, news of the abnormal screen means that two mutations consistent with CF have already been identified by DNA analysis and clinicians have already more or less concluded that the baby has CF.

Almost without exception, parents I interviewed described themselves as poorly informed about NBS at the time of notification, and confused, in one way or another, about what the screening meant, regardless of which laboratory procedures had been conducted.[7] Most did realize that the heel stick, or "PKU test," would occur in the hospital but considered it just "part of the routine"—that "thing they do when a baby is born." Parents who remembered getting information about NBS before the test encountered it as something to "glance over" rather than truly study, since they had "no reason to think that there would be any problem." As Barb put it: "I had read other books and whatnot, and I knew obviously that when he was born they were going to do tests for different things. Did I know exactly which ones? No. I thought they were the standard tests like when you go to the doctor and they take your blood nowadays, you know. But I knew they had to check something and I knew they were going to take his blood. What they were checking for exactly, I thought was just standard testing. I didn't really know."

Other parents too were given no clear sense of what the test was for, and thus were left with just a vague impression that "they were testing for a type of retardation," for blood type, for cancer, or for diabetes. Summing up the kind of impression many parents have, Joan says: "I just thought they tested their hearing, their reflexes, and that stuff. I didn't know that it got into genetics and I had no idea that we would come out of it with a diagnosis for something."

Only one of the parents I spoke with described a meaningful verbal exchange with her health care provider before the blood was taken; the doctor explained "that the newborn screening was to make sure that there were no genetic diseases that were not obvious. And they do that as a precaution just in case, because some of the diseases are pretty bad and hard to diagnose without this [test], just with symptoms. So they try to catch it at birth so they can start treatment right away."

For the rest, those who had any formal notification in advance of the screening remembered only receiving a pamphlet or booklet about the program, or having it mentioned along with lots of other things during a visit with the doctor, at childbirth class, or in the hospital. However, this health information seemed to most of them, at the time, like just one more thing in a pile of pamphlets and paraphernalia. Paige describes how irrelevant and unimportant the material seemed when it was given to her: "When we were in the hospital, somebody had given me a booklet saying 'We test for these metabolic diseases.' And I just kind of glanced through it and set it aside with the other bazillion things that you get when you have a new baby, you know . . . the diaper bag and there's formula samples and the wipes. . . . So, it just kind of got stuffed in the diaper bag and put off to the side. I really didn't pay much attention to it until I got the phone call, and then I was digging for anything I could find."

Other mothers talk about getting NBS information while they are in labor, when "there's so much going on," and "heaven knows I wasn't even listening, if I'm in labor, whatever, 'Just give me some drugs! Where do I sign? What do you need me to sign, because I'm in pain, come on.'" The clinical literature's concession that close proximity to birth "is not necessarily the optimal time for parents to successfully assimilate and understand information" (Duff and Brownlee 2008, 23) does not begin to capture how very laughably bad a time it really is. As Nana puts it, with ironic understatement: "Apparently somewhere while I was having labor pains I signed some kind of form, and didn't really know it. You are kind of caught up in the moment at that time."

Anthony too finds it understandably hard to remember precisely what information he and his wife may have been given before the screening. However, he gives his health care providers the benefit of the doubt, assuming that they did their duty to inform him and even to ask him to sign in consent. "Yeah, part of me says [details about the screening process] could have been offered. I just didn't pay that close attention because I didn't—maybe it's just me, [but I thought] that's all the other people, it never happens in my children. Perhaps they did give us all that information and it was among eighty other pieces of paper they, you know, handed [us] before [and] during the birth process. . . . I don't remember the exact time when we signed [a form], but I knew that newborn screening existed and basically the breakdown of it. . . . I just sort of went with the program."

From a parent's perspective, then, NBS barely shows up on the radar until there is an abnormal result. Parents know little or nothing about it before it occurs, and the heel stick procedure itself usually comes and goes without much particular notice, lost in the maelstrom of physical, emotional, medical, and familial events that surround birth. Like Gladys, parents "just figure everything was fine" once the hospital staff give the baby "a clean bill of health" and send both mother and child home. And like Bess, most parents have no idea "what the heck CF" is, "what it entails," or what a possible diagnosis with it means "was going to happen." As Roxanna relates: "When you walk into your pediatrician's office for a two-week checkup on your beautiful new baby, and you find out you didn't pass a test you didn't even know you had, . . . [it was] like the rug had pulled out from underneath my feet. . . . I had no idea what a newborn screen was. I didn't even know that was something they did."

Once providers of care (the pediatrician, CF specialty clinic, or NBS program follow-up worker) receive the positive screen result from the laboratory, protocols require that they inform the family immediately and set up confirmatory testing. If by chance a well-child visit at the pediatrician's office coincides with arrival of the NBS laboratory report, as it did for Roxanna, the news may be given in person. Most often, however, the first notification of parents occurs by telephone—a life-changing call from out of the blue.

Although Lilly's daughter was diagnosed more than a decade before my interview with her, like most parents who have gotten such a call she remembers every detail. She was out in her barn when it came, and taken completely unawares. The pediatrician, Lilly recalls,

said he was very sorry to have to call me and tell me this, but did I remember that in the hospital they did this heel test? And I remember them doing the heel test but I did not remember them saying what that was all for . . . and he explained to us that she tested positive for, um, indications of cystic fibrosis. And I just broke down and started to cry and my husband was standing right there by me at the time . . . and I ran in the house cause she was sleeping in the house and we had the monitor by her and I just sat by her and said, "Oh, my little baby, there can't be anything wrong with you." And then I started calling relatives and trying to find out about it, what exactly it was. 'Cause I had heard of cystic fibrosis but I didn't know what it was. . . . I was concerned about what was gonna happen, you know, is she gonna be okay, what do I have to do, where do I go, what do I—what steps do I have to take, exactly what is it?

This mixture of absolute surprise and full-throttle panic about what a positive newborn screen means is paradigmatic of parents' NBS experiences. Francesca describes the haze of guilt, fear, confusion, and sorrow that descended after that first conversation with her daughter Tess's doctor.

I don't get how this happened because everything was so perfect; . . . everything seemed to be so right, so it was a big, a huge shock, I guess, after, to find out she has the CF. . . . It took me like two days to quit crying. . . . I cried a lot, I mean that, and I slept with her even for nights before I could let her just go back in her own crib and stuff like that because you just want to hold on so tight because you don't know. . . . It was like a blaming thing, like what did I do wrong and how is she gonna be with it, you know, [and] is she hurting now? . . . I was just bawling and I was there all by myself and . . . calling like half of [the city], it felt like, trying to find somebody that . . . was home and that could talk. . . . They told me it was genetics but I didn't understand what genetics truly meant either, so I was like, well, what did I do and, you know, what could I have done different?

Most devastating of all, yet not uncommon, is the question parents can hardly bear or think to ask while holding the other end of the phone: Will my child live, and what can I do to keep him alive? In the poignant words of one parent: "They call and say 'You have got a problem and you have an appointment on Tuesday.' And we say, 'Is this something so bad that he could die between now and Tuesday?'"

Recounting such narratives about getting NBS results, no parent feels the system is working well. But there are a variety of ways in which even the most frightening kinds of news can be delivered—and some of these ways work better for parents than do others.

Failing the Stealth Test:
Better and Worse Ways of Getting Bad News

Though delivering bad news is a regular job function for many health care workers, receiving such news is—as Rayna Rapp says about prenatal diagnosis—"never routine" for the person hearing it. My interviews also corroborated Rapp's finding that "the circumstances of [its] delivery are indelibly etched into the memory" of each parent (2000, 220–221). The pain of learning that something is wrong with one's child is not easily mitigated; little can be done but to live through it and hope that time and experience will lessen its hold. But the way bad news is delivered—by whom, at what time, and in what way—this is something that can and does vary substantially (Baile et al. 2000; Helft 2005; Helft and Petronio 2007; Cleary, Hunt, and Horsfall 2009; Maynard 1996), and these variations matter quite a bit to people on the receiving end.[8]

Parents with a later diagnosis are generally in the health care provider's office or hospital when the sweat test results come back, or they have agreed with the provider ahead of time on clear follow-up procedures: how to get the result by phone, what to do next if the result is positive. The diagnosis may by then be expected, or it may still be a shock, but in either case it is unfolding in the context of the symptoms that prompted the test to begin with, and of a professional setting that parents are familiar with. Nancy describes learning about CF after her relatively healthy child had a rectal prolapse at age one:

> When we took her in to her pediatrician, she ordered a sweat test and sent us to the GI people to figure out what to do with this prolapse. And they admitted us to the hospital because they needed to lightly sedate her because when they would reduce it, or push it back in, she would, you know, feel it. . . . And so after she was admitted to the hospital, a few hours later the pediatrician came back and said that the sweat test was positive. And she said herself she would have bet a hundred thousand dollars that it would have been negative because other than being a little small, you know, she'd had one respiratory infection but got over it with no trouble and otherwise was healthy. So it was quite a shock. . . . She stayed one night for [the rectal prolapse] and then the next day we got the spiel from the CF doctor and the nutrition and then whatnot on "this is what cystic fibrosis is and this is what things are going to be like."

Erica too was told about her child's diagnosis in a health care setting and was connected immediately with the specialized resources she needed to begin addressing her daughter's symptoms. As a parent confronting CF for the first time, Erica found—as have other parents receiving diagnoses (Taner-Leff and

Walizer 1992, 95; Tluczek et al. 2005)—that face-to-face contact with doctors, "that personal touch . . . the person in front of you," was invaluable. So was immediate access to other resources. "I needed that information at that point, I think, as a new [CF mother]. I think parents need to leave with papers; you need to walk out with something in your hand. Also just an appointment makes a difference because you feel like, after you get your diagnosis, like you are blown away. It doesn't matter what it is. It could be leukemia, anything, but you need to know you are going to another doctor because then you feel like—you feel like it'll be okay."[9]

By contrast, parents of newborns who receive news of a positive screen generally have no way to walk out of the conversation with papers in their hands. What is in their hands instead is the telephone they answered when the fateful, unexpected call arrived—with a nurse, doctor, administrative worker, or newborn screening program employee on the other end. Often this person is a complete stranger to the parent answering the phone; and this is almost always true for parents who get an abnormal NBS result for a first child and thus have no relationship with the pediatrician or her staff. Sometimes, the caller will refrain from giving the positive screen result and instead tell the parent to come into the pediatrician's office as soon as possible so it can be given face to face. But usually, information about the first positive screen is actually given in full during the first phone call, and a date for confirmatory testing is immediately set.

Parents feel keenly the lack of advance warning or context for bad newborn-screening news, and most find this objectionable. Joan recounts her experience like this:

When [my daughter] was about two weeks old, we received a call from her pediatrician and her pediatrician informed us that one of her newborn screenings had come, that her pancreas wasn't working, and that she was presumptive positive for cystic fibrosis and that we had to follow up with sweat test. And he kind of made me mad because he told us over the phone. It was kind of like, "Get her to the hospital because we need to do tests." It just wasn't the correct way to tell us because we were like, "What is cystic fibrosis? Is she going to die?" . . . I think that could have been done in a better way. I think he could have explained a little more what it was. . . . I think he could have done it in person. I think over the phone was a little impersonal. . . . Especially something that is affecting your child and is going to affect them for the rest of their lives. And you can't tell me in person?

Other parents describe their telephone interaction with the person who delivered the screen result to them as "just simply" one of the worst aspects of a painful and prolonged diagnostic process. They go home with their "healthy, full-term" baby thinking that their "biggest problems are [breastfeeding] latch and how to get [the] mother-in-law out of the way, and to get some sleep." As Manny describes it, summarizing the experience so many parents recounted, when the phone rang, the nurse on the other end was "someone they had never met," and she was neither informative nor attuned to what the experience might be like for them.

> The nurse on the phone who gives you the news where she says he has got an elevated level . . . at the time I couldn't even understand what she was saying. I said "08? O-H?" I didn't know, and it wasn't enough of a word for me to say. . . . What is she saying to me? Is that the name of the disease? Or the name of the compound? Is that short for something? I just didn't know what that actually meant, it didn't even have any context for me. So I said, "What is that, is it the name of a disease?" The nurse said, "Well, do you have any medical background?" And I said, "What kind of a question is that to be asking me right now? I really don't want to debate with you as to whether or not I will be able to understand the information; I just want a little bit more."

These parents are voicing dissatisfaction with the standard method of communicating positive screen results, a dissatisfaction shared by most parents I interviewed who had received such a phone call. Other studies in the "bad news" literature also affirm that, "if there is no established relationship and no preparation, a message received by telephone may be catastrophic" (Salander 2002, 730). Newborn screening programs, and many of the medical providers who get screen results from the labs, have developed generic systems for dealing with positive screens that help them cope efficiently with a large number of tests. From the perspective of the system, it is just too costly and work intensive to arrange a home visit or even an office visit to explain every abnormal screening result (as Sally wishes had been true for her) "on a personal level" and in "a more friendly situation," where it would be possible to "have discussion" and ask questions. After all, the number of positive screen results is very large, but the vast majority are false positives and therefore signify little or nothing about the health of the baby. For newborn-screening programs coping with rapid expansion, often unaccompanied by adequate funding for follow-up services (Kemper et al. 2008), it makes sense to focus scarce resources on families with true positives. Yet for each parent getting the news that something may be terribly wrong with his or her child, the statistical likelihood that the positive screen does not indicate a real health problem is usually little comfort.[10] As one mother, (who, ironically, is a statistician by profession), put it, "I know odds are different from . . . reality, what actually happens. . . . I mean at that point I didn't care about one in four, I just cared about my baby." It is also not NBS system practice to differentiate results for emergent conditions that require immediate parental notification and vigilance from those, like CF, that are not time sensitive in the same way. Thus, all parents are notified as if there is an immediate cause for alarm, even when the condition in question is more chronic than acute and highly likely not to have severe (or any) early onset.

These narratives about the unexpected phone call also highlight the shock of receiving unexpected bad news when no interpersonal context exists for its delivery. An office setting alone is no panacea for this distress, as Ron illustrates in recounting what he calls "the most traumatic point we had" in the entire diagnostic process. After being suddenly summoned by phone to the pediatrician's office,

> the doctor picked up a pile of paper and was like, "Here's the information on CF, I'll be back in a bit, read this in case you have any questions." And then they all left the room. And it was [my wife, the baby,] and I just sitting in the room with a pile of papers. And my mind was blown. From the first news, to the [next] morning, to watching him scream as they were trying to get three vials of blood out of a six-pound eight-ounce [baby] . . . and they had had such a hard time, and then to just have this paper dumped on us—"Read through this and I'll be back if you have any questions." It was just really awkward. I don't even know how to describe it.

Sociologist Douglas Maynard has called this way of communicating "blunt informing," and his research confirms that this kind of interaction appears "to maximize the chances of panic . . . going to pieces . . . and otherwise being devastated" (Maynard 1996, 124) in just the ways Joan, Francesca, Lilly, and so many other parents receiving newborn screen results describe. Delivery of potentially life-altering information in the impersonal manner characteristic of NBS programs, with no forewarning, violates practically every accepted standard and commonsense precept about optimal communication of bad news. Patients do best, decades of research suggest, when they have "received some advance warning that the bad news is forthcoming," when the setting for news delivery is "as caring and uninterrupted as possible," and when there is "a reasonable amount of time . . . allotted for questions, answers, reflection, and grieving" (Helft and Petronio 2007, 809). In the case of NBS, these conditions are rarely met not because health care providers are inherently insensitive or uncaring (though this too can be a problem in some instances), but because of how the process has been structured.[11] In a system that mandates screening, does not provide adequate education, requires informed consent only by exception, demands immediate disclosure of abnormal results, involves health care providers who are not conversant with all the conditions screened for, relates results before many families have an established relationship with a pediatric care provider, and produces high rates of false positives, how can bad news but be delivered badly?

The disjuncture created by unexpected news summarily given is increased, for some parents, by the genetic nature of the detected abnormality, since genetic diseases are commonly thought of as already-identified aspects of heritability within families. As Manny describes: "It was definitely a huge surprise, and I think [it was] . . . mostly that this kind of stuff doesn't happen to me or my family, the family as a whole, both of our genetic families. I think mine especially is really sort of devoid—at least at the time let me say I felt like it was very devoid—of health issues." In the absence of a family history of genetic disorders, the positive screen feels preposterous—a violation of every assumption about how things would and should be. "At the time I felt that kids in our family were healthy and grow up strong," says Manny. "So then why is this happening now to us? Like, what is going on here?" For CF, this response is likely common, given that more than 95 percent of babies diagnosed via NBS have no reported family history of the disorder (Massie et al. 2010).

Even more disorienting for families are IRT/DNA screening protocols that result in identification of two known disease-causing mutations, and clinicians who interpret these results as a firm diagnosis before sweat testing even occurs. In such cases, parents have even less time to prepare for CF. As Gladys describes the unexpected call she and her husband received on the Friday evening after they had taken baby Johanna home from the hospital, the person "at the pediatrician's office, that first night they . . . said usually they do a second test, but they don't even need to, that they were positive she had it." Barb had a similar experience. The doctor "told us your son has CF, and he told us what it was sweetly," she says. But the shock made absorbing anything else during that interaction almost impossible.

> I am sure he told us a lot of information, but after that point you kind of shut your brain off. We were devastated. We came home, cried, and honestly stayed.in bed for a few days. . . . Right then that was kind of the

moment, and then after we processed a little bit the doctors called us the next day, and I said, "I am not ready to talk yet." . . . It was absolutely awful—you take care of your body and your baby the best you can and you find out that they are sick, and I just needed a few days to process and grieve. I am a mommy and I need to do what I need to do—this is my baby and this is our life and so it just took me a few days to grieve and get my head back on.

It seems likely that NBS will be etched into public consciousness one day the way prenatal tests are today (Rothman 1986; Rapp 2000). If so, the "devastating surprise" parents describe here will be significantly changed by parents' anticipation of standardized newborn genetic profiling and its results. Meanwhile, the impact of NBS diagnosis is softened only in relatively minor ways, for subsets of the population. One of these ways, which was described by several parents I interviewed (as well as in the published literature; see, e.g., Clayton 2005, S27), is shifting the setting for giving bad news from the telephone to the doctor's office, where communication has a slightly better chance to unfold with more sensitivity, and from which one can at least "leave with papers." Panic still sets in after the unexpected phone call, since it's obvious to parents that being hastily summoned to the doctor can portend nothing good. As Paula puts it: "I got really nervous, because I knew . . . they don't tell you about stuff over the phone if it's bad. I just was not expecting that." She continues, however, with this description of how her pediatrician created a little buffer for her in the diagnostic moment by preparing himself for the meeting and making time for a lengthy conversation about the abnormal IRT/DNA screen results received for baby Celeste.

> We have a good relationship with our pediatrician, and he was very sympathetic and spent a lot of time with us. I think we were in there for over an hour, and he even gave me a hug afterwards. . . . We sat down and he was pretty direct with it and said, "This is what they found." And that's when we kind of said, "Well, is there a possibility that this test was wrong?" And he said, "Probably not. Usually when it comes back with this mutation it's pretty definite." . . . I thought my daughter was going to die as a child and that was kind of my worst fear that any mom would have. And you know, I told him that and he was very sympathetic and letting me know that there have been a lot of improvements in care and changes in the way the disease works and the kind of hopefulness of all the research going on, so it was hard, but . . . it could have gone a lot worse if we had a doctor who was not willing to take the time with us

and explain things. . . . I think he'd even done a little bit of research before we'd gone in so he had up-to-date things to tell us, and he'd already set up the appointment with the CF clinic, taken care of that beforehand.

What the pediatrician managed to do in this case was what Maynard refers to as "forecasting," a "strategy for delivering bad news [that] provides some warning that [it] is forthcoming without keeping the recipient in a state of indefinite suspense (stalling) or conveying the news abruptly (being blunt)." The context thus created for Paula allowed her to begin inching, perhaps more quickly than others in her situation, toward "realization"—that is, the ability to hear about, understand, and begin to accept and effectively inhabit a new social world (1996, 109, 128).

What perhaps most changes parents' initial experience of a positive NBS screen is carrier screening during pregnancy—and a push from the American College of Obstetricians and Gynecologists to screen for CF during pregnancy (ACOG 2005) may make this mitigating experience increasingly likely. In cases where both parents have already been identified with CF mutations, the potential for a problem has already been flagged and the newborn screen result may not come so completely out of the blue. This is certainly not true for all women in this situation: parents with carrier results in hand sometimes forget that the newborn screen will take place or assume that, because—as Marta put it—"she is so big and she is so healthy," no bad news will come. In other cases, though, carrier identification provides a context for the newborn screen that substantially lessens the surprise element. This is how things went for Marta. Although learning about the screen result (which for her baby included DNA analysis affirming two mutated copies of the CFTR gene) was "upsetting" in the extreme, and not something Marta thinks anyone in their family will ever completely "get over,"

> it wasn't something that was shocking, you know, like, "Oh, my God." At least we had the educational piece and we knew that she was a high risk. . . . . And of course we were by no means experts, but we were somewhat educated about the disease, and it was scary but it wasn't as scary as what I first thought it was. It was certainly upsetting but not unexpected, but again I had found out that we were both carriers, maybe like in July, so it was a good five months that we had that knowledge; we didn't know Bethany was affected but we certainly knew she was at high risk, a one-in-four ratio, so we at least had the five months to kind of digest.

Marta hypothesizes that if she hadn't had this sort of advance preparation, she "would have been kind of crazy" getting the pediatrician's phone call, and the whole experience "would have been much, much worse."

"Everything Seemed Perfect":
CF Diagnosis for Healthy and Healthy-Seeming Babies

Most babies with CF are not overtly symptomatic at birth. Therefore, many parents who receive positive newborn screen results are not only completely surprised that the screening occurred, but also jarred—when the news arrives—by the juxtaposition of abstract information about a genetic disorder with concrete evidence of their child's good health they have had during pregnancy and in the days or weeks since birth. As James put it, summarizing the sense of objection and disbelief voiced by many parents I interviewed: "[My son] was born eight pounds two ounces, he was a big boy, he ate constantly; . . . he just wasn't showing anything that could make you think anything could be wrong at all." Even years later, many parents mentally and emotionally play, and then replay, their baby's healthy birth or early days, as Francesca does here: "Even when she was born, there was nothing; . . . she was born and she was seven pounds eight ounces, just, I mean, everything seemed perfect. . . . I didn't know. . . . Even now when I think about Tess having CF, it's so weird, 'cause we taped her birth and everything."

Suzanne had even less time than do most parents with positive newborn screens before getting a CF diagnosis for a newborn she thought was just fine. Because she and the baby's father had both tested positive as carriers for CF during the prenatal period, she had consented before her son Quinn's birth to have his cord blood tested immediately. Nevertheless, it came as a surprise to Suzanne when the test results came back on Quinn's fourth day of life. Aside from some iatrogenic problems with his umbilical cord, which kept both her and the baby in the hospital beyond the time at which they might otherwise have been discharged, she had found him relatively healthy since birth. She had been completely focused on getting to know and enjoying the baby, her firstborn, and she hadn't been focused on the test at all. "It didn't even occur to me [to think about the CF test] even when the doctor came in to tell me. I think I was more wrapped up in the euphoria of having [Quinn]; . . . I didn't really think about it until he came in and told me." However, once the results were in, Quinn's identity was immediately transformed from that of a healthy child who could be cared for primarily by his mother to that of a sick child who needed to be treated by the health care professionals in Suzanne's hospital setting. "I had to learn everything about him," she recalls, "how to treat him. I had to learn the physio and about the enzymes and different medications that he had to take. . . . It was like starting again, really. . . . It was huge. It was absolutely huge." Learning "about him" becomes, with the test result, a process of learning about CF and learning how to begin preventive treatment—a radically transformed context for early parenting. Suddenly, Quinn is no longer seen as, constructed as, just "a normal baby who you were allowed to hold and try to nurse." Rather, he is a newborn with a genetic disorder, a baby who requires expert treatment from professionals and whose mother cannot, at first, be entrusted with his care.

Although Quinn's health at four days of age seemed robust, he soon developed symptoms that required intensive treatment. That he appeared well as a newborn certainly colored his mother's encounter with early diagnosis, lending it the quality of devastating surprise experienced by so many parents. Over time, however, his label of "CF disease" began to align with manifestations of digestive and pulmonary illness in Quinn's life, making Suzanne a member of that subgroup of parents for whom NBS diagnosis marks an early departure from any expectation of normal health for their infant, and the beginning of active caretaking for a symptomatic child.

For another subset of parents, the jarring juxtaposition of disease labeling and good health that begins with NBS diagnosis lasts for months, years, or indefinitely.[12] For these families, CF diagnosis turns out to be a complicated genetic profile that may or may not result in any manifestation of illness. A CFTR mutation has been identified and the result has been given to the parent, but the child is healthy and may well remain so into adulthood or throughout life. In many instances where children manifest no illness, it is unclear whether the preventive care regimen has in fact been essential for maintaining their good health, or whether their particular genetic makeup would have kept them symptom-free regardless of early diagnosis and prophylactic treatment (Botkin 2005; Wilson and Jungner 1968). For some children, the latter explanation clearly holds.

Margo is a child who falls into this category—a little girl with very mild mutations for whom the doctors effectively withdrew the CF diagnosis by the time she was two years old. Her mother, Shannon, happened to be in her pediatrician's office when Margo's newborn screen result came in; she had never heard anything about CF before her doctor informed her of the positive screen. "[Margo was] chunky," she recalls. "She was over nine pounds at birth, so I mean there was no indicators, you know, I mean visually, looking at her there wasn't anything to think there was anything wrong with her." Getting the newborn screen was "very terrifying, you know, and I mean you're sitting there and it's like you're holding what you thought was a really healthy baby."

Shannon and her husband left through the back door of the pediatrician's office that they had entered blithely, from the front, an hour before; it was too overwhelming to contemplate being in public as their "world came crashing down." Margo looked the same after the test as before. She acted the same as well, and her good health remained unchanged. But the positive screen—and subsequent sweat and genetic tests that confirmed that she carries two copies of a CF mutation—irrevocably changed many things for her and her family, sending them on an odyssey of worry, monitoring, medical interventions, and "planning for something terrible that never happens" (Bailey and Murray 2008, 28). Shannon's story typifies scenarios hypothesized but rarely verified in public discourse about NBS (Baily and Murray 2008; President's Council on Bioethics 2008).

As is the case for many parents, the positive CF screen brought Shannon abruptly face-to-face with the contradiction of a laboratory result suggesting that her baby suffers from a serious and potentially fatal genetic disorder, and the very palpable reality of the thriving infant in her arms. Unwittingly, Margo was subject to what Dorothy Nelkin calls "a form of predictive diagnosis . . . [that] allows the anticipation of problems or conditions that are not necessarily visibly expressed in overt symptoms" (1996, 539). Shannon's assumption that her daughter was fine because she nursed well, slept well, and looked well was suddenly called into question, the experiential evidence on which mothers often base their sense of their children trumped by DNA analysis. Instantly, Shannon experiences Margo's identity as radically reconstructed by her genetic test.

Waiting Periods

The length of time between suspected and confirmed CF diagnosis is one important factor in the testing process that varies significantly depending on whether testing was initiated in response to symptoms. All parents feel a sense of urgency about performing a confirmatory test once CF is mentioned as a possible diagnosis. For parents with a later diagnosis, however, the time between a recommendation that the test be conducted and the test's completion is usually very short—a matter of hours or days, rather than the weeks it usually takes when testing is done via newborn screen. If their child has been symptomatic for a long time, as we have seen, these parents may have already suffered a diagnostic delay because of their health care providers' overall failure to take their observations seriously and recognize the reality of a problem. But the time lag for them is in knowing that CF might be the culprit at all, not in getting through the procedural stages between a positive screen and an established diagnosis.

In my interviews, many parents with a later diagnosis described enormous stress before CF was identified as a potential cause, but none of them described problems associated with the testing process itself once it was put in motion by their health care provider. This is consistent with other research about the testing process (Al-Jader et al. 1990; Tluczek et al. 2005), which found that all parents are "extremely anxious while waiting for the sweat test to be arranged," but that those with a newborn-screen diagnosis are far more likely to experience a distressing delay than are those whose children are tested once symptoms have emerged (Al-Jader et al. 1990, 462).

Lorraine was the only parent I interviewed with a later diagnosis who mentioned the possibility of an unplanned delay in obtaining the CF test.[13] Her need to act quickly to circumvent a waiting period illustrates just how strong the need for immediate action is for most parents once they are alerted to the possibility of CF.

> [The doctor] said, "Do you have any cystic fibrosis in the family?" And we said no. And she said, "Well, I want to test [your daughter] just to rule that out." It was a Friday afternoon, though, on the Fourth of July weekend and she said, "Well, you're not going to be able to get a test set up now, though, so you'll have to wait [until after the weekend]." And I was like, "No, we're going to get a test done." So we got on the phone to various hospitals and through a combination of pleading and making our case and tears and all other types of discussion with various lab techs we got some poor guy who agreed to stay late to administer the test to my daughter. So we ran over there and he administered the test on two arms—it was a sweat test.

Parents who receive a newborn screen result generally bear the burden of much longer waits, given the multistage nature of the testing process and the time that inevitably elapses between the steps. The diagnostic process in newborn screening, unlike testing for symptomatic children, begins with a positive screening result that is just a first step toward confirming the presence of genetic abnormality. In some states, that result may reach the parents after just one test, and the baby may then have to undergo a second IRT screening test and subsequently—if indicated—a third test to confirm or rule out the diagnosis. In other states, the child's blood may have already been double tested by a combination of IRT and DNA analysis by the time parents know about it, which halves the number of additional tests and waiting periods. But whatever the next step is, parents are usually told that the first positive screen result does not mean that the child is actually affected; a positive sweat test is needed for that. (The exception, as mentioned earlier, is when pediatricians interpret DNA results as a definitive diagnosis.)

As I have already shown, parents with a later diagnosis are generally most focused on their child's lived experiences with symptoms and what might explain them. For parents receiving an abnormal newborn screen result, however, the disease itself most often has no meaning except in the form of the abnormal screening levels. Consequently, the diagnostic process takes center stage, and parents all agree that the waiting period is terrible.[14] It is full of "tears" and "a lot of sleepless nights," of constant worry and anticipatory grieving; of fervent hope that the "test was wrong" and the next step in the diagnostic process will clear up the mistake. For some, "not knowing is the worst thing of all"—harder even than the diagnosis, in some ways, because of the helplessness and confusion it brings. Paula, whose mother flew in from another state to help her after news of the positive screen result, captures the "shocking and challenging" ups and downs of the waiting period this way: "I think I tried to put it out of my mind because [our daughter] was doing so well. So I just held her a lot. And I would have times where I would just start crying. And then pull myself out of it. And then just start crying. And then pull myself out of it."

One major source of distress for parents with newborns is when they receive a phone call announcing the positive screen and need for follow-up testing, and are then left in limbo to await further testing (Grob 2008). Often, the pediatrician, nurse, or office worker who communicates the positive screen result to the parent provides only the most minimal information about what CF is and what it might mean for the baby. This is partly because the structure of the process does not allow for in-depth interaction, and partly because the provider may herself know little about the condition. The general lack of knowledge about genetics and genomics among primary care doctors is well documented (Faulkner et al. 2006; Greendale and Pyeritz 2001; Kemper et al. 2006), as is their limited familiarity with CF in particular (Boulton and Williamson 1995). Add to that the astonishingly rapid rate at which the number of conditions being screened for at birth is increasing, and the chances that the person informing parents of a positive screen result can responsibly tell them what they need to know shrink even further. Duff and Brownlee (2008, 32) estimate that a typical "primary care unit" for children would encounter abnormal CF NBS results just once every ten to twenty years, and newborn-screening directors echoed concern on this issue. As NBS personnel in one state told me in an interview on May 5, 2009: "A lot of the physicians . . . are not comfortable with some of these disorders because they've never heard of them before."

Parents are often left to research CF on their own, then, after they find out about the abnormal screen—left, as Anthony puts it, "just trying to understand it without having [a] professional guide, or somebody who'd seen it many times before and could give us more concrete information." It was "actually just horrible timing," he continues, summarizing an experience many parents described of getting the call announcing the positive newborn screen for CF when "nobody was around" to provide more information or help. "I actually called some of my colleagues who I know are very well versed in birth defects and so on and they weren't even available. They had left, . . . so it was just, you know, bad timing on that. I ended up speaking to a nurse over the telephone and contacting the San Diego Cystic Fibrosis Foundation [which was still open]. . . . I needed a person, I didn't wanna just look online and speak online; . . . I needed to speak to somebody immediately."

In the absence of "a person," many parents try to learn more on their own. Sometimes physicians warn parents that there is misinformation out there, or information they just don't need to know yet, and advise that they stay away from the Internet in particular. But the need to do something—anything—in the face of potentially devastating news about one's baby is too powerful for most parents to suppress. These parents are desperate to know more, to find out whatever they can as they wait for further tests, and they are therefore often brought abruptly face-to-face with descriptions of the disorder (for which their newborn baby had just screened positive) as terminal and severely life shortening. Deena's description captures succinctly the shock of apprehending CF in black and white. After news of the positive screen, "I got on the Internet," she says, "and that was a big mistake. I actually got to the right site, and then you know, at the time, life expectancy was forty years old, and I'm thinking, Oh, my God, my son's gonna die, and I was just hysterical."

Once the diagnosis is confirmed and parents are integrated into the specialty center care system, medical interpretations of CF focus parents' energy as intensively as possible on the importance of early intervention in preventing or mitigating the disorder's effects. But during the waiting period, parents do not yet have access to this view of CF. Instead, they encounter modal descriptions of the disease, summaries of its accumulated natural history as understood to date, and average life expectancies.

One savvy mother pinpoints, in retrospect, the problem of disjuncture between publicly available representations of CF and the view of CF encountered by parents with early diagnoses who become integrated into early-intervention care systems.

> For me the most important thing is to get people who are learning about
> CF the most accurate current information about the disease . . . in the

beginning. I don't think I . . . got that. I only got it when I went to an Internet web page that hooked me up to other parents. Because . . . when I read official things—even the CF foundation web page . . . started out with something like "CF is the most common incurable fatal genetic disease." That was the first line of the CF Foundation Web page. And in fact as I've worked with them over the years I've gotten them to change that because I don't think that should be the gateway, . . . having you worry about this disease. I mean, you should not have that kind of preconception about a disease that at this point . . . I have a lot of confidence [will] become a highly treatable disease.

A related aspect of the "horror show" parents encounter during the waiting period is outdated information that does not take into account developments in overall CF care that have significantly extended the average lifespan of a person with the disease. "After I got off the phone with the doctor," Paige says, "I had picked up an old medical book. The copyright was like 1982, and it was talking about cystic fibrosis, and life expectancy was eighteen years old and this and that, and it was just very grim." And from Shannon: "The data is changing so much that if you read anything with any age to it, you know, you're gonna read a death certificate . . . ; there's so many people who still have them dying before they're thirteen." Other parents had a preconception about CF's severity without reading anything, because they knew someone, or knew of someone, who was desperately ill or who had died young because of the disorder. Evelyn's waiting period was haunted by images of a client her father had who died at age twenty-two; Paula's by an uncle who lived only to sixteen; Roger's by a childhood acquaintance who had it "pretty rough" and died early in high school.

Many parents turn not just to the Internet and other written sources, but also directly to their own infants in an effort to determine if she or he is really affected. Parents often search online to see "if there are any home diagnostic tests or anything, observations I could make to try to . . . rule it out or . . . rule it in, . . . anything I could . . . observe about our baby that would . . . give myself some more peace of mind that she wouldn't be diagnosed with this." Since there are no official home tests, sight, touch, and taste are parents' only avenues for collecting additional empirical information while they await more data from the laboratory. While parents hold their babies more tightly than ever, or wonder if they should "love them very much" since they may have a very short life, they also search them to see if there can really be anything wrong. Cora describes the experiments and investigations undertaken by many parents during the waiting period with her usual combination of verve and pathos: "We kept licking [the baby] 'cause, you know, all the stuff says if you have CF you have salty sweat. So we end up licking him." She and her husband began the search for symptoms even before the actual diagnosis—a search that later becomes ongoing for parents whose children have early diagnoses and are asymptomatic or only mildly symptomatic. We "absolutely" looked for signs of illness, says Cora. "We checked every poop. We were like, Okay, it's supposed to be, you know, greasy—is this greasy? Does this look greasy to you? How do you know if it's greasy? Oh, everything. Listening to him breathe. Putting my head to his chest. . . . I was just a little obsessive about kind of needing to understand it completely, and I just kind of got a little crazy about, kind of needing to know everything about it."

For other parents, the abnormal screen seems to illuminate, retrospectively, clues indicating that illness had been there all along. One father whose child has remained asymptomatic for more than a year recalls how many small things that had happened in the days since birth began to seem ominous after he got the NBS phone call. "You start to assemble all of these little pieces into some illness that you aren't even sure what it is yet," he says. "I guess when you get some sort of diagnosis, whether your children are symptomatic or not, . . . you are sort of saying that anything that is wrong must be part of this."

A minority of parents describe keeping panic at bay, "holding it together" during the waiting period by avoiding too much direct contact with information about CF and doing whatever possible "not to get worked up" before follow-up testing occurs. Many of these parents focus on the fact—which had been emphasized to them in some cases by the person reporting the abnormal IRT—that the result they have received is a positive screen rather than a final diagnosis, and that the initial problematic reading could be "just a glitch." "So I guess I hung on to some kind of hope that they were wrong," says Paula, "and the sweat test would come back saying that he didn't have it. So I think I was more into denial, saying, He doesn't have it, he's gonna be fine, it's okay, he doesn't have it, they're wrong. I think that's how I got through." Yvette describes the waiting period as "scary" and emphasizes that "even though they tell you not to worry, you're going to worry." Nonetheless, hopes for a false positive and reassurances from her pediatrician's office did reduce her fear.

> [Our daughter] was probably, I want to say she was a week to ten days old when they called, and they just said . . . one of these tests just came back a little high and we just need to redo that test; . . . basically they told me that the state had just changed their testing and it was brand new and it was still getting regulated and everything, not to worry about

anything, that it was just, you know, you just needed to redo it and that a lot of babies have to have it redone, whether it be because possibly they didn't have enough blood or possibly that they did it when the baby wasn't quite old enough, like they say like they should be forty-eight hours old, well, she wasn't forty-eight hours old when they actually did the test. . . . [They said] that it was no concern, that we just needed to have it redone.

A number of parents searched the Internet for information specifically about false positives or pointedly asked their pediatricians how often babies with abnormal screens are actually diagnosed. In several cases, parents "were comforted to find out that . . . as far as screenings go, a fairly small number of . . . the babies that are recommended for further testing actually are diagnosed positive." One father undertook the complicated task of researching the IRT cutoff level in his state and in other states around the country. Since his daughter was "barely . . . above the threshold for to where they recommend further testing, and . . . in fact in a lot of states, [they] wouldn't even have recommended further testing," the information about the nature of the screen resulted in his feeling "a little bit less pessimistic." A third parent, who lives in a state with a pilot NBS program for which consent is obtained before screening occurs, notes that she almost opted not to do the supplemental screen because she didn't "want a false positive and have to go through all the stuff."

For other parents, awareness about the high rate of false positives generated outrage about the newborn screening system. If the screen was much more likely than not a false alarm, then why—as one father phrased it—put so many parents through an "unnecessary . . . roller coaster of emotions?" For Anne, who had a particularly acute sensitivity to the issue of false positives, the roller coaster led from a zenith of optimism to a nadir of anger. After she got the call announcing the abnormal screen, Anne learned a great deal about false positives both from her own research on the Internet and from her pediatrician, who had said that since there was no family history for CF in baby Niko's case, the follow-up test was "not really a big deal," just standard procedure to "make sure everything's okay." However, her anxiety during the "week it took" before follow-up testing was extreme, and this was infuriating. "It was more of the not knowing that made me anxious than the actual disease itself at that time," she says.

It was more of the anticipation of Am I doing all of this for nothing? Am I worrying for nothing? Even to the point of getting angry, because if this is wrong then why do they even do it? If it is not right most of the time, why would you even do that? Just all kinds of different reactions to that. . . . Actually, I found a lot of things [on the Internet] that made me very hopeful and convinced myself that Wow, this really does happen all the time, that they do get a lot of false positives, so it actually kind of helped me calm down a little bit but at the same time it probably magnified my anger. . . . Like why can't they come up with a better way to do this? . . . Like why stress people out for nothing?

The waiting period associated with the NBS diagnostic process does eventually come to an end for most families, resulting in confirmation of a genetic disorder, identification of the baby as a carrier of one mutated gene, or news that the child is not affected. However, for most families with disease diagnoses, other waiting periods then ensue—for some, the period of waiting for older siblings' test results, and for many, the period of waiting to see when, if, and how symptoms will occur. And for families who are told their child has genetic "variants of unknown significance" or who hear other inexplicable news from the laboratory, the waiting—waiting to find out what their child's positive screen really means—extends indefinitely and profoundly changes the life-course of parents and child.

The "Cursed Blessing" of Newborn Screening: Timing and the CF Diagnosis

In her moving essay exploring the effect of newborn screening on the beginning of her life as a parent, Jennifer Rosner reflects on what is lost as well as what is gained from the unsought diagnosis of a disorder during the first hours or days of a child's life. Jennifer's baby was diagnosed as hearing impaired within hours of her birth. "I have . . . had two years to live with my mixed feelings about the cursed blessing of newborn screening," Rosner writes. "At once the grateful beneficiary of information that has enabled Sophia to hear and speak without delay, yet left longing for the pure joy of new motherhood, I cannot help wishing, still, that I had had just a bit more time unravaged by the news, at least more than a meager six hours—time to sing lullabies to Sophia, without worrying about whether or not she could hear them" (Rosner 2004, 21).

This kind of deep ambivalence about early detection is an aspect of newborn screening that is little considered in policy debates, research studies, or public discourse about NBS. By most existing standards (Wright, Brown, and Davidson-Mundt 1992), there is nothing subtle or debatable about Sophia's story. The early identification of her congenital deafness led to early medical interventions, which in turn enabled her to compensate for her hearing loss and to be able to hear in the normal range. According to the most widely accepted criteria for assessing newborn screening (ACMG 2005), this case is a winner: the condition is identified at birth, there is available treatment, and the treatment results in health benefits for the child and the family and in cost savings for society.

For Rosner, though, the immediate diagnosis also deprived her of a relationship with her daughter before she knew she was deaf. In coming to know Sophia and to make decisions about her health care, she had "little else to go on but her deafness," no other dimensions of her identity to counterbalance this early signifier of disability. "Singing lullabies felt idiotic," she recalls. "Indeed, all impulses to make sound were stifled by sadness and anger before they could leave my throat. . . . That I had only six hours of untempered joy at the arrival of my baby was maddening" (2004, 20).

When it comes to early diagnosis, parents care about aspects of NBS that the American College of Medical Genetics and other research and expert bodies generally fail to consider. Mothers whose children were diagnosed after symptoms developed often tell heart-wrenching stories detailing suffering that was alleviated once a diagnosis was finally made, and the improvements in health that occurred once causes were identified and treatment begun. And most parents with NBS diagnoses are explicitly grateful they found out at birth, as I have noted, because they believe that the earlier the intervention, the greater the health benefits to their child, and because they fear that the only alternative to NBS is the dreaded "diagnostic odyssey." As one mother aptly summarized, when it comes to getting the terrible news that your child has a serious disorder: "Never would be a good time! But if never's not an option, then as soon as possible, so you can start treatment." Nonetheless, in a complex echo of Jennifer's lament over lost lullabies and the "cursed blessing of newborn screening," some parents of children with CF also speak of the loss of something precious when diagnosis arrives so soon after the infant's birth, or of gratitude that the newborn period was not eclipsed by the bad news.

Kaya was about ten days old when Paige got the positive newborn screen result. Before the diagnosis Paige had intermittently suspected there was a problem with Kaya's health, but she also had basked in the glow of "falling in love" with her gorgeous new baby. In the four years since Kaya's diagnosis, those ten days have served as a sort of reservoir of remembrance, a memory to return to for emotional refreshment or respite.

Do I wish I would have had maybe a month, maybe two or three months, where she was healthy and we didn't know she had cystic fibrosis? Absolutely! Because I express to my husband, I say this all the time, some days I just wish I could go back to that time, to that first week, her birth, being elated about her birth. She was so beautiful, she seemed so healthy, that first week where everything—we were this little family and we had our first little house, and everything was so perfect and just as planned. It was just so content and so peaceful, and I was so happy, sometimes I wish I could go back to that time, so absolutely I wish I would have had a month of that, or two or three, before the diagnosis.

Other mothers who got the diagnosis either at or before birth speak wistfully about wishing their relationship with their child had not always been colored by CF, wishing they had experienced a time free of the sadness and stress that the diagnosis brought. "I think I would have opted for having a little bit more time," says Evelyn—and then she goes on to talk about how complicated that longing is, given that her child's continued good health might have been contingent on the earliest possible diagnosis. "I think it was our first day back when I got that first call, and that was hard . . . because there is so much going on. It is nice to be able to get to know your baby, but on the other hand I say that because Tyler is doing fine now. But if he had been sick, I guess they would have been doing testing anyway. If he had been a little bit sicker or had something going on that wasn't very apparent or clear to the doctors, and that . . . was doing damage, and wait three months [for the diagnosis]. . . . I don't know, it is hard . . . [but] I do feel it would have been nice to have a little bit more time." Gladys too, despite gratitude that her daughter was spared the possible health problems that a later diagnosis might have meant, wishes she had "had like a week at home" before getting the phone call about Johanna's diagnosis. Crystal, who got a prenatal diagnosis for her son Martin, yearns for "just one day where I didn't know." When I ask her what that day would be like for her, she replies that she doesn't know, she can't even imagine. But that's precisely why she wants it. "I would like it," she supposes, "'cause even when I'm not thinking about cystic fibrosis, it's in the back of my head."

Parents who got a later diagnosis view the question of timing from a different standpoint. These parents did have time with their child before knowledge of CF arrived—sometimes months, sometimes years; sometimes plagued by serious health issues, sometimes virtually without health problems or entirely symptom-free. Their responses to questions about what might have been gained, and what lost, by an earlier diagnosis were complex. They all, each and every one, believe that early diagnosis has beneficial results for the health of children with CF in general. They wanted to go on record as supporting newborn screening as a matter of policy because—as Nana put it, voicing the perspective of nearly all parents I interviewed—her child "is healthy right now, but who's to say he would be if we didn't know." At the same time, many parents spoke eloquently about the emotional importance of the time they had with their child without knowledge of CF.

Nancy and Paul capture very articulately the complex feelings a number of parents expressed about the timing of the diagnosis, that tricky push-pull between their own experience and their knowledge of what many professionals believe is state of the art in CF treatment. Their daughter, Alexandra, had been relatively healthy for her first year. Her growth had slowed some—a phenomenon noted at the time, but given significance only in retrospect. As mentioned earlier, neither her parents nor her pediatrician were overly concerned about her health or development before she suffered the rectal prolapse that led to prompt CF testing. The positive result shocked both the family and their health care provider, since Alexandra had been so healthy up to that point. Looking back, it's difficult for Nancy and Paul to separate out their own experience (both felt the timing of Alexandra's diagnosis was optimal) from what they know is being advocated in the professional world of CF. In Nancy's words: "Newborn testing, you know, they say that that would be best, if she would have been diagnosed, I mean, the earlier the diagnosis, the better, is what they say. But I don't know. I think about this sometimes and I just—it was great having one year of blissful ignorance basically, so I don't think I would have changed it. But I think the diagnosis came at a good time. I definitely wouldn't put it out any further. . . . I'm glad, I'm actually pretty glad for when we got the diagnosis." And from Paul: "It's hard for me to think that any [other] way [of getting the CF diagnosis] would have benefited *us* more. . . . The only thing that I can think of is that with cystic fibrosis, scientifically and medically it is better to be diagnosed earlier, to get a jump-start on treatment and maintaining good nutritional habits as well as eliminating unnecessary exposure. . . . I think only from the scientific and medical standpoint, I would say it'd be better to know at least at birth."

Catherine, like many parents, wishes she had had an earlier diagnosis for Joseph; he suffered terrible malnutrition during his first seven months, and she is certain that at least some of the multiple developmental issues he continues to struggle with at age seven could have been prevented with early treatment. This was a terrifically sorrowful consequence of how the diagnostic process unfolded for her. Even so, she knows she would have lost something precious if she had, like Sophia's mother, experienced only a few hours or days getting to know her son just for himself, rather than as someone with a genetic abnormality. "I'm actually grateful for what I had [with a later diagnosis], because

I did have my moment in the sun. Even if it was that one day in the hospital with all the guests and the flowers and the balloons and thinking I have this beautiful healthy baby. It wasn't robbed from me from the get-go, where other people know right away and they never have that moment in the sun. They always have to be anxious—when is it coming, what's going to happen."

Evelyn, whose asymptomatic baby was diagnosed in infancy after a positive newborn screen, experiences the flip side: yearning, endless yearning, for precisely that lost moment in the sun a later diagnosis buys. Amid the barrage of condolences that poured in as news about Tyler's diagnosis followed immediately on the heels of news about his birth, Evelyn says she didn't want to keep hearing from others " 'Oh, my gosh, I am sorry.' I wanted that support, but at the same time I remember saying to [my husband,] Pete, and everybody, 'I just want to go back,' and that feeling of I don't want to be here where I am right now. . . . I wanted that excitement about having your baby and all of that, but it just stopped."

Not infrequently, an infant's positive newborn screen precipitates the utterly surprising diagnosis of an asymptomatic or largely asymptomatic older sibling—and thus a whole different set of complicated emotions about diagnostic timing. This was the case for Lorraine, whose son Luke was two and a half when she learned his younger sister Jessica had CF. After Jessica's diagnosis, Lorraine and her husband had insisted—over the objections of a physician who resisted doing the test on such a healthy sibling—that Luke be tested too. For Lorraine this always difficult process was made substantially easier coming at a later age, when she already knew that CF need not mean poor health and suffering.

> I was actually really glad that my son was two and a half when they were both diagnosed because my own experience with my son was as a very healthy kid. And so when I got the diagnosis I didn't all of a sudden put him into a category that all of a sudden he's an invalid. And I had with my daughter, because she was so thin and fragile at the point she was diagnosed . . . but having my son being so hale and hearty I knew that that was not necessarily something that was predestined. I knew that we had a CF kid who was perfectly healthy.

Lara's daughter Frida was also not diagnosed until age two and a half, and was also largely asymptomatic during almost all that time. But then Frida began to have puzzling digestive problems, and eventually CF was identified as the cause. For Lara this timing was a mixed bag. On the one hand, Lara believes that if her state had already had newborn screening for CF when Frida was born—as it did by the time her youngest child arrived—Frida might have been even healthier than she was at diagnosis. On the other hand, Lara knows that if Frida had been diagnosed via newborn screen, "there's a lot of things that would have changed in our lives. Like would we have had two more kids if we knew she had that from birth? I don't know. There's a lot of things that might have changed. . . . I think it would have been more devastating." Cassandra's seven-year-old daughter Vera was completely asymptomatic when she was diagnosed after her baby brother had a positive newborn screen. Cassandra has no regrets: Vera's diagnosis "happened the way it happened." Because her daughter did not suffer the diagnostic odyssey Cassandra has heard about from other parents, she is content.

When parents remember their experiences with the timing of CF diagnosis and imagine what it might have been like if the timing had been otherwise, several other life circumstances are introduced repeatedly as important factors.[15] One of these is whether the affected child is a firstborn. Getting a diagnosis in the first weeks when you're a first-time parent—whether you have suspected a problem or not—is perhaps uniquely difficult, for there is neither experience with another child nor a history with the affected child to act as an emotional buffer. Marta describes how she "had no idea how to care for a child, let alone a child with CF." The collision of new motherhood and a little-understood diagnosis is devastating, "especially when you just had a baby for the first time and you are like, Oh, my God, this is so overwhelming." Gladys concurs: "I just sort of felt [my daughter] as like this baby that I had to keep alive. And how am I supposed to do this? . . . She was my firstborn, so . . . I had the stress already there of knowing what to do and how to take care of her, and wondering if I was doing things the right way." The surprising, early diagnosis heightened these feelings of vulnerability so that she ended "just having [my daughter] with me more, . . . like at night, she was with me constantly . . . and, like, all I could think about was CF."

Francesca describes how the combination of new motherhood and surprise diagnosis result in particular forms of uncertainty and hypervigilance: "As a new mom, you're always skeptical. Do I put her down, or should I go check on her? Should I not check on her? And with CF, it's like, Okay, now I have this newborn and I have CF, I can't put this baby down. I have to sleep with her right next to me because I don't know what's gonna happen and what's going on. I think it just—as a mom, it made me a little more paranoid." Paige tells a similar story: "Kaya slept next to my bed in a little cradle, where I would fall asleep and my arm could reach over on her stomach so I could feel her breathing, because I was afraid she was going to stop breathing in the middle of the night, I was going to wake up and my baby would be dead, until she was seven months old, and just that fear is so intense."

Experienced parents on the whole seemed to share the perception that news of the diagnosis is somewhat less shocking if there's a child in the home already. For example, Lilly, who had a healthy four-year-old at home when she got the newborn screen diagnosis for Mia, imagines how difficult it must be to manage when one is a first-time parent. "You're going from no baby ever to having a baby and now trying to work all your life around . . . it, and now you have to do all this extra health care with this baby." After pausing, she adds: "I think if it would have been my first child I would have felt like I missed out on having a normal child." And from Roxanna, who has three unaffected older children:

> Honestly, I feel so sorry for people that . . . it's their first child. . . . Because you're robbed of so much with your first child having CF. . . . When your first child's born, yeah, they're beautiful and they're great, but you already have—you have so much learning to do because, number one, you don't know everything that you're supposed to do, you learn as you go along with your first one. So I think when you throw in the CF factor with that, you know, not only are you learning, Okay, what does this cry mean and how, when, do I feed him? . . . You're having to get up at all hours of the night and you're sleep deprived, then you have to give them enzymes, and how are you supposed to get the enzymes in them, you know, it's just so incredibly overwhelming to have a first child.

Another critical aspect of the timing of NBS diagnosis is the mother's vulnerability in the postpartum period.[16] For most women, this is a momentous and highly emotional time. The physical demands are always significant and sometimes overwhelming. Between 50 and 80 percent of birthing women go through "the postpartum baby blues" during the first weeks after birth, experiencing a range of symptoms such as tearfulness, depression, insomnia, emotional instability, elation, headaches, fatigue, confusion, and poor concentration (Rothman 1993, 311). About 10 to 20 percent also suffer postpartum depression, a syndrome whose "usual symptoms are sustained depressed mood, heightened concern about her own and the baby's health, anxiety, somatic preoccupation, indecisiveness, fatigue, irritability, and sleep disturbance" (ibid.). Getting a CF diagnosis during this alternately fragile and exuberant time, with "all these postpartum hormones going on," presents specific challenges. Cora describes them like this: "I mean, it was a nightmare. 'Cause you're dealing with someone who's completely postpartum, right? So your hormones are all over the map anyway.

You're not sleeping anyway, you have this new creature in your house that you're not really sure what you're doing with, and then it's a Friday and you get this [positive newborn screen result] dumped on you, but you have no answers yet. Especially, you know, if it's something like this where 'It may be CF, but we don't know yet, we have to do more tests.'" Yvette had similar experiences. "You're sleep deprived anyways," she says, "because you're up at night . . . and then you still have your hormones that are out of control from having a baby." Getting the NBS results in the midst of this postbirth time, "hav[ing] that on top of it to worry about . . . did play a lot," for her, into how very devastating it was to cope with the positive newborn screen.

Selena's nightmare involved not only her new, apparently healthy baby, but also a diagnosis for an older child. During the first conversation in which positive newborn screening results were reported, the pediatrician instructed Selena to have her older children tested immediately. "Having a baby is very emotional," she says. "Finding out that this terrible child disease—she has it—and then . . . finding out a second of your three children has it was pretty bad."

Catherine says she has thought about what it would have been like to get a newborn-screen diagnosis, to find out about CF in that immediate period after birth when her son seemed perfectly healthy.

> I think it definitely would have been like a punch in the stomach. . . . You're lying there. . . . I was not well; other mothers might be basking in the glow of their baby. And then you are told that there is something wrong. I think things would have very quickly disintegrated because, you know, there's also postpartum issues there too and it could get really ugly. Cause, you know, the whole newborn thing anyway, you're tired, you're exhausted, you're recovering, you're this, you're that. You don't know what you're doing, you don't know what to expect, and then to get a diagnosis on top of it just seems even more looming and frightening.

Nancy concurs: "[The NBS diagnosis] would have of course been just as shocking and I just think as a new parent that would have been almost too overwhelming for me. I was really overwhelmed with a newborn anyway. . . . When we did get the diagnosis, it almost did feel like we had a newborn again. We had to learn so much about her and give her, you know, enzymes and figure out how to do this and how to do that. . . . I just think with a newborn it would have been—I can't even imagine what that would have been like. To have had both at the same time."

The CF diagnosis brings with it—among other things—a crushing, sometimes disabling sadness, a chronic sorrow. As Erica puts it: "I remember waking for . . . nine months when [my children] were first diagnosed, [and] within two minutes it would hit me and I felt like I was kicked in the stomach. . . . It wasn't a death, but it was the death of a dream of a healthy child." Kim says the depression she fell into after the diagnosis was debilitating. "I don't know how I would be today," she adds, if she hadn't gotten help in the form of medication.

If a child is ill, there can be no question of separating the moment of diagnosis from the postpartum period; the disease is manifest and must be dealt with immediately. But what is the effect of piling the genetic diagnosis of an apparently healthy newborn on top of all the other postpartum issues? We know that young children can be significantly affected by their mother's postpartum depression, but the literature has not yet addressed the relationship between this well-documented phenomenon and newborn screening.

A related theme relevant to diagnostic timing that arose again and again in my interviews is the heartache of being visited by the specter of death in the midst of experiencing birth. Confronted with the possibility that their baby has a fatal disease, most parents are thunderstruck at the juxtaposition between the freshness and fragility of the brand-new life they are holding in their arms, and the idea that this baby's life will be cut short. As Cassandra puts it: "At first when we got the news that he even possibly had it, the first thing I thought was, Well, he is going to die. Here I had this wonderful baby that seemed so perfect and he is not going to be with us for that long." From Paula: "I really kind of lost it. I thought my daughter was going to die as a child and that was kind of my worst fear, that any mom would have." And from Barb (whose newborn, Kenny, appeared "healthy and strong" at birth like the majority of infants who screen positive for CF): "You would never have known" there was anything wrong. But when the call came announcing the abnormal newborn screen result, she—like most parents—immediately imagined her child's imminent death. "You look at your baby and you think 'fragile.' I instantly thought, If you touch him, he will break. . . . When I looked at him, I thought, well, I didn't know how much time I had at that point, I didn't know if this was something that happened within days; I really didn't know much about it at that point. . . . I did not know what his lifespan would be, I didn't know if this was going to change him physically, I didn't know anything."

Of course, there can be no good time to anticipate the mortality of our children. It violates the rightful order of things for parents to imagine surviving their kids, and being made at a child's birth to contemplate that child's early death presents particular challenges. As Barbara Katz Rothman wrote of anticipating shortened life as a result of prenatal diagnosis, this kind of foreknowledge "is incapacitating. We have no framework for handling foreknowledge such as this. . . . All our children are going to die. We birth all of them into the passage of death. But it really doesn't do to think about it. When a woman is forced to confront the inevitability of her child's death, she must evaluate the meaning of her child's life" (1986, 175). When that life has not yet had time to unfold, the meaning of birth is challenged in particular ways. As Paige described, voicing emotions that nearly all parents I interviewed expressed in one way or another: "I had when she was born so many hopes and dreams and aspirations for this child and she is—she is the most beautiful child I have ever laid eyes on and so smart, and I love her so much, and I want so many things for her in this life, and yet it scares the shit out of me, excuse my language . . . to think of, you know, what's it—what's it gonna be like, how sick is she gonna be, how many years does she have, and the hardest thing is nobody can answer my questions."

Going Public with the Diagnosis:
Social Construction of the Child's CF Identity

Children belong, in some sense, to their extended families and communities, as well as to their parents. Most children have several and sometimes many adults in their world who care for them and about them, who want the best for them.[17] These adults have their own spectrum of reactions in the face of substantial threats to a child's health and well-being. CF is one such threat, and parents—particularly those who receive a newborn screen diagnosis—find the process of telling family members and friends about the diagnosis to be a crucial aspect of their own experience.

Parents manage the dispensing of bad news in a variety of ways, of course. Some share with others their fears and suspicions, the worrisome signs or medical news they receive, right from the beginning. Others wait until test results are in and the situation has been more fully clarified before bringing even intimates inside their trouble. Some look to people outside the nuclear family for support, assistance, advice; others feel that they have to manage the reactions of other people and that giving them information is therefore a burden. Part of this variability is attributable to personal and interpersonal style and psychology; to how physically and emotionally close the parents are to family and friends; to what else is going on in everyone's life at the time. But also important is how, when, and within what context parents themselves receive the news.

Parents whose children have had chronic health problems over a period of months or years before the diagnosis are least likely to be alone with their sense that there is a problem by the time the diagnosis comes. Often these parents have already talked with others about their concerns, asked for help, sought referrals to health care providers, and otherwise gone public with their knowledge that something is wrong—or that they suspect something is wrong—with their child. Sometimes other family members and friends have seen evidence of the child's poor health or impeded development firsthand. By a process of accretion, the child has already begun to be constructed both within and outside the household as someone with health issues. The CF diagnosis is thus more often a confirmation than a surprise not just to the parent, but to the extended family and community as well. Knowing that CF is to blame can still be a shock for everyone involved, but it is unlikely to bring with it a complete reconstruction of how people understand and perceive the child. Parents of children with a later diagnosis may therefore focus less on the challenges associated with telling others the news, and more on the role of people beyond the nuclear family in connection with caregiving; on the impact of the diagnosis on relatives' reproductive decisions and sense of self; and on the dangers of contagion at family gatherings and in other shared settings.[18]

Parents who receive a positive newborn screen for a child with no or only few and nascent manifest health issues are in quite a different position when it comes to telling family and friends the troubling news. With the call from the doctor's office, a set of complex interpersonal dynamics is set in play. Parents wonder, Do we tell other people about the positive screen, or wait for the confirmatory sweat or genetic testing? Do we wait until we know more about the condition and its implications, or ask others for help navigating this new terrain? How will family and friends respond to the news, and how will their response color my own as I adjust to my new knowledge? And underneath all this, implicit yet palpable: Will telling other people make this unreal news more real? Will it make my baby forever a sick baby instead of a well one in the eyes of the world, and thus in actuality?

Shannon, the mother of a well child with CF, articulates the difficulty and confusion of going public. She describes wrestling with what to tell people, when to tell them, and the subsequent need to cope with their responses as "the hardest part of [the] entire process"—quite an assertion for a parent going through an experience so profoundly difficult in so many ways. In the time between the positive screen and the confirmatory diagnosis, she and her husband "didn't tell anybody what was going on because we didn't have enough information, as far as—not because they didn't provide us, but we didn't want to tell people, a bunch of people, that there might be something when there might not be. . . . Why get everybody worked up, and also, too, it is [a] very . . . hard thing to explain because nobody has any experience with the disease."

Again and again Shannon returns to her reluctance to share the screening results, to get other people involved. Partly she was being self-protective, wary of their reactions. "I've got enough to keep my own emotions in check right now," she says. "I don't need to have to try to . . . take care of y'all, I need to take care of myself and my kids and my husband and that's it." But also during the time between the screen and the test Shannon felt deeply hesitant about putting her daughter Margo's public identity in question, bursting the bubble of congratulatory joy that accompanied the baby's birth and replacing it with—what? The idea of a daughter who seems healthy, adorable, and chubby, but is actually carrying a potentially deadly genetic disorder within her week-old body? A future that suddenly seems ominous yet is unclear in terms of actual implications? Shannon and her husband, like many parents in this situation, were themselves vacillating between hope and fear, between a sense that nothing could possibly be wrong and a deep foreboding that something was. Why encumber the process with the weight of other people's responses until, as another parent put it, they themselves actually "knew what was going on"? Why give other people the power to participate in constructing the child's identity while they are still struggling to do so themselves?

In contrast, Evelyn and her husband decided to let a wide circle of family, friends, and co-workers know about baby Tyler's positive newborn screen. "That was emotional too," she recalls, "just getting all that support." But as the news spread and calls of concern began to pour in, all that worry did in fact make the positive screen feel like an inevitable diagnosis.

> We were getting calls from people, and calls from people . . . and I started getting a little scared about it, like I was thinking, Is somebody preparing me for the worst? Why are we getting so much support before we really know definitively? But I still in the back of my head [was thinking], I really don't think he has CF . . . but I was in the back of my head going, Why are we getting so much support? And then again I felt all the support we were getting. . . . [Does it mean] Tyler going down a bad path, and I know that is not logical, and is that why we are getting all this support? All of those weird things were going through my head.

After the confirmatory test, going public brings another set of issues. The reality of the genetic mutation is now irrefutable from a scientific standpoint, but the process of understanding what this means, of conceiving who this child really is and what role CF will play in her life—that has just begun. Parents must begin at this point to cope with the diagnosis themselves, to hold this shocking news about their child's life and identity in whatever way they choose, or are compelled, to hold it. Other people told about the diagnosis and therefore included in this process can disrupt the parents' own modes of adjustment in a number of ways. Parents of newborns sense keenly how fundamentally the baby's identity is "socially bestowed, socially sustained and socially transformed" (Berger and Luckmann 1966, 98), and they endeavor mightily to protect both themselves and the baby by controlling this process during infancy as much as possible. However, their capacity to manage the responses of other people is limited, and the resulting distress can be significant.

Joya recalls that telling other family members about the diagnosis was most difficult because others would react more strongly than she. They would see CF as more dire, and her daughter Ariel as more vulnerable, than Joya herself did. Waiting a while to tell the hard news "probably had to do with that I didn't want people to feel bad for me," says Joya. "I think I didn't want that bad vibe or bad energy. I just wanted the love and happiness and I didn't want them to worry, and [my husband and I] both agreed that we thought it would be better to keep the good as long as we can, and hope for the best the way everything turns out."

For Joya, going public presents the risk of having her child's situation immediately construed as disastrous in that tender time when the baby and the diagnosis are both new. For parents reeling from the news themselves, parents with "little else but the diagnosis to go on" in their perception of their infant, it's not helpful to have others predict or foresee a bleak future, a limited life span. It's not helpful for parents to "get people calling and saying, 'We hear your baby's dying'" (as one mother reported), while they hold and tend their newborn. It's not helpful when relatives who knew someone with CF who died young begin to assume (as another mother put it) that "that is going to be my path." Such responses, or the fear of them, force families inward, changing the newborn period from a time of shared joy to a period of self-induced isolation, a time when you "don't wanna . . . talk about [the baby and the diagnosis], not—I shouldn't say not being able to, but choosing not to."

In some families with asymptomatic babies, the diagnosis remains undisclosed to others for months, years, or indefinitely after the positive newborn screen. The prolonged silence is sometimes motivated—at least in part—by loving consideration of others and the wish to spare them pain. Baby Marin's grandparents, for example, are no longer young, and her father, Roger, can't bear to give them news that he fears will worry them unduly.

We just think, . . . Why put this burden on them, you know, when we could wait a little while longer and let them know, when we do tell them, they'll know that we've known for a while and we're okay and, they'll just—they'll worry about her, Marin, of course, they'll be heartbroken, and they'll worry about us too, [but] I feel that if we wait a while, perhaps they'll . . . feel better about us . . . because they'll know we've dealt with it and we've adjusted and they'll worry a little bit less about her because they'll know she's doing well and not a little infant, you know. . . . We want them to accept it a little bit easier as she gets . . . older and less fragile looking.

As this articulation of Roger's reveals, the desire not to worry others is often inextricably linked to the desire not to be worried by others—to hold, instead, an optimistic interpretation of the future. Marin has a little-understood mutation and is asymptomatic; in other words, her diagnosis in no way portends a particular prognosis. Better for Roger to suffer the distance that secrets impose between him and his parents than to tip the emotional equilibrium he has struggled so hard to establish in the face of potentially devastating news, and thus to impose a perhaps unnecessary sick role on his thriving newborn.

When diagnosis as well as prognosis are uncertain in the wake of a positive newborn screen, the difficulty of telling others can multiply exponentially. Abby has struggled for well over a year with this situation. "No, we did not tell anyone else," she says, "because we figured at first why get them upset, we don't even know what is going on. [But] that feeling sort of never went away, and we still don't really know what is going on." The silence will become untenable at some point, she projects, and they are "getting to the point where we are going to have to get out of the closet a little more, and that is hard, too. It is really hard." Hard because it means coming out as the parent of a potentially sick child; because it may change the way others regard that child; and because divulging the news at this late date might incite anger, hurt, or worse. "I have a sick kid," says Abby, "but not really. I don't want to be the mom of a sick kid and . . . I don't want him to be perceived differently. Until there is a point where I have to stop the playgroup and say, 'Okay, it is time to take your medication,' I don't really feel the need to put it up there. At the same time I do run a huge risk, because if he does get really sick a lot of people are going to be like, why didn't you tell us something about this? You know we could have helped you or we wanted to know."

When disclosure does come, it can often bring relief. Cora, for example, describes herself as "the kind of person" who needed a lot of people to know "what I was going through." Happily, she has been gratified by an outpouring of empathy and assistance. "The response has been so supportive, and so terrific." Paula too remembers how "supportive and positive and hopeful" her parents were when she called with news of the diagnosis. Nana and her husband found solace in telling their pastor, so he could pray for them.

In Barb's case, telling family was crucially important yet complicated by her sense of being at fault for the diagnosis. "It's almost like a guilt thing," she says. "And you have got to go through the whining of it. What did I do? Did I drink soda and I wasn't supposed to? Did I walk through a smoky restaurant or something like that? Like what did I do? So you go through something like that, you feel a little ashamed, like you did something wrong, but you get over it, you know. I needed my mother, my mother and I are very close, and my husband's mother, she was amazing." Barb and her husband made a point of trying to normalize their son Kenny's diagnosis, reassuring family members that it was best not to avoid the topic. "People tiptoed for a little while and didn't say much, but Irv and I would bring it up, and we would talk about it kind of randomly to people just to show them it was okay to talk about it, and that we were okay, and it was a good thing that they should know about [it]."

For many parents, though, the diagnosis creates a dividing line between themselves and the realm of normalcy in which they formerly dwelled. Paige captures the sense that others cannot truly comprehend the seismic shift the diagnosis has caused, or how profoundly it has transformed what it means to mother the new child.

> In the beginning everybody's in shock. And your whole family hears about the news, and there's . . . visitors pouring in to visit, and . . . sympathy cards of "I'm so sorry," and phone calls of "Oh, my gosh, I can't believe this is happening," and family members who want to buy air purifiers for the home or give money for this or make you meals. But then after it settles in, . . . everybody goes on with their day-to-day life, which is normal. But your life isn't normal anymore . . . not normal, per se. And now you're doing—people don't know—you're getting up in the morning, you're doing breathing treatments, you're doing chest physiotherapy, and you're dealing with emotional issues and financial [issues]. I mean, the dynamics of the disease are huge, and those phone calls stop . . . and the in-kinds stop, you know. And that's normal, but it's just so lonely. . . . I can't tell you how many times I would have just loved to just pour out all of my feelings and cry about it, and I think people are hesitant to ask. . . . It's just very—it's just very lonely, with cystic fibrosis.

Like the mothers who find themselves taking a self-protective turn inward after the diagnosis, those who experience the awkward falling off of inquiries and support end up feeling very much alone, walled off from the physical presence of loved ones and community at a time when support—not just emotional, but also material—is critical. As a parent interviewed by other researchers puts it: "One is never more alone than after one's child has . . . been found to be ill or disabled. One encounters rejection and distancing from others—even those from whom one has a 'right' to expect better. One withdraws, bruised and hurt" (Taner-Leff and Walizer 1992, 98). When the diagnosis becomes, as it inevitably must, a public as well as a private event, it affects all the "embedded contexts"—household, extended family, community, social support systems—in which early childhood unfolds (Bronfenbrenner 1979).

Only a few mothers in my study described "an act of social recognition" (Taner-Leff and Walizer 1992, 99) that helped them feel less rather than more isolated after an early diagnosis. Evelyn was one of these. Her initial grief, after an NBS diagnosis for her second child, was utterly debilitating. She was "totally sobbing," she says. "And then just looking at Tyler and just disbelief, I just couldn't believe it. . . . I just got home with [my husband] and I just cried and felt like I was crying for three days straight, and just looking at Tyler that was all we could think about. Then feeling sad for [our daughter India] and how this was going to affect her, that was one of my biggest fears too, that was hard, . . . can we be here for her just emotionally, we were so distraught that I was like, Can we get through this?" Pretty soon after the diagnosis, though, Evelyn got a call from Alice, the mother of an adult child with CF who was a friend of her sister. That call, which was both compassionate and well timed, bore very precious fruit.

> When Alice called me, and she woke me and said congratulations on Tyler, that was like the first thing she said. It was so nice to hear that. . . . The one thing that Alice did tell me too, which was great, she said, "You know how you are probably starting to put India in a naughty corner or a time-out or whatever, or thinking about that she's getting to that point?" I said, "Yes, she isn't quite there yet." But she said, "You will be doing those same things with Tyler. He will go to the naughty chair; he's going to be driving you up the wall on certain days and will be laughing on some others." So she was putting a really nice normal human address on it. So that was really important to hear. Like, it is not always going to be me feeling devastated and sorry for him?

As I have shown, the experience of parents who encounter illness before a diagnosis differs from that of those who get a diagnosis at the very start—sometimes long before any symptoms, but always before the child's identity has been clearly established apart from CF. The latter experience became increasingly common as prenatal diagnostic tests were introduced and quickly became the norm more than twenty years ago (Rapp 2000; Rothman 1986). Now, with the rapid growth across the states of newborn screening for CF and myriad other genetic conditions, mass screening and presymptomatic testing affect ever-larger numbers of parents. As a result, the relationship between parental knowledge of the child and scientific knowledge of the child, between the experience of CF as a physical illness and the experience of it as a diagnostic prediction, is shifting again. As I will now discuss, this shift has profound effects both on parenting practices and on relationships between parents and health care providers.

Chapter 3

Specters in the Room

Parenting in the Shadow of Cystic Fibrosis

A diagnosis of CF is unquestionably a shock and a sorrow, a critical moment in the lives of parents. They remember it vividly even many years afterward. They relive it often, recalling every detail of who was kind and what was hurtful as it unfolded. It is the moment that ends the parents' pre-diagnosis existence and marks the beginning of their careers as parents of children with a genetic disorder. Once on the postdiagnosis side of the divide, parents can never go back. Facing a present and a future shaped by the diagnosis, they have much to say about going forward—about the impact the CF diagnosis has had on how they connect with and view their child from infancy onward, and about how their parenting practices and styles unfold once they know about the disorder.

Living with the Ghost of CF

Any diagnosis of disease occupies the forefront of parents' lives when it is new. Most are utterly preoccupied, at first, with understanding and responding to the news. Over time, as with any seminal event, there is a process of acclimatization; the disease begins to take its place within the family context, no longer occupying every nook and cranny of available time and space. However, it is never far below the surface, even in times when the child is healthy or when other major life events—the birth of other children, divorce, career changes—are occurring. As one mother puts it, CF is "nothing I can just put in the back of my mind. . . . I know every minute of every day." Another describes her pain over the diagnosis as constant, something she thinks about "every time" she looks at her son. A third describes knowledge of CF as "just a burden, there's just a weight, . . . there's just a little shadow lurking around. . . . It's almost like there's a ghost in the room you need to live with, . . . and that ghost is cystic fibrosis."

For most parents receiving a CF diagnosis during their child's infancy, that ghost transforms their perspectives on their child and haunts their dreams of what the future might hold. The context in which their parenting unfolds suddenly feels like a bounded one, one that might no longer be able to hold the grand dreams or the lavish hopes that come with a sense that you are caring for the next generation, the one that will outlive you. Suzanne describes the change she underwent during Quinn's infancy this way: "I think beforehand you sort of think about—like you have certain dreams and expectations of what life with your child is going to be like and . . . that they are gonna live a normal life and be happy and healthy and everything else. But afterwards it's all different. Like you sort of think about, well, no, it's not always gonna be healthy and maybe they're not going to live for as long as you think that they would've before knowing about it, and I . . . think it just changes your perspective on things."

Paige's dreams for her baby were also radically altered when she received the newborn-screen diagnosis, her taken-for-granted optimism also suddenly shattered. "I was going to do everything to make sure this child would grow up to be a great individual who—you know, with a great childhood . . . that thrived so well. I was going to do everything in my power to make sure everything went well for her, and all of her dreams were coming true. When I found out she had cystic fibrosis . . . , a lot of my dreams for her—I felt like they very well could die, because CF might take her before she can attain these dreams."

For Kayla, diagnosis when her son was a newborn felt like a violation of every assumption she had held about what it would be like to have a baby and become a parent. "You don't expect to have to deal with something like that," she says, "knowing that through your whole pregnancy you are so excited about this beautiful healthy baby." The arrival of the diagnosis obliterated this excitement, replacing it with grief, denial, confusion, and the sense that maybe she got the wrong baby. "That wasn't supposed to happen," Kayla observes. "This is a healthy baby, we are young healthy parents, . . . we don't know what this thing is, this CF thing—we don't know what this is. . . . Nobody in our family has it; this is an impossible-type thing. It's not us."

The responses these mothers describe influence many aspects of life: the ways parents bond with their child, how they try to safeguard the child's well-being, the shape of their caretaking practices. They influence family priorities, the shaping of children's lives and identities, and the day-to-day parenting and household routines that form the context of childhood.

This Isn't the Baby I Thought I Had:
Bonding after the Diagnosis

For parents getting a positive newborn screen at their infant's birth, profound gratitude for information that may result in better health and development for their child often coexists with a sense of loss and sadness about how the process of connecting with the baby was irrevocably altered by an unexpected diagnosis during the first few weeks or months of parenthood. Deena, for example, experienced the newborn-screening diagnosis as a clear interruption of the bonding process she had begun with her baby. It was harder to connect with him, she says, "because during that time I thought, . . . Why should I bond with him if he's not going to be around for years to come? Why bother?"

Joan had to undergo an extended process of adjustment both to the routines of preventive care, and to the idea that baby Isabel had a CF diagnosis, before she could establish intimacy. "It seemed like it was six months to a year before I felt, Okay, I know what I am doing now and I really feel close to this baby. . . . I think I had to mourn the loss of the healthy child I had. You know, I had to go through that mourning process of, Okay, I don't have a healthy child. This isn't the baby I thought I had."

In some cases, one parent has a more difficult time than the other bonding with their baby after diagnosis. This was true for Gladys and Al. Gladys got over the shock of the diagnosis relatively quickly. Her husband, Al, however, "just had it in his head that . . . we're going to raise her and she's just going to die" for nearly a full year after the diagnosis. "He only saw her as someone who was going to be weak and sick all the time," says Gladys. "He could only see Johanna as like a sick kid. . . . So we finally got into some counseling for it, and our counselor [told] . . . him how much he was missing out on because he wasn't really present, because he had completely just kind of shut down, and so finally he started to actually enjoy her."

Francesca also found the first year of her daughter's life dominated by CF; for her, too, it was only when Tess turned one that she began to regain the confidence and ease she had felt that first month of Tess's life, before the pediatrician called with the positive screen. "It took me . . . [until] her first-year birthday where I actually felt like, Okay, we're not dealing with CF, the CF is gonna have to live with us." The shifts Francesca experienced were radical: from not suspecting anything could be wrong with her apparently healthy baby, to having Tess's identity dominated by an unknown and invisible disorder, to coming out the other side with a synthesis of the two—a clear sense at last that the lives of the family and the child are primary and the diagnosis secondary, rather than the other way around.

Shannon, whose apparently healthy baby had been diagnosed by newborn screening, found the diagnosis made her self-protective, afraid to love a daughter who might die young.

> The hardest part about that whole time, . . . it's just knowing that this is something that . . . could potentially take her life. Having been a mom already, the hard part was that at times I felt like I was scared to fall in love with her because I didn't know how long I'd have her and so that was the hardest part, because I mean those [weeks and months] that we were waiting for the information back, um, I have to say I did look at her a lot and think about it, and it's hard to look at her and go, Well, . . . nothing's wrong with her 'cause she's beautiful and she's, you know, just the epitome of healthy. . . . [When she was a newborn I wondered], Okay, who are you? And then to find this out a week and a half after she's born, so then that compounded on top of it . . . it's kind of like, Okay, . . . I'm trying, now's the time when I'm supposed to be falling in love with you, but I'm scared to.

Reflecting on what it was like to connect with her baby in those early days, another mother with an early diagnosis comments: "We had to get to know her as somebody with CF, not just to get to know her for her and then figure, Oh, she's got CF." These mothers feel keenly the effect of never having known their child before the diagnosis. Thus Jennifer Rosner's observation that the "excitement of having a new baby was entirely eclipsed" by the early diagnosis (2004, 20) was echoed by parents receiving a diagnosis of cystic fibrosis during their child's first few weeks of life. They too felt grief over every experience their child might not have, over the struggles the child was already encountering or might encounter when older, over the loss of the "baby they thought they had." Some were immediately confronted with the diagnosis because the child manifested illness, but most lost the ability to get to know their baby first just as a baby—not because the baby was sick, but because of the early test.

It is customary for research looking at the impact of early diagnosis on bonding to discount shorter-range effects, seeking instead to determine whether there are long-term outcomes in terms of behavior or attitude and how these outcomes compare to those associated with other forms of diagnosis. The underlying questions have usually been these: Are measurable difficulties with attachment that parents may experience after NBS greater than those associated with clinical diagnosis? And are bonding issues related to NBS diagnosis temporary and ultimately resolved, or sustained and significant enough to cause lasting harm to the child or to the parent/child relationship? Although psychometric studies have documented some temporary rejection of infants (Al-Jader et al. 1990), most NBS commentators characterize the published research as concluding "that diagnostic distress, although considerable, is no more extreme following a newborn diagnosis than a later clinical one, nor is the mother-baby relationship more negatively affected" (Parsons and Bradley 2003, 287).

The narratives recounted to me by parents do not refute these findings. Rather, they highlight qualitative aspects of experience not easily captured by other forms of measurement—the residual sorrow, guilt, and regret that come to mothers as a result of having ever kept at a remove children to whom they are now so passionately committed. Every parent I spoke to, no matter how hard that initial period was, found a way to get through this, a way to profoundly connect with the child. Some of the most moving moments in these emotion-filled interviews came when parents described this process. Listen, for example, to this mother, who began the work of bridging the distance she felt from her infant very soon after the diagnosis. Imagine you can hear the tears in her voice as she speaks. "I went up there [to her room] . . . with my camera and I sat there and I held her, and I dressed her up and we took pictures and I just talked to her for a while and it was—it helped. It helped a lot just to tell her that I'm her mom, and it's okay, and we're gonna take care of her, and, um we're gonna have a lot of fun, and not to worry about whatever's gonna happen 'cause we'll take care of it. And um I just kinda sat there and explained it all to her, and it kinda put a perspective [on] how I felt about her, 'cause obviously I cared."

Of course she cared. Each parent cares, and each also tends her or his child with tenderness, competency, and abundant love. As one father told me, they eventually lean down over a sleeping child and whisper, "Don't worry, no matter what happens, I'll always take care of you." But this does not mean that the bonding issues raised by an early diagnosis weren't both devastating in the short run, and also resonant over a much longer period of time. In fact, it's precisely the contrast between what they felt at first and what they came to feel later that remains an open wound for these parents. As one father expresses the sequence of emotions, at first "you have this feeling that is like I shouldn't get that close to this baby because he could be gone in a couple of days." Later, though, you are "super, super guilty" about having felt "you shouldn't spend any time with your child, . . . because . . . he doesn't deserve not having me because he might be gone or something."

Nicole communicated the pain of this contradiction in all its fullness. She told me in detail, weeping, about how right after birth, with the pending diagnosis and a host of treatment issues to attend to, the work of parenting was numbing, devoid of the emotional connection she grew to feel once her daughter got older and she came to know her. "I think in the beginning it was such a—it was a job," she recalls. "I loved her but I was so busy caring for her that it was almost kind of routine almost at the beginning. And [then] she grew and she became stronger and I guess you just have to know her, but she is so happy and loving." Nicole feels regret and guilt for having at first experienced her care for baby Jenna as numbing and technical rather than joyful and heartfelt. How could she ever have failed to love this baby as she deserves to be loved? How could she have seen her as coextensive with her diagnosis rather than as the full human being Nicole now knows her to be? None of the parents I spoke to could recount their version of this contradiction without similarly deep emotions, even if many years had elapsed since initial estrangement melted into absolute devotion. A CF parent blogger summarizes powerfully what I heard from women in my study. When the doctor told her about the positive CF newborn screen, she writes: "I looked at my baby. She felt foreign to me at that moment. I wanted to get out of that office. It is hard to admit, but at that moment I wanted to get away from her. Not because I did not love her, . . . but because I suddenly felt like I had let her down. I felt guilty that I had made her and she was not perfect. That moment in time is burned in my memory forever. Just writing all of this is making me cry."[1] Another source of parents' concern and regret is the impact their own grief might have—whether transient or lasting—on the child. Parents worry that their strong emotions about the diagnosis may create a toxic environment for the baby, disrupting, as one parent put it, "such an early time and such a bonding period, . . . feeling heartbroken instead of overjoyed." Roger describes his struggle to cope with the diagnosis while taking good care of his baby daughter:

> It was really hard, you know, because it's such a bonding time with your child and to be upset during that time—I knew that that's just not good, that hurt . . . , in the first few weeks of the baby's life, to be upset, you know. . . . It's so much preferable to be in a good state of mind during that time, you know. I'm sure the baby picks up on those things, if you're upset about something, and feels instead of seeing. . . . I got home from work one day and looked at her and I was just heartbroken, thinking about it, and . . . I know that that's not good, I know that it affects . . . her in the long run, psychically somehow, deep down, it's affecting her, and so I tried to put on a good face and tried not to let her see, you know, me upset or anything like that, but . . . babies can feel, they can sense your mood when you're holding them and stuff.

Sally too tried mightily to buffer young Stephan over the first year of his life and beyond from what she describes as an "overwhelming" response to the diagnosis. "It was really hard for me," she says.

> I couldn't talk about it, because in my mind, it really put me in a depressed state where what my mind focused on was, My kid is sick and going to die. That's where my mind went to. Not the fact that he is hardly affected by it, but there's no cure for this and he could die as a child. . . . It just was overwhelming for me, I had a problem dealing with it, . . . the thought of my kid dying, I'd get to the point where I'd break down in tears. And I tried my hardest not to do it in front of him because I thought, Here's a kid who is probably for the most part happy and it's not his problem to deal with my emotions so I don't want to do it in front of him. So I would make sure not to be doing it in front of him. I'd go into another room and have my breakdown for a few minutes and then be fine.

And from Evelyn: "I know when you have a baby you feel like all you do is spend your time to survive for that person. However, I just felt like we were inside crying and stressed for the first—I don't know how long."

These parents try heroically to shield their newborns from the emotional trauma unfolding around them in connection with the diagnostic process and its results. As Abby notes with such moving modesty: "It was like the worst moment in my life, but I was trying to make it okay for my baby." Still, parents wonder if they succeeded well enough, and what the impact on their children will be.

Well before NBS's vast expansion, Clayton observed: "No one has determined . . . whether the benefits to the child of avoiding parental uncertainty exceed the impact on the child's bonding with the parents when serious disease is diagnosed in the newborn period" (1992a, 642). Some studies have demonstrated that high maternal anxiety during the newborn period is associated with "adverse interactive behaviors" in later infancy and decreased sensitivity on the part of mothers with respect to their babies (Zelkowitz et al. 2009, 56), but little research has been done about the effects on children of anxiety related to newborn-screening diagnoses per se. The experiences of Sally, Roger, and others suggest that it is essential to keep asking Clayton's question if we are to grapple fully with the implications of newborn screening.

Whatever I Do, It Will Affect My Child: CF and Parental Vigilance

Anxiety, watchfulness, and the intense desire to provide an optimal start in life are all well-documented characteristics of contemporary parenting—especially middle-class parenting—in the United States (Marano 2008; Stearns 2003). However, early diagnosis of a genetic disorder heightens these tendencies exponentially. Evelyn put the matter succinctly: "I knew he could become sick, and I was worried about whatever I would do, how it would affect him, like the whole germ thing and keeping people away who were sick." And from Manny: "The world of newborns says everything you do right now is going to have lasting effects forever and ever. So we thought just because we were supplementing some formula, Am I losing five IQ points [for our baby] every time I do this?"

As CF moves to center stage in the drama of family life during the baby's first months and years, vigilance emerges as perhaps the central parenting motif. Ordinary awareness that children are influenced by everything around them morphs, for these parents, into hyperawareness. What naturally follows is an effort to control every element of the child's environment that may impinge on her health.

Now We're Germophobes: Minimizing Exposure to Risk after the Diagnosis

One significant change many parents experience after a CF diagnosis is increased protectiveness toward the child. As they learn about or experience the pulmonary and nutritional vulnerability CF can produce, parents of the newly diagnosed baby find themselves trying to mediate their child's exposure to germs of every kind. This can take the form of becoming a "hand-washing Nazi" in the home, as one parent said, or as another put it, of sprinkling sanitizer over every surface and feverishly scrubbing every toy and appliance. "[You become] very protective, very overprotective," says Meredith, wanting to guard your child "from anything, . . . be it the insane world we live in, or the bugs that some kid next to him sneezes and wipes his snot on his arm." "I was like the mother bear," Paige remembers. "I just became so intent and almost worried and obsessive about some things, pouring bleach down my drains every other day because pseudomonas could live in my drains, cleaning like crazy, almost to the point where I was driving myself nuts. . . . I mean, since then I have calmed down a lot, and I've learned a lot more about cystic fibrosis, but it was just very intense [in the beginning]."

Acting a "little freaky" about germs means not only "scrubbing the house constantly, disinfecting this, disinfecting that," but also preventing contact between human purveyors of infection and the diagnosed child. Barb sums up parents' efforts to wage a two-fronted war on germs this way: "I have done a lot of things; I have become a massive germophobe. . . . I do a lot of cleaning. I own every antibacterial product on the market. I find myself very into illness around me, because I am very careful what situations I put Kenny in. Malls at Christmastime does not happen. . . . He doesn't know McDonald's has a play place. He has never been to any of those things. . . . I carry a thing of Purell on my key chain, things like that."

Parents who already had a child or children before the one who got the positive newborn screen are aware that they cope with exposure to germs in substantially different ways for the diagnosed child. Selena's reflections are illustrative:

We are more cautious about things [with Jana]. Like with [her older brother] Rich, we never thought twice about things, we would just take him and pick up and go take him wherever. Now with [Jana] being diagnosed, . . . we were very careful, we didn't let anyone in the house, . . . we were very leery about going anywhere, and I carried a big bottle of sanitizer before anyone could touch her, anyone who smoked wasn't allowed near her, like even outside because I didn't want the smoke, anything, getting near her. . . . It pretty much became a germ issue after Jana was diagnosed. Even the boys, they weren't allowed to touch her, take your shoes off before you come in, wash your hands. It was rough. . . . [The doctors] kept saying, "The best medicine is preventive medicine," and all they kept saying was "preventive, preventive, preventive." That is why we do physical therapy twice a day, that's why we do [medication] twice a day, so I said, "Okay, no one sneezes the air or breathes the air and everyone's hands are clean."

For some families, doing everything possible to keep the diagnosed child healthy also results in significant restructuring of household arrangements and approaches to family life. How the baby is cared for, and by whom, is one primary focus for many parents in the wake of unanticipated CF. Anne, for example, recounts that for her and her husband, being "germophopes now" meant the decision not to send baby Niko to child care as they had envisioned. "You know, [at the CF clinic] . . . in that first initial thing, they stressed very few little things—but the one thing they stressed was, keep Niko away from sick people. . . . You have to protect him from getting sick." Instead of group child care, Niko stays home with various family members who reworked their schedules in order to make this possible. Marta and her husband also created a different child-care structure after the diagnosis, significantly revising the system they had set up during the first few weeks of baby Bethany's life when (first child though she was) excessive caution about her exposure to other people seemed neither necessary nor optimal.

Mothers for whom staying at home is a financially viable alternative may decide after the diagnosis not to return to work after all, opting instead to care for the affected child themselves full time. "With Eben," Kayla says, unlike with her older child, "I carry five bottles of hand sanitizer with me. [And] we made the decision for me to stay home because I didn't want to put him in day care." She wants to be home with him to keep him away from germs, certainly, but also because she doubts the competence of others to carry out the prophylactic regime with adequate rigor. "In the beginning I was very sheltering with him. I didn't even want anybody else to hold him. With his care I am reluctant to let other people care for him when I am not there because I know how to do it, I know I can do it right, I know I am going to do it and I won't forget. . . . It has been very difficult for me as far as trusting other people to care for him the way I do. Even grandmas, even people that I know might take care of him, I even watch [his dad] sometimes because I want to make sure he is doing it right."

Relationships with immediate and extended family are substantially affected by an early CF diagnosis, given how challenging it can be to stay close with relatives while remaining vigilant about germs. Parents yearn for the joy of sharing their child with grandparents, aunts, uncles, and cousins; in many cases they also want the support that these family members can provide. At the same time, each contact with other people represents a threat to the child's health that some parents feel just isn't understood or adequately accounted for by even the most trusted relatives. As Yvette sums up the dilemma: "We have a big family who like to do lots of things together and . . . they don't really realize. . . . They just think, Oh, I just have a little cold that's not going to hurt anybody, I'm not contagious, or whatever. But we're always like calling, Is anyone sick over there? Anyone have a runny nose or anything? 'Cause we can't come if . . . they do. And so that's been kind of difficult, but I'm sure it will get better."

Holidays, which hold so much meaning and also entail so many people gathered in one spot, are particularly problematic. Like Anne and her husband, many families find themselves "altering the way we're going to do our holidays now, because of [the diagnosed baby]." In some cases, this means forgoing time with family altogether and just staying home. In other cases, parents opt to attend gatherings but enforce infection control practices with rigor. "I got everybody into the kitchen and I said, 'Guys I have to tell you something. The last time you were here [the baby got sick], and I am not trying to blame anybody for anything by any means, but he did get a virus from somebody that may have not known that he had it, so I am asking everybody to make sure that before you pick him up, even if you have already done it, every time before you pick him up, just use the hand sanitizer.' So only about two people held him."

This sort of strategy may result in less exposure to germs for the baby, but it also makes others "more held back" from the baby—a response that parents recognize, and one that causes sorrow. "Before that, everybody wanted to hold him," says one mother, "but since they have seen how serious I am about [preventing infections] it has kind of changed them a little bit as far as how willing they are and how much they want to handle him." Another mother reflects on how bad she feels that she can't share her CF-diagnosed baby with loved ones the same way she was able to share her older children.

Yet another approach to significant holidays is to attend and to watch closely so as to be well positioned to intervene just before unwanted contact is made. Roger and his wife have gone this route. "Thanksgiving," Roger says, "we had a bunch of family together and [we were] worried, just watching her, wondering when those kids are going to start grabbing her face or something like that and perhaps giving her a cold." It was good to be with family, but being "paranoid about people" and beset by "constant worry" made the holidays entirely different from how they had been envisioned before the diagnosis.

Not surprisingly, being germophobes in the postdiagnosis period can result in significant physical and therefore social isolation for mothers, since keeping their affected child away from people means that the mothers too must avoid contact with others both in public and at home. There is satisfaction in guarding the baby's health so thoroughly, and relief from the anxiety of watching over the child in public can be huge, but the costs for the mother herself can also be significant. As Evelyn recalls: "You feel kind of isolated anyway when you first have a child, you are at home and nursing and doing all that, and this kind of isolated us even more, because I was concerned about people coming over, taking him out. I remember that being a hard thing, and relationships changing a little bit because of that, or not spending as much time with other people." In particular, Evelyn's being separated from her sister, with whom she is close, at the crucial moment of combined new motherhood and unexpected CF diagnosis was "just a huge thing." This aspect of the newborn screen diagnosis—the imperative to keep the baby away from germs as vigilantly as possible—puts a significant and growing group of parents with NBS diagnoses in precisely the situation a parent interviewed by Patricia Taner-Leff and Elaine Walizer describes about the experience of early diagnosis: "Laura's pediatrician wanted her kept away from everyone with their wintertime germs—'don't take her shopping with you, don't take her near other kids'—and of course both the season and the presence of a new baby made it harder for me to get out anyhow. I had been used to working closely with adults and teenagers every day—literally having a couple thousand interactions—and suddenly I was locked up in the

house with a . . . newborn and a cat. The telephone helped some, but my physical isolation echoed the isolating effect of Laura's birth defects" (1992, 139).

Many parents are well aware that there is a danger in becoming too protective, both in terms of the child's healthy all-around development, and in terms
of their own need to "have some sort of social life." However, arriving at that
balance between minimizing the risk of infection and getting out into the world
a bit is not always easy. As Andrea puts it:

> I was kind of torn. I wanted to make [my son] really healthy, wanted to
> put him in a bubble. . . . People used to joke that they would almost have
> to go in the bathroom and shower before [touching] the baby. . . . We
> cleaned out the house, we scrubbed it top to bottom and just set every-
> thing up. No carpeting in his bedroom 'cause I wanted to make sure—
> I mean, I knew that there were respiratory things, so I wanted to make
> sure that there was no chance of asthma-related things. . . . I wanted to
> wrap in him in a bubble but I still was logical enough to know that
> that would not keep him healthy; what I needed to do was make him
> active. . . . The whole thing is keeping his lungs strong, . . . keeping him
> active, to let his lungs grow strong and his heart grow strong.

Additional contact with medical professionals, continued good health for
the diagnosed child, or simply the passage of time can begin to ease the intensity of parental vigilance in many cases. For other families, competing family
priorities intervene. As Cora recounts, she and her husband are "really conscious" about exposure to germs for their asymptomatic toddler. "The Purell,"
she says, "we do all that." However, "the reality is that I have a five-year-old
and a two-year-old, and they love each other, and I can't possibly stop the
germs from going back and forth between the two of them, and frankly, it ain't
worth tryin'! You know what? There's only so much energy you can expend in
a day, and that would take all of it. . . . To tell my daughter she can't give her
brother a kiss? Not worth it!"

Parents whose children were older at the time of diagnosis are generally
more sanguine when it comes to issues of vigilance. They protect their children, and a number of them mentioned specifically and with regret how connecting in person to other families with CF is impossible because of the high
risk of cross-infection between kids. At the same time, they see a substantial
difference between their own parenting practices regarding infection control
and the practices of those diagnosed early. As Erica puts it:

> Well, one thing I have noticed [is that parents with early diagnoses] . . .
> become more like lunatics. A lot of these people, they will share different

stories. They are putting, like, plastic on the shopping carts. I guess they are so young when they are diagnosed that they are so concerned about bacteria and stuff. They become more overprotective, I guess that would be a good word. And I guess I'm more relaxed with things. I mean some people are, "I can't come into contact with other people." One girl, I wonder what happened to her. She had two kids with CF, and her sister had it. She wouldn't let her sister see her kids.

Parents who have a healthy older child diagnosed with CF after a younger one is diagnosed via newborn screening are also much more sanguine than those whose only knowledge of CF is shaped around an early-diagnosed baby. This was the case for Lorraine, whose older child was a completely healthy two-and-a-half-year-old when both he and his little sister were diagnosed. "If I had known when he was a brand-newborn, I might have been a little bit more alarmist [and] concern[ed] than I was knowing he had made it to two and a half without any real misses and had CF," she says. "I honestly think [if I had known earlier] I would have been way more protective than I ended up being." However, with the diagnosis coming later as it did, she is emphatic that CF didn't change how protective she was or much of her feeling about who Luke is. "My son had done so well. . . . I was just determined that he was going to be fine and I really didn't become overprotective. I mean, at that point we were in, we had a nanny and she was watching my son and another boy and they went to the park, and he went to preschool and little art classes and gym classes and that kind of thing."

Lara too found that having an older child diagnosed later provided useful ballast in the face of the NBS diagnosis of her baby. "We have to be more concerned than the average family about somebody coming into the house with a cold or whatnot," she says. But the difference in household routines from before to after the diagnoses is not extreme. This is because by the time her older daughter "was diagnosed, we could already look back over two and a half years and say, Well, she's obviously got a mild case of it." If she had been diagnosed at birth, however, Lara says the diagnosis would have been "more devastating" and her reaction more extreme, because "at eight days I couldn't look forward and say, She's obviously going to have a mild case of it. We would have been reading all the awful things and, you know, been told all the awful things about CF and would have feared the worst."

Waiting for the Other Shoe to Drop: Anticipating the First Symptom
Vigilance about germs is greatly intensified for parents of NBS-diagnosed children; however, it is by no means unique to this group of parents. By contrast,

hawkish monitoring of asymptomatic children is specific to those who receive early news of CF—via either prenatal testing or newborn screening—for children with no signs (or at least no obvious signs) of illness. Even in instances where the child's CF mutation has been identified as a mild one, and even when health care providers and/or the most up-to-date literature suggest that no symptoms are likely to emerge for quite a number of years (if ever), parents can't help but watch anxiously for telltale signs that the much-dreaded first symptom is arriving.

Crystal's child, for example, has a very mild CF mutation, yet her knowledge that he is unlikely to be displaying symptoms during babyhood feels largely theoretical in light of his grave diagnosis. "I think that if we had not had this testing," she says, "I don't think he would be diagnosed right now. . . . He doesn't have symptoms." Nonetheless, for this third child of hers,

> there's things about him that I just pay much more attention to. . . . I mean all this stuff about poop, it's kind of funny—what do babies do? They eat and poop. And the twins, . . . they were just healthy; whatever they did, they did. But with him, I'm like calling, you know, every time I visit a doctor, . . . it's like talking about how often he poops and et cetera, and I'm concerned about it. . . . He's really gassy, and . . . a lot of times, I'm like, I don't know if his gassy problems are just from being a baby or [from] cystic fibrosis. . . . I'm worried. I just want him to be normal.

Francesca describes how the early diagnosis changed her experience of parenting from one dominated by an assumption that all was well to one dominated by a preoccupation with what might be wrong:

> When I just had her those first four weeks [before knowing about CF], I would have never have thought she was different than anybody else. But then I don't know if it made me more paranoid after the sweat chloride test, but then you would hear her breathing heavier or like her chest sounded like . . . more kind of gunky and just, you know, like it didn't sound clear, it always sounded like it had a rattle to it, and I don't know if some of that is just paranoia that set in or if it was truly that she had these symptoms and just being a new mom, that Tess was my first one, I just didn't know different.

Parents of asymptomatic children say they wonder what "the slightest cough means." They are "watching out for any symptoms—a lung infection, or malnutrition." They listen to how their child breathes, "listen for wheezing sounds or any kind or indication that something might not be right." Any sort of sound, real or imagined, makes them "start to worry right away" and to "freak out." Even when there is no appearance of illness and the child seems entirely healthy, they "look for signs—every day" and wonder, "When is it going to happen? How is it going to happen?" For some, this is "the hardest part," this living always with "that elephant in the room," wondering if sickness will arrive tomorrow, or "six months or six years down the road," or never.

Hypervigilance and the search for symptoms are unavoidable sequelae of the diagnosis for almost all parents. As Kate puts it: "I analyze everything. It drives my husband nuts. When I come home and the babysitter's there, 'When did she poop, what time, what did it look like?' . . . 'Cause I feel like I have to stay on top of it." And from Cora:

> We're also always listening to, you know, is he wheezing? Does he get
> out of breath? . . . Any time when he starts having stomach problems,
> I start, Okay, is this it? Is this finally, you know, the thing? . . . Even
> though I know logically it's not digestive problems because he gains
> weight, and he's doing great. . . . I'm also constantly on the lookout, Is
> this going to be the thing? . . . This could be it. This is it. This is the other
> shoe dropping. And it hasn't been . . . but just knowing that this is out
> there, and . . . not knowing when that cold's going to be *the* cold . . . it's
> kind of like the sword of Damocles is always hanging over your head.

Cora has not yet found anything truly worrisome to report in the two and a half years she has been mothering and monitoring her son; since his mutation is extremely mild, and his case of CF has been described as "borderline," the other shoe may not in fact drop in the foreseeable future, or ever.

For some mothers of asymptomatic babies, vigilance takes the form of tracking not only potentially worrisome signs but also growth, developmental milestones, and other indications of normalcy. These accomplishments are memorized in detail, and filed in memory (and sometimes in writing too) as evidence that the child is not completely defined by his disease. As one mother puts it:

> There is definitely an increased vigilance, just a real sort of hawkishness
> in terms of when he was not gaining weight, I counted every calorie that
> went into his body every day until he started gaining weight again. I can
> tell you the day of every single one of his developmental milestones, not
> because I care about those kind of details, but it seemed important to me
> in the face of all these doctors who are saying, You have this kid that is
> messed up, and then I would be able to say, Well, he did this and he did
> that, and on this day and that day, and he sat at five months, and he

crawled at seven months, and he is incredible. You want to be able to say something to people when they say that your kid isn't good, you say, Yes, he is. So, there is the vigilance both for the good things and the bad things. I want to be able to tell you he knows twenty-two words, not like more than twenty, but twenty-two, and that means that he is smart. . . . Maybe I would have been like this with a normal kid, but I don't think so, I don't think I would have been as mindful, . . . because I could also tell you every single time he had a cold, when it started, whether or not he had a fever, and how high his fever was.

Shannon is yet another mother whose preschooler is completely asymptomatic. Shannon doesn't feel she treats Margo differently than she does Margo's older sister, in particular, but at the same time, she describes her own version of the monitoring, the vigilance, and the uncertainty voiced by others who had an early diagnosis without symptoms. "There's never been anything to show, or anything scary or tarry or mucusy-looking or foul nasty-smelling," she says. "I mean they said there's so many ways on that end that you would notice something was up, but you know, it's hard, 'cause I've always been like, Am I missing something?"

Am I missing something? Is there a symptom here I might fail or have failed to catch early enough? Is what I'm seeing normal, or is it a sign of CF? These questions are most common for parents with early diagnoses and completely or relatively healthy babies. Children who get a later diagnosis are already known: symptomatic or not, their mothers have developed some sense of their children's bodies, their patterns, how they work. Although it is true that many parents of children with a later diagnosis become more protective after they find out their child has CF, for most of them the change is markedly less dramatic. They may be vigilant about germs and contagion for a time, their hearts may skip a beat when they hear their child cough or see her clutch her stomach, but anxiety over the unending hunt for not-yet-visible symptoms is one heartache they're spared.

Carol Boland and Norman Thompson, in a study looking at effects of newborn screening for CF on maternal behavior, found that mothers of screened children who were asymptomatic scored significantly higher on an "intrusiveness" scale and higher on a "fostering dependency" scale than did mothers of screened symptomatic children (1990, 1242). Similarly, Kevin Southern, in a 2004 analysis of the implications of newborn screening for CF speculates that parents of asymptomatic children diagnosed through newborn screening may find their situations "stressful," since "in some ways it is more difficult to be living with the anticipation of future deterioration in condition" (2004, 59). Other researchers observed the same phenomenon with respect to testing for hereditary breast cancer, noting that women acknowledge that access to genetic information can be potentially harmful because it can make you "sort of doomed to a life of checkups going on and on and on, and always worried that it's going to come out at any moment or the next year after, and [thinking] would I have to plan for the future because you may not have one" (Hallowell et al. 2003, 77). For parents of asymptomatic children in my study, hyper-vigilance is pervasive, even for those who sometimes wonder if it is warranted. As Manny summarizes, with an asymptomatic child you feel like "a super hypochondriac parent. . . . You are always sort of at these two extremes where it is like, Am I really doing the right thing? Or am I just being overprotective, because there is actually nothing really wrong with him?"

This summary of parents' experience with vigilance is by no means meant to suggest that anticipation of symptoms is more difficult than coping with manifest symptoms; framing the issue in comparative terms is not the point. But as a matter of empirical verification, it is clearly the case that parents caring for asymptomatic children wait for that first symptom nervously, look for it vigilantly, and sometimes doubt their own competence to detect it early enough. And even while they wait for it, as I show below, they also try with all their might to avert it.

Is Hovering Most Harmful?
Asymptomatic Children and the Risk of Stigma

Many parents of asymptomatic children are wary about the impact disease identity may have on their kids in much the same way they were loathe to disclose the initial news of a CF diagnosis. Parents are aware that their caretaking tends to focus on keeping the child healthy, but at the same time they are determined that their child not be "perceived as a sick child" or "miss out on something because somebody else has decided that [she] can't do it." As with so many things in the ambiguous realm of child raising, parents can only try to walk a middle line. James describes the balancing act this way: "I try not to focus on [CF] or treat him differently. Obviously we are going to have to, but I don't want him growing up feeling like he is different or can't do things that other kids can. . . . I just don't ever want to start that, because I want him to feel as normal as possible and have the life—as much as he can—as he would have if he didn't have cystic fibrosis. I don't want him to ever think that he is different or not as good as other kids because he has a disease. Especially as a kid, because they don't understand that kind of stuff."

Timmy too is adamant that his son be considered "just a normal two-year-old." He himself, however, had to pass through what he describes as "a journey, psychological and emotional," before arriving at his conviction that this is so and at a parenting style to match. "The first reaction is, he's different," Timmy says.

> So, you know, it definitely changed the dynamic for a while, until it did become routine. Until everybody knew, Okay, well, you have to have your treatment at this point. But . . . it definitely changed the dynamic of everything's peaceful, everything's normal, it's okay. He is, for lack of a better word, he's "special." He's different. . . . [But] then it's like, Okay, let me actually learn something about CF. And let me see how it's affecting my son. And it's not. So he's not different. You know? God forbid if he showed symptoms one day, then he'll be different than other kids, but . . . we'll deal with that as it comes. You know, he'll need more treatment or whatever it is. But right now, yeah, I mean, he goes to school and he's the life of the party. Runs around, nobody knows any different. It is mild, he has no symptoms right now, he's perfectly healthy right now. . . . And we obviously have gotten to the point where we don't treat him like he's different. He's normal. He just happens to have CF.

Cora's focus is most on how to protect her child from the stigma of being regarded by others as ill when he is entirely asymptomatic. She has networked with other parents of diagnosed children who are dealing with the same issue, and who have voiced concern as their children get older, even "about doing fundraising or making an issue of [CF], because you don't want your kid to be 'That's the sick kid.' 'Cause he's not. And even if his—even if something happens and he gets hospitalized, he's still not the sick kid. There's nothing he's not going to be able to do. You know, he'll be able to play sports, he'll be able to do some things. And so you don't want him to be labeled as the sick kid, and people to treat him different. . . . As he gets older, I think that is going to be more of a concern, that I'm going to want him, in his world, to be looked at as normal as possible."

As children get older and parents continue to get to know them and to see the impact of their parenting practices, some begin to feel concerned about the risk of overprotection. Manny is adamant on this point, though it's one on which he and his wife do not entirely agree. "I have sort of a 'Que sera, sera' feeling about it," he says. "If I don't treat him like a normal child, I think I am going to do much more harm than the possibility that something I do will cause him to trigger some [illness]. I [worry about] the possibility that if I treat him with kid gloves his whole childhood, that he grows up to be sickly and unable to sort of deal with the real world. I think that is a much bigger danger than [if] we are at the park and he catches a cold and then he gets really, really sick. I guess that has sort of been my experience with him thus far." More specifically, Manny doesn't want his son to be constrained by parental anxiety. "This feeds into this thing where I don't want him to feel like everywhere he goes, he has constantly a hovering over him," says Manny, "and that we are keeping him from experiencing the highs and the lows of the world because we are afraid that it might trigger some sort of illness."

Keeping the Child as Healthy as Possible: Parenting and the Prophylactic Regime

Protectiveness and vigilance are means to an end—tools parents use to keep their child healthy in the moment and to keep CF at bay for the long term. However, as already suggested, the role of parents in CF prevention is by no means limited to tactics of germ avoidance and intensive monitoring. Starting at their first CF clinic—which for parents with a newborn-screen diagnosis most often occurs within the first few weeks of the infant's life—parents are taught to implement a rigorous daily regime of preventive care that almost always includes medications, manual chest percussions to prevent mucus buildup in the lungs, nebulizers, a high-calorie diet, digestive enzymes taken orally, and more—even if the child is asymptomatic (Elborn, Hodson, and Bertram 2009; Prasad, Main, and Dodd 2008). The CF diagnosis immediately propels this pro-phylactic regime into the center of family life, where it has a significant impact both on parent/child relationships and on overall household dynamics.

Although learning about CF always feels daunting at first, generally those whose children were diagnosed later not only experience relief at finally knowing what is wrong, but also take satisfaction in learning about and embracing whatever interventions are recommended. As already noted, after the helplessness of tending a sick child with no diagnosis, there is enormous comfort in at last having something concrete to do. Erica talks about the introduction of CF-related home treatments and preventive therapy for her children, ages six and four at diagnosis: "With my [six-year-old] daughter, I always knew something was wrong. And I think sometimes . . . finding out something, it gives you . . . , not peace, but at least you have a name and you know how to treat it. As opposed to nonstop coughing, that worry, that uncertainty or worrying. At least . . . you feel like you're doing something, you're treating them, you're doing something."

Many of these parents—particularly those whose children were quite ill at diagnosis—see their new regime of treatment and infection control rewarded by marked improvement in their children's health. Administering enzymes to children who have pancreatic insufficiency, and have become malnourished as a result, helps them begin to gain much-needed weight at last. Treating pulmonary symptoms with a combination of medication and chest percussions often brings them under control: lung function and thus overall health begin to improve. Some children who had been in and out of doctors' offices and hospitals before the diagnosis stabilize, and these visits become a rarity rather than a routine. "She was terribly malnourished and underweight without us realizing it," says one mother. But after she began getting treatment, "she became this totally different little girl."

The gratitude of parents with a later diagnosis for being able to "do something," and for improved health and quality of life, is enormous. It can also, however, be bittersweet. These parents had already established routines and caretaking practices with their children before the diagnosis, had already developed their parenting habits and styles. Just as a CF diagnosis creates a clear "before" and "after" in parents' perception of their child and in their dreams for the future, so also it creates a clear "before" and "after" in their career as caretakers—and the adjustment can be substantial. Here is Erica's description of the transition:

> One impact of [the diagnosis] was, like with the kids, everything is before and after. I mean, I really truly view things as before they were diagnosed and after they were diagnosed. In terms of? Everything. How our social lives changed, . . . 'cause CF varies. . . . It's all involved. At times we'd have up to three to four hours a day doing treatment. So before that we never had that. So it's a lot different. Like I would say I was more carefree. I always remember that it wasn't until about two, three years ago was the first time we had gone out at night since the kids were diagnosed. But just for a walk round the block or something because their treatments . . . take from 7:00 to 8:30, then they go to bed. . . . When [kids] are born with it, they don't know any better, and I think for me as a parent you fight it more when you find out later because you knew what normal life was. . . . You deal with it, but I think later on you fight it. You just remember how things were. That sort of before-and-after thing. I mean like every picture in the photo album, I can look at it and see whether it was before or after. . . . Your concerns change and it's a very isolating feeling because there is nobody who can really relate to you.

Nancy too described the enormous divide marked by the diagnosis. For her too the shift was both emotional and practical.

Our whole focus, our whole perspective, everything has changed since we had the diagnosis. . . . We don't say, "This won't happen," or "That's not gonna happen." We don't have that kind of thinking anymore because we just, we don't feel so secure like we used to, or so immortal I guess. Yeah, I definitely think there's a division. . . . It [also] take[s] a lot of time, just [feeding my daughter]. I mean normally you'd just hand them the sandwich. And now we're like, "Okay, . . . we need to get the enzymes. How many enzymes does she need for this meal? How much is she gonna eat? Is it a high-fat meal, or a regular meal? . . . Does she need her vitamins at this time or does she not?" . . . And just cleaning the nebulizer cups and sterilizing those and everything is just—it's very time consuming. When we were on the month without [medication], it's like, "Ahhh [we're so relaxed]," and then the month of [medication] is "Urgghh. You do the [meds] and I'll clean, I'll boil the neb cups and hang them out to dry and then I'll get them ready for the morning treatment." So it's definitely very time consuming, it's extremely life changing just in all those ways, everything that I took for granted.

Parents whose children are diagnosed later work diligently to keep them as healthy as possible; new parenting practices in the service of health are a prominent aspect of the "after" side of the diagnostic divide. And they, like parents with earlier diagnoses, recount with pride their successes: children able to participate in sports and other ordinary childhood activities; children who have been hospitalized only minimally or not at all since diagnosis; children who keep up with or surpass their unaffected siblings or friends.

These narratives are powerful; parents' investment in improving and maintaining their children's health cannot be overestimated. But this aspect of their parenting takes place within a broader context.[2] For some parents, this context includes the normal life that came before, with its as-yet-unaltered parenting styles, priorities, and expectations that the child would live an average life span. For others, it may also include the abnormal health problems their child suffered before the diagnosis, and the feeling that things have now begun to get better. Parents feel enormous anger at the delayed diagnosis, and sometimes guilt as well. But the physical and developmental signs they monitor with their diagnosis-inspired vigilance most often mark an improvement rather than a deterioration in health, at least in the short run. They aim to influence the course of the disease as much as is humanly possible, but they have generally already learned, through the difficult experience of seeing their child show symptoms, that they cannot mitigate its effects entirely. Furthermore, they have some degree of confidence that they'll recognize CF when it manifests; the disease is after all an old foe already, even if it only recently got its name.

Attitudes about and experience with controlling the child's health are quite different for parents who get an early diagnosis, and whose parenting has therefore always been focused on maintaining good health despite CF, at least for the affected child. For these parents, vigilance, protectiveness, and preventive treatments are the norm that substantially defines what it means to parent that child—without any sort of "before" to act as an outside referent.

For parents of children with newborn screen diagnoses, the various daily preventive care routines seem normal and have always defined what it means to be a parent. Andrea, for example, recounts (with a chuckle) how very taken for granted these parenting practices become after a time. "I really don't even remember how to feed a normal baby anymore," she says. "I was watching my nephew when he was a newborn and caught myself getting ready to give him enzymes. . . . It's automatic: you see it's a baby, you give 'em enzymes!" For Andrea, there is no parenting of Bobby without these practices. "Now, six years later, there's no remembering a time without it. There's no remembering a time before the treatments, and before the chest percussions and before the enzymes and the antibiotic rounds every few months. It's just normal to us now and we try to make it as normal as possible for Bobby, 'cause then he doesn't feel like he's different." For Barb, too, it's impossible to envision parenting without medication and other preventive care routines. "This is motherhood to me; this is what it means," she says. "Being a new mother you don't know anything, and therefore this is how I learned to live my life. We take pills and we eat; I don't even think about it anymore. I mean, he has always had them every time since the day he was born."

Preventive-care routines become very normal, but at the same time many parents regard them almost religiously. As Kayla notes, the prophylactic regime is nonnegotiable: fidelity to it, down to the last detail, is mandatory in order to keep disaster at bay. "I am a little on the OCD side here, just very particular with his feeding, . . . very strict about the way things get done, because I want to make sure that we don't forget medicines, and that we don't forget to put salt in his milk, and we don't forget these things, because if we forget something bad might happen."

Though her child remains entirely asymptomatic at age two and a half, Cora is also emphatic about maintaining the routine each and every day. "We try to be as incredibly conscientious as we can," she says. "There has been a day or two where we've missed it, but . . . we were at my in-laws for Christmas, and in the middle of everybody sitting there opening Christmas presents, [my son] was sitting there on my lap with a nebulizer mask over him opening Christmas presents." Roxanne's son is also totally healthy, a child the doctors have said would probably have been, without NBS, "one of those kids that [CF] didn't show up . . . for years." Nonetheless, she does "everything, 99.9 percent of the time, to the letter for him. He gets enzymes every time he eats, he gets two doses of salt a day, he gets two treatments of albuterol just to keep his airways open, and then he—we have a breathing vest, actually he's actually the youngest patient in the U.S. . . . to have a breathing vest."

Thus, like parents with later diagnoses, those who learn about CF early often find enormous comfort in having something to do on behalf of the affected child—a reality noted also by researchers, who emphasize "the psychological benefit to parents of their infant receiving prophylactic treatment" because of the "high level of confidence" most people have in medicine and the importance of partnership with health care professionals in "developing coping strategies" (Parsons and Bradley 2003, 285–286). In some instances, the newborn was already showing early signs of pancreatic insufficiency, so parental gratitude for replacement enzymes is based on observed improvements in the newborn's health. Anne was one such parent. "I was upset that he was sick," she says, reflecting on the CF diagnosis she received when baby Niko was about eighteen days old, "but relieved that we could help him. You know, I was concerned about his poop . . . and how he was little, and now I had an answer to why. And as soon as we started the medicine, he gained a pound in a week. It was unbelievable." Sally's experience was similar: newborn Stephan lost a pound at birth and didn't gain it back until after the diagnosis (at a couple of weeks of age) and the beginning of treatment. At that point, "he started gaining weight [and the medication] just became part of life."

Most parents whose babies receive a newborn screen diagnosis, however, begin the prophylactic regime with asymptomatic babies. For this group, no manifest problem exists. Their enthusiasm about preventive care stems, therefore, from relief at being able to take decisive action in the face of a frightening abstraction that leaves them feeling otherwise helpless. Marta, for example, observes that despite Bethany's apparent good health, "we had to start the therapy right away [the same day as the sweat test], with the enzymes, and then the chest therapy." There is no doubt, she continues, that "it kind of sucked, but I kind of felt like the sooner we could . . . get started with her care and treatment that we could try and keep her as healthy as possible. . . . It was overwhelming, [but] . . . I am just more an aggressive person." In Deena's case, treatment began even before the confirmatory test results came back. At first she was shocked to be swept into meeting with the CF treatment team when she thought the

diagnosis was still in question, but the doctors argued persuasively that immediate intervention is most advisable. "They gave us enzymes that day to start
him on. And I said, 'Well, what happens if the sweat test comes back and shows
that he doesn't have it? Will these enzymes hurt him if he doesn't have it?'
They're like, 'No, they won't hurt him if he doesn't have it. It's not going to hurt
him at all.' But they're like, 'If he does have it, even a few days earlier, it's
better to start him on it.' So I said, 'Okay, that's good to know.' So they went
over how to give it to a baby and they got us all signed up."

Other parents with asymptomatic babies and early diagnoses may see the
preventive care regime—at least in the beginning—as foe rather than as friend.
When the baby is chubby and content, and when the newborn period is unfolding without a hitch apart from the diagnosis itself, preventive treatment is the
sole reminder that all may not be as it seems. This is how it felt to Joya, who
says she wept every time the doctors gave her a new treatment for baby Ariel.
"Even though I knew I had a child with this illness, it was just [that] in my
mind she seemed great. Everything was fine, and then she needed the treatment
and then I said, Yeah, there are real problems. I guess there was some denial or
whatever . . . going on, and just getting used to this whole thing. My husband is
really great when it comes to things like this. He says, 'Don't hate the treatment,
hate the disease! Be positive about the treatment and taking care of her and
looking for the cure!' . . . So little by little we started doing everything that we
have to do now."

For Selena too, accepting some of the prescribed treatments was difficult.
"Her bowel movements were fine [and] you didn't hear any wheezing or anything, and so I think that is what made it so hard too, because they kept saying
she was sick and I kept saying I don't see it. Even if I heard the wheezing, . . .
at least I would have some solid proof that something was wrong, but they
assured me something was wrong." The diagnosis is very hard to accept "even
to this day," she continues. "Does she really have it? Or could it be one of those
things? No one else in the family has it," so it is difficult to be sure "they didn't
just mess up. Hospitals mess up all the time, they amputate the wrong legs, . . .
[and] even to this day my children are super healthy."

Even for parents with "super healthy" children, however, the diagnosis
retains a central place in their view of the child, in the structure of their relationship to health care professionals, and in the routines of daily life.

Even at SeaWorld: Doing Every Treatment, Every Day

Although the preventive care regime becomes routine for families over time, its
effects are substantial both in terms of what it produces and in terms of what it

displaces. Some parents regard this daily investment of time as a straightforward fact of life, since there is no way it can be wished away or minimized. As one mother summarizes: "The doctor basically told us, you don't miss them. You do every treatment." Other parents, such as Timmy, hold a more positive view, emphasizing that prophylactic treatment for an entirely asymptomatic preschooler is usually "just part of life, and it's one-on-one time with the kids." He and his wife collaborate on the routine, so "one of us gets to hold him and, at least lately, his big thing is, Let me watch TV while I'm getting treated, but he sits on our lap. So I'll hold his hand, I'll tickle his feet, you know. Whatever it is. I'll rub his head, I'll give him kisses. And the other one of us is helping our daughter with her homework or hopefully getting a chance to play a game with her or giving her a shower. But it is what it is; it's life. It's what we have right now." For Cassandra's child, Neil, the routine is much more difficult—a twice-daily struggle she cannot relish though she believes in it with all her heart. "We do a lot of things that he doesn't like and that make him cry, and you feel like you are torturing him, and it is no fun for anybody. But you know you have to do them, because they teach now [that] the more preventative things you do now, the better things are going to be in the long run."

Because the breathing treatments, in particular, are so time consuming, their daily implementation often precludes other kinds of activities and routines both for the affected child and for his or her siblings. As Cora comments, with a combination of humor and exasperation, if she gets home from work even a tad late there's little time for anything but the prophylactic regime. On those occasions, she walks in the door saying, "Okay, hi everybody. Love you. Let's play for fifteen minutes, and then we have to treat Jim, because that takes forty-five minutes." A particular concern is the effect of the treatment on her older child, who suffers no genetic impact from CF but experiences the emotional ramifications. "I know how unfair it is to my daughter that I'm spending forty-five minutes holding [Jim and] doing his treatment," says Cora with regret. "And she's stuck by herself. And how do we compensate for that? How do we make that fair?"

For Evelyn, too, the lost opportunities associated with time-consuming treatments are substantial. Here's her meditation on how the care routine mediates her parenting, rendering it an experience substantially different from the one she had with Tyler's older sister: "You do your breathing treatments first, and then you follow it up with the chest therapy, and then making sure he is gaining weight, so . . . his diet. I feel like so much of my day is surrounded around him, [but] I have less time to be with him, and playing with him. . . . I am sad that I don't have time like I did with [his sister], and like any second child, you don't probably have the same kind of time obviously as you did with the first, but it is even more so now that he has CF."

Even family vacations, as several parents note, are not exempt. "We're planning a trip out to [an amusement park] this summer," says Timmy. "And we have to make sure that we have a room that has a refrigerator, because one of his medications needs to be refrigerated. Then we're going to have to make sure we have all the notes that say we can carry his vest and it's not a bomb. And we can carry his nebulizer. And it all has to come on the plane with us and all that sort of fun stuff." At SeaWorld, or anywhere outside the privacy of one's own house, administering treatments can be even more challenging than it is at home—not to mention embarrassing. It can be "really frustrating," for example, to give enzymes to a baby in public. Lara elaborates: "Because you have to try to hold him and you've got to set the bottle somewhere, to get the applesauce—I'm talking about, like if I'm sitting on a couch somewhere. You gotta pull all this stuff out. And then if you're really in public, you have people wondering what the heck you're giving your kid. I hear people say, like, 'What is she thinking?' They probably think I'm giving him some New Age vitamins." Kate concurs. "I'm at the gym giving her enzymes, so people see it and they ask me questions about it and 'Oh, my God, you're giving your baby applesauce, it's too early.' It's so funny, because people start to go berserk, and it's like, 'She's been doing this since she was three days old, I think she's fine, thanks.'"

It's a Way of Life: Children's Adjustment to the Preventive Care Routine

Children as well as parents must adapt to the routines of preventive care at home, and to the frequent clinic visits that follow CF diagnosis. Parents speak often about the phases children seem to go through as they grow, noting that their willingness to do what needs to be done can change over time. However, it is clear that parents whose first diagnosed child is diagnosed early see the immediate establishment of care practices as advantageous in several ways. They, like all parents, invest in the prophylactic regime as a long-range strategy for minimizing the impact of CF and improving health outcomes. In some cases, immediate relief of symptoms is apparent and serves as its own reward. But for parents of asymptomatic children, other logic is also at work. For these families, the prophylactic regime is valued not just as a means to an end but also as a process that will weave a fabric of habits and expectations children need for the long haul, so they are prepared if CF in fact rears its head. As one mother quipped: "Drink milk! Take your vest!"

James says the "chest-thumping" therapy prescribed for his son beginning at two months of age was "to prevent the build up of the mucus." However, since the baby had no pulmonary symptoms or issues, "the thumper" was even more to "get him used to it, because he will have to do it as he gets older." There may not have been any mucus in there at the time to break up, James continues, but it was essential to "get him in the routine when he is younger, so when he gets older it is not such a shock to him." Roxanne, who had a lengthy battle with Medicaid to obtain a breathing vest for her child when he was one year old—below the age at which such devices are usually prescribed—concurs wholeheartedly. "This is a child, you've got to remember, he's not coughing up anything yet, but I wanted the vest because, you know, if you wait until they're two years old—this is just my feeling as a parent, and I know that I'm kind of a pioneer in this with babies having the vest—but my feeling is, number one, it's not going to hurt anything for him to go ahead and be on it. Number two, it prepares him and conditions him for when he is two or three, and I'm not going to have to fight him then, he's not going to be afraid of it, and it's going to be something like brushing his teeth every day."

For Yvette, instituting chest therapy for a baby with "lungs that always sound clear"—so clear that Gloria has not been prescribed the pulmonary medications Yvette knows are given to so many babies with CF—seemed objectionable at first: "I just kind of felt like, if she doesn't have any problems, you know, why are we doing this?" Yvette understands that "to cough or clear away" any extra secretions may prevent breathing problems in the longer run but seems to have made her peace with this element of the prophylactic regime largely because she believes it's a healthy behavioral pattern to establish while Gloria is young. "It . . . helps to help them get used to it in case they ever do have—when she does have some kind of infection, you have to [have] more therapy, you know, and so hopefully she'll already be used to it and be on a routine. And then hopefully, if I'm doing it now . . . when she's so young, then she'll also be used to it for when I can't hold her down. Who wants to run around? . . . So at first I didn't really want to do it, but now I'm okay with it."

Cora feels similarly but emphasizes how for her religious regularity about the preventive care regime is motivated in substantial part by the need to establish a protocol that preschooler Jim cannot wheedle out of or understand as susceptible to compromise. "Occasionally he gets a little, you know, a little 'ugh'" about doing the routine, she says. "But mostly he doesn't fight treatment, because it's a part of his regular life. If we skipped a bunch of days and all of a sudden tried to go back to it, would he be that good about it? Maybe not. And since it is going to be a regular part of his life, you know, let's keep it that way. . . . Because he's definitely stubborn enough that if he thinks he can get away without doing it, he's going to try to get away without doing it. We don't want him to realize that he can go without it, because he can't; . . . it's good for him."

For other parents whose only experience with CF is with a newborn-screen diagnosed baby, having begun preventive care at birth is simply a way of instantiating it firmly into the life of the child from day one. As Joan put it: "When they are diagnosed that young, it's nice, because it's a way of life for them, they don't know anything else. Versus if you have an eighteen-month-old and all of a sudden you have to do all these treatments and medicines and it's all new to them. So it's kind of nice that [our daughter has] never known anything else." Andrea has a similar sense that things are easier for her son because treating CF has been normalized since birth. At age six, "he doesn't ask a lot of questions," she says. "He's so used to it, he doesn't even notice that his classmates [don't] have to go to the office for medications before lunch, and he doesn't even notice that his classmates don't have to eat extra food or don't get practically a meal for snack in the morning." Paula shares this viewpoint and reports with a laugh that the preventive care regime figured so prominently in baby Celeste's life that it provided inspiration for her earliest orations. "She's got a vest now, so we call it 'tappers,'" says Paula. "And her first complete sentence was, 'I don't want to do my tappers now!'"

However, parents who have an older child also diagnosed with CF when the younger one got a newborn screen diagnosis tell quite a different story about adjusting to preventive care regimes. These parents, who have experience establishing the preventive routine both with a newborn and with an older child, observe that it's actually less difficult to begin treatment with an older child. As Cassandra puts it: "It is easier with her being seven when she was diagnosed. She knew when we said you have to do the vest, you have to do your treatment, and she does [it] because she knows she has to. . . . She does say, . . . 'I wish I didn't have CF,' and I say 'I know, I wish you didn't either, but you do and these are the things that we have to do to take care of it.'" And likewise, from Lara: "It was easier starting with Frida at two and a half—we made a game of it. She thought it was funny that she could sing or say the ABCs and have it sound funny, you know. We took pictures of her. We just made it a positive experience. And with [our newborn,] Peter, you can't do that. You can't make it fun for him, so he just feels tied down and we give him toys and stuff but at his age, there's nothing that's a good enough distraction that he doesn't remember that he's being pounded on. So. It was easier to start it at her age, at two and a half."

As children grow older, parents begin explaining to them directly why familiar care routines and precautions are necessary. At this point the parent begins teaching the child to take more direct responsibility for the never-ending routines of illness prevention. Francesca describes her efforts to keep her daughter and her nephew, who also has CF, apart when one of them may pose a danger to the other: "When one of the kids gets pseudomonas, it's hard, because you have to try to keep them apart, and it's just—it's trying at some points because they're close. . . . It's hard to tell Tess that [she can't] . . . go play with C. [I say,] 'Well, you can't.' 'Why?' I'm like, 'You're sick.' 'Well, I don't feel sick . . . I'm not sick.' [I say,] 'Honey, but you're always kind of sick, you just don't realize it.'"

Parents with early diagnoses are relieved that they don't have to suffer through a transition with their children, going from normal life before the diagnosis to an existence full of treatments and precautions afterward. They feel the child has been spared the pain of losing prized freedoms, and they themselves have been spared the frustration of introducing new routines into a life already built without them. But, as Francesca's observations illustrate, the formation of precautionary habits and schedules of care at birth also signifies the development of an illness identity right from the start. Children are "always kind of sick," even when they "don't realize it." Parents of children with newborn screen diagnoses can't, as Kate puts it, think of the child as "a baby first and then she has CF" because it's impossible to "divorce the two. It's like, my baby has CF; . . . it's so tied to me as who she is." And it seems highly likely that's how Kate's baby Erin, and all her peers who were diagnosed with CF at birth, will think of themselves as well—regardless of whether or not they develop symptoms.

Is My Sick Child Healthy? Measuring Parental Success by the Child's Health

Because early CF diagnosis so significantly influences parents' perceptions of their child's identity, and because their parenting is then so significantly shaped by vigilance and preventive care practices, it is only natural that parents also begin to assess their success as ongoing custodians by measuring the status of their child's health. Diagnosis with genetic disease at birth can thus transform a general parental intention to "do everything in my power to make sure everything is good" for the child into a specific commitment to keep the child physically well and symptom-free.

Lilly speaks with passion about how after the newborn-screen diagnosis, it became her explicit goal to "make sure [Mia] stayed healthy." Further, she is careful to measure her own success in this most critical of parenting arenas. "[Mia] never has been hospitalized, she's never had intravenous antibiotics or anything." Furthermore, she rides horses, plays the saxophone, and is extremely physically active. In fact, "she's healthier—my sick child is healthier than some healthy kids."

Kayla is aware that she is vigilant about guarding Eben's health "to a point of where I am overbearing and overprotective probably." Her confidence that this is the right way to care for him, however, is absolute. "I don't want him to be sick," she says emphatically. "So if I can save him from one cold or one hospital trip, and I have to be anal, . . . then people are just going to have to understand that I am going to be anal with him. So that's all there is to it, and I am not going to stop doing it and risk him getting sick." Kayla is duly modest, but she's also sure that her hard work to safeguard Eben's health is "a lot of the reason he is doing so well." "He is still in the seventy-fifth percentile for his age," she reports with pride, "and that is not typical at all for babies [with CF], because usually they don't gain weight. But that is definitely not his problem."

Selena is also proud of her vigilance, even while ruefully acknowledging the impact it has on her toddler with CF and on his younger sibling. "Derek absolutely hates me in the wintertime," she says. "Hats on, scarf on, gloves on, . . . they look like snowmen when they leave; they have on two shirts and a sweatshirt, a jacket, and Derek goes, 'I am sweating to death,' and I say, 'Well, you have to wear it.'" At times, the kids' protestations lead her to relent a bit, letting them go out without a scarf or gloves. But then she's immediately subject to a sense of guilt and failed responsibility, because "if they get sick and didn't have their gloves on, then it is my fault because they should have had their gloves on." She tries hard not to overprotect them or make them feel singled out as different. Further, her common sense tells her that some childhood illnesses are inevitable. Nonetheless, she knows that if illness follows a change in her preventive care practices, she will feel "maybe I should have tried harder, maybe I should have been more on top of it, . . . maybe they didn't wash their hands enough, something of that sort."

Like so many other parents, Kate describes her success as a parent in terms of keeping her baby, Erin, healthy. "I feel I'm succeeding if she's doing well," she says. "If she doesn't get sick, I'm doing the right thing as a parent. If I can tell you every time you call me, 'She's doing great! The enzymes are working!' . . . then I'm doing the right thing." Clearly, though, as anticipated by Selena, there's a problematic flip side of this way of defining parental success: the heavy weight of guilt that descends when something goes wrong, even something as banal as the onset of a mild cold. If the child's health is a defining measure of a parent's success, then there's an awful lot riding on every fluctuation in the child's physical well-being. As Kate says, "When [Erin] caught the cold, I felt awful. . . . I should have kept her away from people, 'cause I took her to my sister's baby shower . . . and then she got sick. . . . And so I shouldn't have brought her to the baby shower. Well, of course I should have brought her to the baby shower, you know what I mean. . . . But I felt so guilty and awful, you know, like that I was failing her and that I was failing as a parent." Bess expresses a similar sentiment, but her focus is more on the future than on the present—and she is determined not to feel guilty about baby Jill's health once she grows up. "We do [the inhaler and face mask]," says Bess, "more for preventive reasons, because I don't want in twenty years for her to be sick with lung disease and know it was because I didn't do enough for her as a child."

One Step Ahead of Trouble: CF and the Illusion of Control

Kate's situation illustrates a critical issue for all the parents I interviewed: the possibility of control and the limitation of control in the face of CF. Nothing can be done to alter the genetic make-up of the child. Despite continued research in the troubled field of gene therapy, the chromosomal mutations themselves are a reality parents must accept for the foreseeable future. The clinical expression of CF, though, is immensely variable. It remains unclear—at the population level, as well as in the individual case—how much of this variability is attributable to the specific nature and combination of the CF mutations a given person has, and how much can be influenced by active medical, behavioral, and environmental interventions (Moskowitz et al. 2005; WHO 2000). As Lara, the mother of two CF-diagnosed children, puts the point—which she understands intimately since she lives it every day: "There's no way to know what the future holds. . . . You can't say, 'Because he has this, this is the outcome.' I still don't really know what she will end up doing with her future, with her life." However, since prophylactic interventions offer parents the only hope they have of altering outcomes, their only opportunity to exert control over a disease they know is capable of ravaging and cutting short their child's life, it is not surprising that they channel so much energy into seeking out and implementing them. As anthropologist Myra Bluebond-Langner and her colleagues observe with respect to parents' commitment to pursuing every possible avenue of treatment for children with cancer, mothers and fathers will choose options with even "infinitesimal odds because the prize they [seek is] of immeasurable worth" (2007, 2419).

It is also unsurprising that parents struggling with the meaning of their child's diagnosis—particularly when that diagnosis is early and/or the child is not symptomatic—are extraordinarily susceptible to the public health establishment's emphasis on the advantages of early diagnosis. Newborn screening programs represent the disorders they screen for as imminent dangers to the child, and the knowledge gained through testing as a means of minimizing that danger. The New York State Newborn Screening Program pamphlets, for example, tell parents that the screen is done to "help ensure that your baby will be as healthy as possible," and that "early treatment is very important," since if left undetected and untreated, these diseases can be life threatening, or may "slow down the baby's physical development or cause mental retardation." The pamphlet notes that "none of these disorders can be cured" but goes on to emphasize repeatedly that "the serious effects can be lessened—and often be prevented completely—if a special diet or other medical treatment is started early."[3] Diagnostic testing of newborns is, like all such testing, "conceptualized as offering control, [as] being a way of 'doing something' in the face of the incipient disorder created by the presence or potential of disease" (Lupton 1995, 78).

On a conscious level, nearly all parents accept this view of early diagnosis. They believe it has given or would have given them the much-coveted capacity to protect the child and substantially mitigate the effects of CF. Again and again, they talk about how important it is to be proactive, to have known about CF before symptoms began so as to forestall them, or soon after they've begun so as to reduce their effect. Anthony, for example, says he's "definitely grateful that we found out before she was symptomatic, and we could start treating this beforehand rather than taking the child into the hospital." Francesca agrees: "I just think to be proactive on things is important, so finding out when we did [via newborn screen] was just a good time for us." Lilly, who got confirmation of CF at four weeks after a positive newborn screen, regrets those several weeks of prophylactic treatment that were missed before the diagnosis, even though her daughter Mia has grown and developed just fine. "Mia could have started taking enzymes sooner," she says, "so she could have grown better right away from the beginning rather than waiting." Even Leslie, whose son was quite sick when he was diagnosed first with meconium ileus and then with CF right after birth, finds herself oddly grateful for his early illness because it led to such a rapid diagnosis. The seriousness of his immediate manifest symptoms pales, for her, in comparison to the potential harm she thinks might have come to John had his disease remained undetected. "I mean, we were fortunate that he did have the meconium ileus," she says. "Even though he had to have major surgery, we were able to find out immediately and we were able to start his treatment. . . . I mean, it's still a horrible diagnosis, but . . . I feel fortunate that we found out immediately . . . rather than risk lung damage and not have treatment." These testimonies are just a few of many that illustrate parents' internalization of the assumption "that individuals must have 'knowledge' of their hidden disease, or its precursors, to be able to act to protect themselves against it" (Lupton 1995, 78).

But there are problems, too, that come with knowledge of the hidden disease—complexities troubling to parents even as they work to forestall every symptom and comply with every element of the prophylactic regime. Despite efforts to identify and meaningfully analyze the CFTR gene's multiple mutations, the "clinical course" of cystic fibrosis remains very difficult to predict, even when both of an individual's mutations are clearly identified (WHO 2000; Moskowitz et al. 2005). It is therefore a case (as suggested in chapter 1) where correlation between the biomedical definition of the disease (i.e., abnormalities of structure or function) and the lived experience of illness (i.e., the person's perceptions and experiences of the disease) is remarkably low (Conrad and Schneider 1992, 30; Hill 1994, 12; Kleinman and Seeman 2000, 231–232).

A newborn screen and follow-up diagnostic tests give parents information about the disease, the fact of CF, but the course of the illness, if there is in fact to be one, remains unknown and unknowable, at least for the time being. However, once parents learn that the genetic mutation lies within their child's body, it becomes impossible for the identified disease not to impinge on the life of child and family, even if no symptoms are manifest. As sociologists Peter Conrad and Joseph Schneider point out, drawing on the classic work of their colleague Eliot Freidson: "Calling something an illness in human society has consequences *independent* of the effects on the biological condition of the organism. . . . Medical diagnosis affects people's behavior, attitudes they take toward themselves, and attitudes others take toward them" (1992, 31).

For parents whose child had an early diagnosis but ends up being asymptomatic or only mildly affected, or asymptomatic for a long period of time, it is illness, not disease, that shapes their parenting practices from the beginning. Yet the illness is not one of physical symptoms. In the absence of manifest signs of the disease, the only "illness" affecting child and family is one of preventive routines, vigilance, and the construction of a CF identity in response to the diagnosis. Parenting is substantially defined by knowledge that the invisible disorder exists, and by an understanding of the disease and of how it can be mitigated, acquired through a combination of medical visits and self-education (Grob 2008). Just as CF diagnosis is a different animal for those who receive it as an abstract test result than for those who receive it in response to manifest symptoms, so too the diagnosed child's actual state of health greatly influences "perceptions and experiences of the disease."

I have already shown that parents with early diagnoses embrace the promise of control offered by the early diagnosis with tremendous energy, significantly shaping their early parenting around prophylactic regimes and defining their success or failure by the child's state of health more absolutely than do their peers whose children were diagnosed later. A study of newborn-screened and clinically identified children with CF and their parents concluded that for parents of asymtomatic children, "the ethos of 'always being one step ahead of trouble' . . . developed to a greater extent" than it did among the group of parents whose children have symptoms. This is because, as I have shown here, mothers of healthy children often feel that "the child's continued symptom free health (and hence his longevity) [is] dependent upon [his] competence" (Boland and Thompson 1990, 1243). The experiences of parents who receive newborn-screen diagnoses for as yet asymptomatic CF also resemble in certain ways those of parents whose child is diagnosed with PKU. As summarized by researcher Schild, for these parents "the early diagnosis takes on an illusive, somewhat nebulous quality, as [they] . . . watch the treated newborn PKU child grow and thrive without apparent pathology." But the watching can be fraught with tension since "the parents operate under a constant threat that if they fail in maintaining the diet, their child will become brain damaged. They tend to respond with excessive monitoring" (Schild 1979, 135, 145). Although the extent of the damage that can be caused by a break in prophylactic vigilance for CF is less dramatic than in the case of PKU, the focus of parental energy on preventive care is nonetheless intense.

Parents' competence is surely formidable, and many feel certain that their care and vigilance is resulting in better health for the child. At the same time, a substantial and growing group of parents find themselves practicing all that vigilance for a child who is unlikely to get sick during childhood, or at all. This leads some parents to realize—though with gratitude for felicitous outcomes sufficient to outweigh resentment over false alarms—that the shadow cast over their families by the specter of CF was likely just an illusion. This was certainly the case for Shannon and her daughter. "With the information that we have [now]," Shannon says, "I don't think she'll ever have any health issues with cystic fibrosis, and pray to God she doesn't. But the thing is, yeah, I don't know if she's ever going to have anything to deal with, with it, so therefore it's like, okay, the tears and the worrying, what have I gotten for it?" In this case, the only illness present seems to be the one manufactured by the diagnosis. And Shannon's vigilance, clinic visits, and preventive routines almost assuredly have nothing to do with the blessing of Margo's good health.

Other parents also wonder about the utility of the early, intense prophylactic regime for their asymptomatic child. However, when it is impossible to know for certain how healthy the child would have been without treatment, most parents remain convinced that preventive routines play a crucial role. Timmy, for example, has questions about the impact of prophylactic care on his asymptomatic toddler, Jim, who has a mild mutation of a type described in the medical literature as highly unlikely to cause manifest symptoms until mid to late childhood at the soonest. "I couldn't tell you at this point," Timmy says, whether Jim's good health has to do with "the treatment or not." But since he can't be positive that Jim would have been healthy in the absence of all that care, Timmy opts for a positive view of the situation: "I am very grateful that we are doing it, because of the future. It definitely helps me stay more optimistic about where this is going." Paula expresses a similar sentiment, noting that "it's hard to say" if things might have been worse for Celeste if she hadn't begun treatment so soon. In the face of uncertainty, Paula continues, "I'm just going to assume it would have been worse if we hadn't started earlier." Why? Because, as Paula succinctly summarizes on behalf of many parents in similar situations, "that makes it easier." The path of least resistance and greatest psychological comfort for parents is to presume that early diagnosis and intervention are helpful—even essential—to a symptom-free childhood for their child. This is true even though before newborn screening, an asymptomatic child might never have been identified as potentially ill (Botkin 2005).

Most parents with asymptomatic children live with a vivid sense of uncertainty about whether their child will develop symptoms or not, and an acute worry about when the first sign will come. These parents can only hope their experience will resemble Shannon's and Timmy's, since a child who never gets sick is what every parent wants. At the same time, uncertainty itself can exact a heavy toll. Rayna describes her ongoing struggle with the unknown this way: "I'm just one of those people that always has to know everything because I plan and I organize and try to get prepared for everything. So I hate that I don't know what it's going to be like [for Riley]. But then I think it's probably good too, because I'm a hopeful, optimistic [person], so I just hope it's going to be mild; . . . then every time he gets [a cold or infection] I feel some of that hope just disappear." Evelyn had a similar compulsion to know, and to predict the future, during baby Tyler's early life. "I think I was looking for answers about Tyler and hoping that they could tell me more about him and what his prognosis or course was going to be. . . . I was always searching for, Is this going to be mild or severe? And I think I came to the conclusion that even though there is a continuum, you just don't know, because there are modifier genes that can change things. . . . I wanted to say, 'Tyler has a mild phenotype and he is going to be fine.' . . . [And] he is fairly healthy, but I know that could change, but hopefully not." Though the compulsion to predict remains, for Evelyn it has abated substantially with time. "I am just finally sitting back and saying I can't control all of that . . . , what the course will be. [In the beginning] . . . it was just more about the fear of getting sick, and what his lifespan would be, and the treatments he would have to do. It is just all those unknowns, and I have just come into the point where it is okay not knowing, I am fine with not knowing the outcome, and I think part of that is just being hopeful, and just getting to know him better too."

Abby, too, is caught between being sanguine and driving herself "crazy" trying to resolve the diagnostic uncertainty surrounding her son. "Like he could be fine for the rest of his life," she says. "He could be fine and that is the truth of the matter, and that is the thing with all the new newborn screening and all this stuff showing up, . . . so you have to sort of have two completely different sort of minds, and it is sort of Dr. Jekyll and Mr. Hyde . . . and the two just sort of can't meet. . . . I have got this kid, and he has got to be fed, and he has got to take his naps, and he has got to go to class, and has got to have a good life. And then you have this universe that something terrible could happen." After a moment's thought, however, she observes that to some degree, uncertainty is a predicament we all share. Her son could also, she says, "get hit by a bus."

For parents of asymptomatic children with CF, constant exposure to the clinic—with its cadre of visibly ill children—can shine an inescapably bright spotlight on the paradox of their commitment to preventive care and the uncertain future their children face. Roxanna describes how exposed she sometimes feels in its glare.

> Every time he coughs, it's like you just shudder inside. I don't know how to explain it. . . . I mean, it's just maybe one cough, it could be that he swallowed the wrong way, but every time I hear that cough. . . . I'll tell you what's so daunting about it is when you're in—sitting in the examining room with your baby and a kid walks by the room that you know has CF because you're in the CF hall, and they're brought into the room next to you, and in the office with the walls, and you hear that CF cough, that is the most daunting, horrible—it's just, all it is is a reminder to you of what's—what's the reality . . . going to eventually be for us. And that's tough; . . . you can't run from it.

For parents who got an early diagnosis and are now beginning to see undeniable signs of CF despite their every effort, the discourse of control presents a different kind of challenge and heartache. Parents' devastation at the diagnosis is heavily mediated, if the diagnosis is made early, by the promise of prevention and risk reduction: repeated assertions by newborn-screening programs and health care providers—assertions that it is best to know early because useful interventions are at hand—breed an inevitable hopefulness. For many parents, though, the hard truth is that the degree to which any real "protection" from the disease can be offered through early intervention is minimal, and that their own power to protect their child is woefully insufficient in the face of her deteriorating health.

Paige feels the anguish of this helplessness in every fiber. On the one hand, she is grateful for the early diagnosis, and enthusiastically invested in early intervention. "Kaya's lucky that since day one she's been getting treatment; we've been doing everything since day one. . . . We've always been able to know that she has it and we've been very aggressive in her care. . . . Rarely there goes a day where we don't have her do her chest therapy or her medications. We're very diligent, very aggressive. At the first sign of cough or illness, I call the physician after I've kind of examined her myself to say, Okay, this is what I think is going on, and what's helpful; . . . I'm happy that [the newborn screen] was done, that it was caught early, that we could start treatment early."

At the same time, however, she articulates how impotent she ultimately feels when it comes to protecting her child from CF. "The hardest thing is as a mom, you're supposed to fix everything, you know. You're supposed to fix the owies and the booboos, and you just can't fix this, there's nothing you can do. And I think that has been so hard for me, 'cause I can't control it at all. I have no say in how this disease ravages on her body. I can do what I can with treatments and medications, but other than that I have no say in what it does. . . . [It's] like [CF is] taking away my chance to give her everything I wanted to give her."

Expression of two conflicting emotions on this topic, two realities, is not uncommon. Parents feel, at once, powerful determination to protect the child from the disease, and extreme helplessness in the face of what may eventually prove, over the course of any given child's life, an unconquerable opponent. As Yvette puts it, "You can do everything that you know to do to try to keep her healthy, but you still can't . . . prevent everything from happening. . . . You hope that you can keep them healthy and . . . they don't have to spend a long time in the hospital ever or . . . anything like that." Ultimately, however, so many things are just "out of your control, pretty much."

Both of these sentiments undoubtedly reflect an important truth about the complicated matter of parenting a child diagnosed at birth with a genetic disorder. But the latter part of the story, the part about how hard it is to have knowledge of the disease and not be able to "fix everything," is often drowned out—in the popular press as well as in the research literature—by the dominant narrative of progress and improvement, of extended life-spans and enhanced quality of life.

Even for parents who find out early, and who have access to high-quality health care and adequate financial resources, control over the disease has definite limits. In many cases, substantial suffering and a substantially shortened life span will be their children's reality, no matter what. Paige captures here how very painful, how really excruciating, it is to know that this could be the case for her daughter.

> I could flash, like flash in my head, seeing my daughter, my daughter coughing like [others I have seen with CF], my daughter struggling to breathe, . . . and how [am] I gonna handle that? I struggled with questions in my head of how are you gonna handle this when it's Kaya. . . . It's so scary, and you read things too, I just can't imagine how it feels, you know. I wish I could be her. I think right now she has very normal— she doesn't have normal lungs, but she has normal lung capacity, and I think she . . . does not struggle to breathe, I think she feels that she gets enough air in. But I think, when she gets older, how is that gonna be? What's it like? Is it, you know, I've heard people describe it's like suffocating, it's like you can't get enough oxygen, you can't get enough air, like you're starving for it. And how awful that has to be, . . . you know, how awful, it's just, I'm just so sad, and so scared for her.

"What If Tomorrow Don't Come?": The Preciousness of Time

Knowledge of CF makes parents more vigilant, more watchful. It opens them up to the grief of possible suffering and death for their child. It thoroughly reshapes their parenting routines if they already had them before the diagnosis, and shapes them from scratch it they did not. But parents also emphasize that the diagnosis can serve to highlight how precious time is, and how important it is to live well in the moment instead of squandering it. Like those whom sociologist Arthur Frank describes as adopting a "quest narrative" in order to make sense of their illness, parents often speak about how they have used their child's CF, making it "the occasion of a journey that becomes a quest . . . [and] the quest is defined by the . . . belief that something is to be gained through the experience" (1995, 115).

Regardless of when the diagnosis comes, parents can gain from it determination to live fully in the present. As Rayna says, the newborn-screen diagnosis "taught me to . . . appreciate [Riley] all the more. He could die tomorrow, but I'm just happy for every day that I have with him." Plans for trips and for engaging in favorite activities should be acted on right away; postponement suggests the luxury of an indefinite future, and parents whose children are diagnosed with CF know better. Francesca puts it this way: "If we plan on doing stuff, we kind of make sure we follow through on stuff like that, just knowing that our days aren't always guaranteed. And not even the worst-case scenario that she would pass on, but just sicknesswise we don't know what's gonna come. So let's just take what we have now and do what we can with it. Maybe if she didn't have her CF, . . . we wouldn't put such a priority on doing some things, 'cause it just makes you think, like, what if tomorrow don't come? What if we can't put it off for five years? 'Cause we don't know where she'll be at with things."

Some parents feel that this appreciation for the preciousness of time and for the wisdom to cherish the child each day is the compensatory gift of CF. Paul describes it this way: "When the diagnosis was made, I definitely feel that in me I gained an additional sense of appreciation and attention, specific attention to just, you know, everything that made her her. You know, everything [that] made [Alexandra] who she was. . . . I definitely appreciated the time that we had with her [before], but I think I appreciate the time more now when I look back in retrospect . . . because of the fact that we now know she has cystic fibrosis. It's also changed the way I spend time with her as well. I spend more time with her."

For some parents, the desire to get the most from every day with their diagnosed child becomes entangled with a temptation to become too permissive and lavish. This urge to overindulge the child is fleeting in some cases, a phase parents go through on their way to settling into a more normal routine and a steadier state. This was the case for Nancy, who quickly reined in her impulse to overcompensate for her child's CF because of her health care provider's admonition that "you don't want to spoil CF kids because, and basically this sounds horrible, but nobody is going to like a child who is sick a lot and coughs a lot and then acts like a brat." Annie had the same experience and feels the best advice the doctor ever gave her was not to treat her son any differently the day after she learned about his diagnosis than she had every day for the past seven years. "If you do, you're going to ruin him as a human being," the doctor told her. "If he's bad, you crack him on the butt, and when he does something good, you hug him and kiss him."

For other parents, overindulgence just becomes an indisputable fact of life. As Sheri says of her son Jasper, reflecting on what changes the newborn-screen diagnosis occasioned: "If anything, he's more spoilt than he would have been." Barb also recognizes her own tendency to treat the diagnosed child differently. "I do sometimes feel a little more generous," she says, "giving him that extra cookie or whatever, because, you know, I guess I love him a little different. . . . I am just a little more patient with him than I think some other people are, because I do look at him different." What's different about young Kenny? That Barb read the words "CF is life shortening" when he was first born, and has never forgotten them.

Overindulgence, however, does not seem to be the most crucial issue even for those who raise it. Far more important is the transformation of priorities that can occur with the CF diagnosis. "I really cherish my son," says Roberta,

> and I do wonder how much it has to do with the diagnosis, through thinking, you know, the time really is precious. . . . He's really healthy, he's doing really well, he's bigger than most kids his age, he seems healthier. But . . . I think we decided right after he was diagnosed that because we didn't know what could happen, we still don't know what could happen, we decided that we were just going to make his life the best life that we could make it. And . . . that's still—that's still how we live. . . . If he hadn't been diagnosed, if he had just kind of been normal, I mean, maybe there wouldn't have been that. . . . Maybe there wouldn't be a lot of the attention.

These responses to the CF diagnosis show a remarkably resilient side of parents—their ability to learn something important, to create something worthwhile, even while experiencing grief and devastation. Here's how priorities changed for Judy, who like many parents became increasingly involved in raising money for a cure as a way of "fighting the disease" after her children were diagnosed: "One day my oldest one, it was within the first year she was diagnosed, she came downstairs and . . . she asked me if the doctors had found a cure yet for CF. And I said, 'Oh, not yet, but I'm sure we'd be the first to know if they did.' And she says, 'But Mom, you're not even looking!' And I thought, You know what, you're right, I haven't done anything to help the doctors try to find a cure. . . . At least [now] . . . I'm trying to raise money so that they can get all that they need to try to find a cure." Anne finds solace the same way: "It feels like—you're like, completely helpless, when you have a child with any serious medical condition, I think—you know, as a parent, I would think that any parent feels like they're helpless. You do as much as you can, but your child has a very serious medical condition, and the thing that makes me feel better is supporting the one thing that is trying to cure the disease that my child has . . . the [Cystic Fibrosis] Foundation. . . . It almost feels like my fight against the disease, you know?"

Chapter 4

Encounters with Expertise

Parents and Health Care Professionals

For parents, a major feature of newborn-screening diagnosis is the immediate and pervasive contact it brings with health care providers—first with those who are involved with screening and testing, then with the "army" of professionals who make up the treatment team. Getting the diagnosis, and then learning to live with it, are not private family matters. Rather, they are heavily mediated by those who test the baby, give the news, impart instructions, provide education and treatment, answer questions, make referrals, see the baby in clinic, monitor compliance, and generally interpret the condition's meaning. I have shown how the diagnostic process—its timing, structure, and delivery—has an impact on intrafamilial relationships and practices. Here I examine the effect of that process and its sequelae on the power dynamics of relationships between parents and professionals; on the development of parental know-how; and on the way parents come to construct their own CF-related beliefs, critiques, and practices.

"You Guys Are the Doctors": The Power of Professionals after an Early Diagnosis

All parents, no matter what the state of their child's health, gain confidence as caregivers over time. Some start out with more confidence than others when tending a newborn, but none are as sure of themselves at the beginning as they are later on, after learning from trial and error, putting in countless hours parenting, and receiving guidance from family and friends. The same trajectory of growing confidence holds true with respect to caring for a child with a genetic condition. As one parent put it: "As you deal with a disease, you become educated. You become educated about the disease process, [and] you become educated about your particular child."

I call this knowledge—which is based on experience, observation, experimentation, and consultation with other people rather than on what is codified in books or professional systems—"parental knowledge" instead of "lay knowledge." In so doing, I follow sociologist Meg Stacey, who favors the term "people knowledge" and writes that the term "'lay' . . . tends to be what is used for those people who do not belong to a specific profession. In referring to people who lack particular qualifications," she goes on, "'lay' suggests the absence of something valuable or prestigious, and may imply less competence, or even less moral worth" (1994, 90).

My interviews with parents illustrated beautifully how people who find themselves in unfamiliar situations often develop and deploy useful knowledge, and reaffirmed that the technical expertise of professionals—while invaluable in many situations—is not superior per se to other kinds of specialized capacity. Professional knowledge draws on a cumulative literature and body of clinical experience that is (at least ideally) assessed and reassessed over time. Parental knowledge, in contrast, usually has far more depth, since parents are saturated in the particulars associated with their own children more intimately than most professionals could ever be. Rather than "drawing lines between these realms," I join sociologist Sarah Wilcox in asserting that "experience and expertise are not opposites, because tactile skill can be a form of expertise . . . [and] lay knowledge is not simply 'experience' but is collective and shared, albeit not necessarily systematic or logical" (2010, 55). My intention here is to convey this view of the multifaceted relationship between parental and professional forms of expertise.

"How Good Can We Do for Him?": Parents' Loss
of Confidence after Unexpected Bad News

Though time is certainly one important factor in the development of parental knowledge and confidence, the diagnostic process also has tremendous influence. It is this process that most often initiates parents' connection to the health care system, complete with its array of professional definitions and norms.[1] As Taner-Leff and Walizer note, what occurs at this time "sets the stage for all future parent-professional encounters" (1992, 69). Further, "parents *never* forget what is said at the time of diagnosis. . . . It is at this intensely painful point in the parent-professional relationship that issues of trust, caring, and mutual respect are emblazoned in bold relief in the family's memory and consciousness" (ibid., 96, 69). The timing and structure of the diagnostic process also affect the confidence parents have in their own power, instincts, and competence, and correspondingly the degree of dependence they feel on health professionals.

When the diagnosis comes early, before the parents have gotten to know their infant, no substantial parental expertise has yet been developed. The baby is brand-new and, as discussed earlier, learning how to care for an infant even in the absence of any identified health issues—particularly if she is a first child—can feel overwhelming. This is a time of vulnerability, of trial and error, of just trying to learn—as one mother put it—"how to be a parent." Professional advice of all kinds therefore exerts a particularly powerful influence during this time.

And there is no shortage of such advice directed at all new parents; child rearing in the twenty-first century is heavily mediated by professionals of all kinds. As sociologist Nikolas Rose summarizes: "Childhood is the most intensively governed sector of personal existence. . . . The modern child has become the focus of innumerable projects that purport to safeguard it from physical, sexual, or moral danger, to ensure its 'normal' development, to actively promote certain capacities or attributes such as intelligence, educability and emotional stability" (1989, 123).

Expert parenting advice in the present era focuses on an ever-broadening array of themes. These include, among others, the need for bonding versus the need for discipline as the parent's guiding principle (Hulbert 2003); the importance of cognitive development (Wrigley 1989); and—most relevant here—the imperative to identify and protect against multiple intellectual, developmental, moral, and physical threats (Gill 2007; Marano 2008; Stearns 2003).

Using early diagnosis of genetic disease via newborn screening as a technique for identifying potential physical threats has now become an accepted part of newborn medical care for well infants, and its influence will only continue to grow as testing panels continue to expand. In the best-case scenario, the tests promise greater control over health outcomes for the child in the long run—and what parent wouldn't want that? In the case of CF, parents make every effort to use diagnostic information in just this way. But when CF is first added into the newborn picture, parents themselves feel ironically even less qualified to be in charge of the infant than they did before. At that crucial and vulnerable moment, parents see professionals—the ones who have decided that testing was needed and who have made the diagnosis—as best positioned to understand the situation and chart a course of action. As Joan describes it: "Well, I would say in the very beginning [when we got the newborn-screen diagnosis], we were kind of like—me and my husband—we were both kind of like, What do you [doctors] want to do, what do you think we should do, what do you think is best? You guys are the doctors, you know."

Newborn-screen diagnosis had a similar impact on James. After getting the results, he says: "I was really scared about how to take care of [our son] or if we could be good enough for him and what special needs he would have, and if we could meet those needs. Just a lot of different things really made me question . . . how good we could do for him." What he needed to begin resolving these feelings was time with the professionals, who could show him and his wife what to do for baby Eben and "help give us confidence that we are doing a good job."

Deena's confidence was so shaken by the positive newborn screen and subsequent rapid-fire diagnostic process that when a social worker was introduced during the sweat test as part of the CF team, Deena immediately assumed the worst. "You know, at first when they said to us that a social worker was going to come in and talk to us, I'm thinking, Oh, my gosh, they're going to take my baby away from me and I didn't do anything," says Deena, tears in her voice as she recalls the moment. "I thought I had done something wrong, or we had done something wrong, [but] they're like, 'No, it's just part of our team and part of the way we help you.'"

A diagnosis by newborn screen, as these vignettes suggest, produces an unusual dynamic between parents and providers. The medicalization of childbirth in the United States has created a situation where birth itself is considered a medical problem that must be managed by health care professionals in the institutional setting of a hospital (see, e.g., Ehrenreich and English 1978; Rothman 1989). Indeed, 99 percent of babies are born in hospitals (Martin et al. 2009). In this environment, obstetrical specialists structure the birth experience itself, and then pediatric specialists step in to structure the care of newborns. Mothers may have more access to their babies while still in the hospital than used to be the case, since many hospitals now allow the baby to stay in the room with the mother most of the time, if that is what the mother requests. Even in such an instance, however, the infant is still in a liminal state. She officially belongs to her parents, yet she remains predominantly in the care of the hospital's medical staff. She is therefore subject to their rules, schedules, routines, and diagnostics—including newborn-screening tests.

NBS as it unfolds in the hospital setting is not a parent-driven process: how can it be, when many parents don't realize it is happening or understand it only vaguely, and when hardly any parents are asked for consent?

A child who turns out to have a positive screen for CF is generally not actively ill in those first days or weeks. She may be entirely without symptoms, or she may be showing some early signs of illness, usually digestive in nature—but in any case, she's not (in most cases) in a medical crisis. Thus she is usually released from the hospital into the care of her parents, who begin learning what it means truly to be in charge of their new baby. But then when the infant, already at home, is found to have a positive screen, the health care establishment once again asserts its dominance over the fragile new family dynamic by remanding parents to a role of simple compliance with instructions coming from the professionals. In the words of New York State's newborn-screening pamphlet, the parents' job is to "make it easier for the doctor to help the baby."

What parents confront when there is a positive screen, then, is a clear instance of the process (so thoroughly documented by sociologists) by which "medical interpretations of conditions . . . acquire cultural legitimacy . . . [and] become the dominant frame for understanding a large range of . . . human problems" (Litt 2000, 4–5; see also Aronowitz 2009). By mandating the heel prick, professionals signal the importance they attach to finding out about and addressing all screened genetic disorders as early as possible in infancy. That parents are not informed or consulted about the procedure establishes that the well-being of the child in this important respect "is committed to the judgment of medical experts" (Wieser 2010, 932). But let's look at it from the perspective of the parents: they receive news of the abnormal result at a time when they are just finding out for themselves how to care for their baby. Now they must learn from their doctors what to look for and see in the child—how to recognize, forestall, and address symptoms; how to minimize the impact of CF; how, in essence, to parent in the genomic age, when part of having a new baby is knowing about and responding to the child's genetic endowment. And they must learn all this while continuing to care for the child at home, in an environment with restricted access to those very professionals who have just (re)constituted themselves as indispensable to the health and safety of the infant.

"I Called So Many Times": Parents Rely on Providers for Help

Once the diagnosis of CF is officially made—or, in some cases, at the very moment it is made—parents generally have a first clinic visit where they meet an interdisciplinary team of professionals: nurses, nutritionists, genetic counselors, pulmonologists, gastroenterologists, social workers, and more. Most often they arrive thinking they are attending, as parents put it, "a typical doctor's appointment," only to find "a conference room full of people" ready to initiate them into their new role as parents of a child with CF. They receive large amounts of information and instruction and then they go back home, where they alone are responsible for carrying out the daily preventive care regime.

Parents describe these first weeks and months with the diagnosed infant as a time when they struggle mightily to understand what CF is and what it means for this newborn whose already-inherent fragility—by virtue of her small size and recent delivery—now feels to them like actual peril. In order to manage this stressful situation, many parents rely extensively on contact with professionals via frequent office visits, or via the telephone.

Parents experience these contacts as vital connections to expertise, advice, reassurance, instructions. Unsure now whether the infant is okay, whether their own caregiving techniques are adequate, they contact professionals often, looking for help. Anthony describes how things changed after the newborn-screen diagnosis like this: "I guess our biggest concern is that she goes to the doctor often and my big—my concern and I think my wife's as well is [that] the day that we kind of are relaxed and go, 'Well, it will pass, let's give it a few days,' is the day that something major happens. So we always err on the side of caution. You know, we'd rather be a pain in their side."

Deena might be more likely to second-guess her own reliance on the providers but, like Anthony, describes uncertainty and hence a desire to remain in close contact with the professionals. "If [our son] didn't have [CF]," she says, "I'd be, like, Okay, he has a cold, give him some cough medicine and wait it out. He'd be on his merry way. But with CF it's like, well . . . that cough doesn't sound so good. Maybe we should call our pulmonologist and get some antibiotics or see what they want us to do. So it's hard to decipher when to call and when not to call, and I think sometimes we maybe call too much but it's hard to really know when to and when not to, especially when you haven't ever been around it before."

And from Barb: "He would cough like a normal person would cough and I panicked, thinking, Oh, my God, this is it, because I didn't know. He was a brand-new baby. I never had a child before, he is the first one in the family so, so he would do the slightest little cough, and I thought, Okay, what does this mean? . . . Is he going to get a fever, and does he need medicine, and do we have to bring him somewhere? You don't know."

For Francesca, the fear after the positive screen and subsequent confirmatory test was intense, unremitting. "Once I found out that she possibly could have the CF, I called so many times in the middle of the night. I'm like, 'Oh, my God, she's breathing really heavy, I don't know if this is right.'" Fortunately, Francesca's health care providers, particularly the nurses, were compassionate and comfortable with making themselves available to her as a resource. "The nurses that were on call," she remembers, were "my biggest help because you could call these people up anytime and even if it would've been a dumb question to them they were very kind about answering them and just, you know, like assuring me that I was doing everything okay and everything was fine. . . . There was just a lot of follow-up that came from the hospital that helped."

Paige had a similar need for help from professionals, a similar reliance on them for guidance in caring for a baby whom the diagnosis had made suddenly strange and vulnerable—a baby Paige could no longer know based on her observation alone. But for her, the process of getting assistance was complicated by her sense that her health care providers regarded her as overly needy.

> What was hard, I think, in the beginning [was] being new as a parent for one and not knowing what was normal for children . . . and then dealing with the disease, the health care. . . . The people in health care were somewhat hard to deal with, because I sometimes would get the feeling that I'm a little pain in their ass, excuse my language, . . . because I would call a lot because I didn't know, because I was so scared, because there was such a fear. . . . I would call, I would call the nurse a lot and say, "I don't know if this is normal or not, this doesn't seem right." And a lot of times, you just felt like you were a real pain or like you were kind of a nuisance, and that was hard.

It is clear that during this period parents perceive the locus of control over their child to lie with professionals. Joan says: "I remember thinking, I can't believe they are going to let her come home with us, at the clinic. We have no idea how to take care of her. I can't believe they are going to let us walk out of the door with her." She had, of course, already walked out the door with her newborn when she was discharged from the hospital after birth, had taken her daughter home and cared for her just fine. But once they got the diagnosis, "it just seemed like everything changed. . . . It was like there is so much more now to taking care of her, and are we really fit to do that? . . . It was just so overwhelming. I mean the first time we went to the clinic they were like, Well, you have to do this and this. And we met with nutritionists, respiratory therapists, and pulmonologists and social workers and, you know, it was just all so overwhelming, all this stuff we were going to have to do. I remember leaving there thinking, How am I going to do all this stuff in one day?" The dramatic decline in Joan's self-confidence as a parent, in her sense of the adequacy and value of her parental knowledge, couldn't be more clearly expressed.

Cassandra's experience was similar to Joan's. "We had everybody come in and introduce themselves and tell us what they were going to do for us. It was just really overwhelming," she says, "and you didn't feel in control of anything at all. That has gotten better now, because at first you just felt like you couldn't do anything without calling somebody and asking if it was okay." In Cassandra's case, however, the doctors wanted her to use her own judgment right away about administering pulmonary medications. But she had neither the experience nor the confidence as yet to take on such a responsibility, especially since the sudden close contact with a large team of medical professionals "just made you feel like someone was watching over your shoulder all the time," monitoring to see the ways "we weren't doing something right." The doctors prescribed a breathing medication three times a day, Cassandra continues, "so I was doing it three times a day, but then I didn't understand; . . . then they are telling me, 'You just do it whenever you feel he needs it.' So I am like, 'Okay, is that daily? Is that not at all? What is it?' The doctor kept telling us, 'Whatever you think,' and it was like, 'I need a yes or a no.'"

It is scary and difficult to be immediately responsible for an infant's complex new care regimes at home, but it may be even harder to get a diagnosis for a nonsymptomatic or minimally symptomatic child while still in the hospital. Suzanne had this experience; she is the mother discussed earlier whose baby was at known "high risk" for CF because both parents had carrier-tested positive, and who was delayed in the hospital because of iatrogenic problems. For her, "everything changed" in the most literal sense after the test result came back. The hospital staff, who "were not used to dealing with babies with anything wrong," took charge of baby Quinn, no longer allowing Suzanne to hold or to nurse him. "They just got a little bit over the top," she says, "'cause he was having feeding problems so they sort of attributed everything to him having CF. Which we later found out wasn't the case at all. So they were, 'He's too tired for you to hold him,' or whatever, so that was their decision." Suzanne says that "a lot of Quinn's symptoms, like he didn't appear to be sick when he was born," yet the hospital treated his diagnosis almost like a medical emergency, controlling every aspect of his care minutely and marginalizing Suzanne. "I got really depressed," she recalls. At the same time, she was grateful for the early diagnosis. Like other parents in her place, as a young, first-time mother she was in no position to counter or question medical authorities when they recommended immediate testing. "How it had been explained to me, the sooner you find out about it, the better the outcome for the child. Which I could understand once he was born. That it was important to know, 'cause it meant they could start treatment straight away instead of having to wait for two months to find out whether he had it or not [via the regular newborn screen]."

Quinn's at-risk status before birth, and his quick diagnosis afterward, firmly situated him as a medicalized infant from the beginning. Suzanne is unhappy with the way events unfolded at the hospital where he was born. It was emotionally devastating to lose control over him when the test result came in at age four days. Yet on balance she is still glad to have gotten the diagnosis immediately. She fervently wants what is best for Quinn. How could she help but have faith that "they" who had advocated an early diagnosis were also in the best position, ultimately, to assure the baby's well-being by "starting treatment right away"?

After an unexpected diagnosis, parents hold very tight, at first, to the lifeline of contact with professionals. Some begin to loosen that grasp a little—at least with one hand—after they recover from the initial shock of sudden diagnosis. And once they have their bearings, parents often reflect on their relationships with the health care system and its representatives in new ways.

Should the "Cookie Cutter" Crumble?:
Routine and Variation in CF Care

It is axiomatic that clinical care can easily become routinized in response to underlying uncertainties about best practice and to pressures on the system that arise when large numbers of patients need care. It is also axiomatic that various consequences then follow for the lifeworld of people who receive this care. In the face of inexperience with CF newborn screening, coupled with what for some newborn-screening staff, treatment centers, and even individual pediatricians may be a sudden increase in demand after NBS expansion, many providers gravitate toward routinized ways of educating families and treating affected children. Here we see what happens when what parents characterize as "cookie-cutter approaches" collide with highly individualized parental experiences in initiating and providing treatment. Parents also give examples of what can unfold when providers *do* ask "what our philosophy was, how we wanted to do this."

The "Positive Stuff" or the "Dirty Truth":
Learning about CF after the Diagnosis

How information about CF flows between parents and providers is a critical aspect of the postdiagnosis period. Professionals are presumed to possess, or to have facilitated access to, medical and scientific knowledge about the disease.[2] Parents view providers as a crucial resource in this regard. At the same time, parents have a detailed sense of their own coping mechanisms, their own psychological balance and how it can best be maintained in the postdiagnosis period. This is knowledge providers don't have, and when they try to apply a generic approach to communicating information instead of taking cues from parents about what they want to know and when they want to know it, there is trouble.

Parents do not all want the same amount and kind of information about CF during and immediately after the diagnosis. For some, no matter how they discover their child has CF, it is critical to know everything there is to know, every detail, fact and statistic, no matter how sobering. "Give me it all; I want to know every possible [detail]," said one parent. Another put it: "I wanted to know everything, which I'm still that way. I'm like a sponge when it comes to CF stuff. . . . I was reading all this literature which was pretty heavy to read when you have a brand-new baby."

For this mother, as for most parents, information about average life expectancy for CF was particularly "hard to swallow," yet she wanted to know even that from the get-go. So did Cora, although at first it was impossible for her to process information the doctors were trying to give her about "what [CF] was, and how it worked," because "I was more like, 'Is he going to die? I need to know that. . . . What can you tell me here about that?' "

In some cases, parents' thirst for medical details and statistical information is motivated at least in part by a determination to build optimism—if any can be marshaled—on solid ground rather than on denial or illusion. Nancy's description is illustrative: "I'm the kind of person, I'm really proactive, so if I find out about a problem or an issue I want to dive into it and figure out what's the best way to do this, or what should we do? So I want all the information I can get. . . . I don't just want to be clueless and think, Oh, she'll be fine, she'll beat the odds. I want to know the dirty truth. I want to know what these people [with CF] go through so that I know how I can prepare myself and how I can prepare [my daughter]."

For these parents, it is infuriating when professionals try to shield or protect them by withholding information or meting it out slowly. As Andrea said: "One problem I have with some doctors is that they talk down to you and don't explain things thoroughly." This form of condescension breeds mistrust of providers, as illustrated by Kim's description of her communication with professionals at the CF clinic not long after the diagnosis. When her daughter, Sarah, cultured positive for pseudomonas, a bacterium that can attack the lungs of people with CF because of chronic airway inflammation and lowered pulmonary defenses (Moskowitz et al. 2005, 9), her providers tried to manage Kim's reaction in a most infuriating way.

I'm like, "What is this pseudomonas?" "I will have Frances call you back in a couple of days," the nurse said. And I'm like, "What?" Well, apparently they needed to give me time to let this sink into my head. So of course I call for two days straight and then Frances called to see how I was handling it and to tell me all about it, this thing that could kill my child. If you don't catch it soon enough, it colonizes and causes lung damage and gets worse and worse and pretty soon you're needing a [lung] transplant. Or the child is needing a transplant because, you know, all her lungs collapse. . . . Well, thankfully they got the pseudomonas in time so it didn't colonize. But this is one of the things where they wait to tell you about . . . and you're just horrified that this is happening to your child and they never even warned you. So of course, in my moment of— I don't know if I should say the word "grief," but whatever, I kind of scolded this lady, saying, "What else could I expect? Tell me, so I can prepare, that this might happen to my child. Because I need to know. So that I can prepare myself, so that I can prepare myself so that I'm not devastated like I am right now."

For Lorraine, medical paternalism was most grievous as she was trying to get her healthy older child tested for CF immediately after her baby daughter was diagnosed. At first, the doctor wouldn't do the test.

He was entirely dismissive of whether or not my son would be affected. He actually refused to test him. He said, "We're gonna want to focus on your daughter, you can't handle having two right now. So we're not even going to look at him." And my husband and I were very concerned that if my son did have it then we wanted him to start treatment immediately 'cause it had been two and a half years and he hadn't gotten anything. We were just very concerned and he took one look at him and said, "I can look at him and see how big he is and know he doesn't have CF. We're not worrying about him."

Lorraine and her husband persisted, and the test was finally ordered. When the positive result came in, the doctor said, "Oh, I knew all along that he had it, but I didn't [think] you could handle it." Lorraine continues:

My husband and I are just not accustomed to being treated like we're stupid, so that was just infuriating beyond belief. . . . When parents are being confronted with a genetic disease and they have a sibling, they are concerned about both kids. And so I think that to try to shield them from the diagnosis is just really patronizing. If a parent were to say to the doctor, "I can't handle it. Please don't test the other child, let's deal with them one at a time, let's deal with the sick child first," that's fine. But we weren't saying that. Everybody's different. I mean, we're people who just wanna, let's get this straight so we can start working on it.

Lorraine echoes here one of the parents interviewed by Taner-Leff and Walizer, who said that providers who attempted to shield him from information about his children were, "in keeping the 'bad news' from us, . . . also exercising power over us and the circumstances that we find ourselves in. This is unacceptable to us" (Taner-Leff and Walizer 1992, 77).

Lorraine is correct in imagining that parents pace themselves differently when it comes to learning about CF and what it means for the family. A "one day at a time" approach is much more comfortable for some. Here's how Barb describes the need to learn about CF at her own pace:

> You hear the word "life shortening" with your four-day-old baby, and then for me I didn't want to know and I still don't, I don't want to know everything about it, I don't want to know what is going to happen on day thirty-six, I don't want to know what could happen, I don't want to know any of that. I want to know what is happening now, and I still live like that. My husband and I still do that, we don't do all the research and find out about everything, because we feel like what we want to do is deal with the immediate symptom, or treat it. . . . We don't want to know anything that could happen, . . . because it is overwhelming and it is too much and it is depressing, so we deal with immediate symptoms. That is how we get through.

For parents focused on the near rather than the far term, the phased accumulation of information provides the time they need to assimilate little by little, to get used to general ideas and feel competent to judge how relevant they are to their own child. As articulated by Joya: "Anything can happen to a child by the time they are thirty. I want to know what my first week is going to be like, I want to know what the first year is going to be like, what the day-to-day is going to be like, the management of the child, that is what we want to know. You are not helpful telling me what is happening ten to twenty years down the road. . . . I just want to know what this is about."

These mothers, like three out of four in a study of parents' experiences with genetic counseling after the birth of a baby with CF, found themselves struggling with "information overload," altogether "[too] much information to absorb in a short time as well as coming to terms with the diagnosis" (Collins et al. 2001, 59). Yvette summarizes here the experience many parents have in connection with their first visits at the specialty center. "When you go to the CF clinic, it's kind of overwhelming," she says. "Just so much information in such a short period of time; . . . it's hard to remember when you leave there what they said, the different things, . . . and you also have your baby there and you're trying to take care of them and make sure that they're happy." To compensate for potential problems with information overload, Yvette deploys several strategies. "I tried to take a notebook with me and write down any questions that I want to ask them," she says, "and then write down . . . their answers to those questions and then anything else that they say." She also tries "hopefully every time" she goes to "take somebody with me just so, you know, they can hear too, and then they can hopefully take care of the baby while I'm listening to the doctor . . . [and] hopefully remember as much as I can."

For many parents, what is hardest to absorb, and what they don't want to be forced to confront in a bald statistical way, are data about life expectancy and descriptions of the natural history and progression of the disease. They know, of course, that this information exists, and they may even have encountered it on the Internet or elsewhere. But they don't want it held in front of them, don't want it to feel like foreknowledge of their children's fate or "crystal-ball predictions of what our children won't be able to do," as a parent in Taner-Leff and Walizer's study commented (1992, 93). As Timmy states, it's "information I don't want, . . . [and] that's purposeful." Being confronted with it unbidden, then, is particularly wrenching. Suzanne describes the disjuncture this way:

> We had one doctor, . . . and we walked into the room and she sat down and we sat down and she said, "Having CF is not a good prognosis." And I sort of thought, I don't really need to hear this. I'm well aware of what it does. I didn't really think that was very thoughtful to say to someone while holding their new baby. . . . This one doctor . . . could be quite callous. And not really think about how you might be feeling as a parent. . . . [What I needed was] the basics for the moment. You can find out everything else as you go along. It's not necessary to know everything right from the start.

And from Judy: "I think I—at first I don't wanna know everything, just wanna deal with things as they come. . . . They threw everything at me and I wasn't ready for that. . . . I didn't want to know the bad things, I just wanted to know as of today what would happen today. . . . I don't wanna know the lungs are expanding and, you know, . . . the organs, all the organs, it's gonna affect all the organs eventually. I didn't want to know all that. I didn't wanna know the life expectancy of it. I just wanted to know what we were dealing with today."

But Judy's CF center—like many centers—has a policy of sitting down with parents and giving them an overall education, a comprehensive overview of CF and all they can expect. "They gave me pamphlets," Judy said, "and all kinds of stuff, you know, a big book about [CF, they] gave me that book and I guess I needed to know those things but I wasn't ready for those things. . . . It was too much to handle at the time. . . . I just kind of sat there and I didn't know what to expect. . . . I just thought that they were gonna give us medicine and, you know, go home. . . . I wasn't expecting it. I guess I didn't realize how much there was to it, really."

Parents who pace themselves in learning about the disease are not in unhealthy denial, nor are they looking for a paternalistic model of care which presumes that providers have an obligation to protect parents by deciding what information to give and what to withhold. They agree with Lorraine that it should be the parents who determine how information is shared, not the providers. What they want is for professionals to check in with them about the education process, to ask them how much they want to know and when they want to know it, rather than adopting a "one size fits all" approach.

Francesca's description of her own needs postdiagnosis, and of how well her providers met them, serves as an example of how meaningful it is for families when professionals can attend to their individual experiences and preferences. "We wanted to know, Where's the positive stuff? We don't want to know all the negatives right away, we just want to . . . hear stories about people who are living with this, who are doing good with it. . . . We try to really focus on some of the positive information about CF. . . . I don't even think at first we even asked about life expectancies and stuff like that, or hospitalizations. . . . We just wanted to know, Who do you know who is living it, making it just part of their life, it's not controlling them, and stuff like that."

Unlike Kim's providers, and Suzanne's, the professionals working with Francesca in the postdiagnosis period took their lead from her, responding to where she was at each point and remaining both respectful and available. "We would just ask them, 'What about this?'" Francesca says. "And they would come back with stuff. Or we would say, 'We're really getting stressed out, there's a lot going on right now.' And they'd be like, 'Okay, you know what, you let us know when [you're ready] and we'll follow back up with you . . . and see how you're doing. . . . ' So they were really good at listening to us, and hearing about what we wanted. They just cared about how we wanted to deal with this. They never told us like how we should deal with it or what to do next or anything."

Sally too found the health care team responsive and sensitive in the face of irreducibly difficult circumstances. "And they could see very well when it started to get overwhelming," she says. "They would change the subject and talk about related—but not of the same level—. . . information. So they were very well in how they handled it. But it was overwhelming. I won't say overwhelming. It was devastating."

Variation in how parents want to become educated about the details of their child's diagnosis is not necessarily connected with when and how the diagnosis was made. Other researchers who have conducted qualitative interviews with parents of children with disabilities have also documented a range of preferences on this issue without identifying any particular pattern based on the timing of the diagnosis (Hill 1994; Taner-Leff and Walizer 1992). However, the rapid expansion of newborn-screening programs that is now underway means more and more parents will be contacted by providers in the period right after birth with a diagnosis of some kind. To meet parents' need to control the flow of information, to get as much or as little as is right for them at any given point, newborn-screening systems and follow-up services would have to become highly individualized. Providers would have to spend enough time with each family to find out—as did Francesca's health care providers—"how parents actually feel by listening and not project how they would feel onto the parents" (Taner-Leff and Walizer 1992, 43).

"There Is No One-to-Ten Scale Here": Preventive Care for Everyone

Education and information about CF are not the only things about the CF health care system parents often find packaged as if one size could fit all. Despite wide variations in CF's phenotypic expression and wide variations in CFTR mutations, the practices of CF management are often quite standardized within a state or specialty center, and most often these practices are oriented toward aggressive intervention. In many states and at many specialty centers, standardized practices include prescribed preventive treatments, clinic visit routines, and protocols for treating emergent symptoms.

As I have already shown, this interventionist standard of care is often a source of comfort for parents, especially immediately after diagnosis, because it provides authoritative instruction about what should be done to optimize the baby's now fragile-seeming health. When providers act with confidence, setting families up with aggressive care regimes designed to keep their babies healthy, parents tend to attribute their child's day-to-day good health to the care they receive and are "very thankful" that the most conservative measures are applied across the board.

This gratitude for intensive prophylactic treatment is shared by almost all families—even those who, like Nana, were told from the beginning that prognoses for CF vary greatly, "that every case is not the same, that one kid with CF is not the same as another kid with CF, and [our son] could turn out to just have something like allergies, or he could turn out to be in the hospital all the time." However, variation in prognosis does not for the most part correlate with variation in disease management; generally, medical experts' acknowledgment that CF can result in a range of outcomes does not extend to making predictions about outcome for any given child. "There is," Bess observes, "no one-to-ten scale; there is no 'She's going to have it this bad.'" As a result, treatment according to the worst-case scenario is most often the norm.[3] As one mother puts it, though the providers have told her that her child will "probably have a more mild form of cystic fibrosis," they "can't treat it that way, because you don't really know. Because the genetics don't actually determine that, . . . so they treat everybody, . . . you know, as if they have it, and . . . the whole thing is to take all these preventative steps to keep the lungs as healthy as possible for as long as possible. . . . So even though he's asymptomatic in all this stuff, he still is doing every treatment. . . . It's the standard preventive regime."

A second mother offers a variation on this theme. In describing why her child was hospitalized despite appearing only mildly ill, she notes that the professionals' strategy for CF is to treat every child with the long-range future in mind. "I am not treating him for today," says Barb's doctor, summarizing the CF center's approach to all NBS-identified children with CF. "I am treating him for twenty-five years from now."

Over the course of my research, as CF screening continued to spread rapidly across the country, an increasing number of parents in my study expressed concern, consternation, or downright outrage over routinized approaches to CF treatment, despite their gratitude for early intervention. As one father put it: "In some ways I think it is a cookie-cutter technique. That this is the way they deal with all patients. I don't feel [it's as] specialized as other forms of medicine at this point. . . . [Now, it's] like you have CF, so you need to be treated this way and only this way."

As fear and lack of experience with the diagnosed infant give way to everyday parenting routines, some families begin to question whether blanket protocols for prophylactic care actually align with their child's needs. Sally, for example, staggers her visits to the CF clinic and to the pediatrician so that her child is seen somewhere every three months, but not necessarily by the specialists every time. She's aware that this is a violation of the clinic's standard procedure, but since she sees the recommended frequency of on-site visits as an artifact of the center's data collection and monitoring needs rather than as a recommendation designed to maximize her particular child's health, she feels free to improvise just a bit. "I don't make a big deal about not going as often as we should," she says,

> because they have us on four times a year and I don't feel it's necessary
> given the way we monitor and take care of him. I know they do it for data

purposes as well, but given the fact that the visit doesn't entail much besides weighing him and measuring him and checking his lungs—the pediatrician does that too. . . . I don't see that going to the pulmonologist makes any difference if he goes to the pediatrician. I figure if I get him somewhere every three months, that's good. And if he was sick, of course I would take him, in a minute. I think they just want the information and I don't blame them but we're busy.

Another family's critique of routinization focuses on the dietary recommendations made for their child, which they don't see as individualized for their child's needs. Like Sally, Ron rejects the medical orthodoxy about how to get his child to gain more weight. He rejects it, however, based not only on the impracticality of what is prescribed, but also as a principled form of resistance to being treated like one more cog in the CF treatment machine. As he puts it: "You have a young man running around that just doesn't like to sit still 'cause he's hopped up on sugar and junk food, he burns as much as he eats anyway. We've kind of learned, I think, ourselves, what he needs, you know, to be healthy, to gain weight properly, for him. And not—not a cookie cutter, this is what you need to do because that's what we're telling everybody."

No Definitive Answers: Parents Confront
New Procedures and Medical Uncertainty

As sociologist Renee Fox has been pointing out for decades, uncertainty is an unavoidable part of medicine. While "progress" often "dispels some uncertainties, it uncovers others that were not formerly recognized, and it may even create new areas of uncertainty that did not previously exist" (Renee Fox 2000, 409). In the case of newborn screening for CF, the lack of clarity parents formerly experienced when they had a symptomatic child but no clinical diagnosis has now been replaced by unknowns of other kinds.

One of these is at least in part a byproduct of NBS's rapid growth. When health care policy results in abrupt change, both systems of care and individual providers are inevitably called on to render services for which they are unprepared. When expansion comes quickly, there is often little lag time for providers to gear up: as soon as screening starts, families with abnormal results begin lining up at the door for follow-up testing, orientation to the NBS system, an introduction to their child's disorder, a plan of care, and ongoing treatment.[4] Despite NBS capacity-building efforts in the public and private sectors and the hard work of many state programs, the pediatricians and specialists who interface directly with families are often (as parents put it) "not comfortable with some of these disorders because they've never heard of them before," or because they are just "learning about it."

In 2005, when I began interviewing families about their experiences with newborn screening for CF, all were from the few states that had already been doing CF screening for a number of years. Between 2005 and 2008, however, as CF screening rapidly spread, I began to talk with parents from states that had just started CF screening programs for newborns. For these families, the relationship with medical authority is often complicated by direct and sometimes dramatic encounters with uncertainty in the health care delivery process.

In addition to the uncertainties caused by professionals' unpreparedness, uncertainty is inherent in the complicated nature of CF, which renders unclear the significance of CF diagnosis for each identified child. This is a characteristic feature of much of the new NBS, of course. But the rapid spread of DNA newborn screening for cystic fibrosis in particular has caused accelerated changes in what the label "cystic fibrosis" signifies.

These kinds of uncertainty can be difficult for families to manage, and parents had a good deal to say about them. Some "understand that medicine takes a little time to evolve with changes." But those who encounter disorganized, poorly coordinated care, or who begin to suspect that even the experts don't have or won't share good answers to pressing questions, are also distressed, angry, and frightened.

"There's Not a Lot Out There on Treating Infants": Frustration with Medical Uncertainty

Newborn screening has had specific consequences for CF treatment because when the disorder is identified so early, protocols for treating symptomatic children may not apply. Although most families feel comforted by the existence and expertise of CF clinic staff, some remain skeptical about their providers' capacity to treat asymptomatic newborns when "they are used to only seeing kids who have symptoms, because that was the only way that kids got to them previously." As Paula put it:

> It's difficult to get answers because there's not a lot out there on treating infants, and that's kind of what I was looking for specifically. You know, they kind of talk about lung function tests and you can't even do those until they're five and a lot of the treatments are for school-aged kids and adults, and it didn't give us a lot of information on what to do, so that was probably more frustrating. That made us think even more, maybe they don't know what they're doing 'cause there's nothing out there

telling them what to do and they're just kind of testing everything on [our daughter]. It was a little scary for a while.

Paula's daughter, Celeste, was only the second child in her state to be diagnosed with CF after a newborn screen, and her doctors—like many doctors around the country grappling with incomplete or even contradictory evidence about effective care—were in significant disagreement about how aggressively to treat her when she developed respiratory symptoms. "They were still trying to figure out how to treat infants," says Paula, and Celeste ended up "in the hospital just from kind of miscommunication between the doctors—how aggressive they're going to be with treating her." The divergent viewpoints of Celeste's doctors resulted in what Paula and her husband perceived to be less than optimal care. Even more significantly, they were distressed and outraged at the doctors' lack of certainty. "We just wanted them to do *whatever* to keep her healthy," says Paula. "But we expected them to know what that was! . . . Part of what drove our questions was trying to make sure they were answering our questions with confidence, that this is what they knew they were going to do, and sometimes we didn't get that, it was like, 'Well, maybe we'll try this,' and we thought, 'Well, that's not good enough.' We need to know that this is going to work and have more definitive answers."

Another set of problems arises when CF providers step outside their areas of expertise to look at the child's overall health. When infants are diagnosed via NBS, they are referred for specialty care right away. Many parents also establish and maintain strong connections with a local pediatrician. Others, however, can come to rely on the specialty center as a significant or even primary source of medical care, displacing the pediatrician and his or her network of associated specialists from center stage in the care of their CF-diagnosed child. The particular training CF specialists have does not always prepare them well, however, for the complexity of the child's overall care. This was true in Lara's experience, and she notes with distress that in her state the specialty service is "called a CF clinic, but really, it's just pulmonologists [who] don't know anything about the GI arena, so they assumed [the cause of the abnormal liver function identified in my daughter] was CF related" when in fact the problem had nothing to do with CF.

Newborn-screening administrators articulate concerns similar to those voiced by families about consequences of the new NBS: the fact is, it isn't clear to most program directors and clinicians how to treat all identified children, even for a relatively well studied condition like CF. "I know with cystic fibrosis," says one director, "we look for one mutation, but there's . . . a thousand out there, and some of these mutations, and some of the variants of some of these disorders, I don't know if the treatment and management is so clearcut. That's a bit of a danger, because if you're identifying something, you know, you're going to upset a family and, and if you don't have any clear . . . direction or management to give them, that's a problem, and we certainly don't want to do that."

In some states, the lack of clear direction is evident in the way approaches vary among CF centers. The centers make an effort to collaborate, yet families attending one clinic are likely to encounter procedures and recommendations different from those in another. As one newborn-screening administrator commented:

> The CF center knows that . . . they get those [mild] mutations so they know this is a kiddo who may end up with either totally no disease or atypical disease. . . . It's kind of up to each individual CF center exactly whether they call it atypical CF or whether they call it normal, but the CF centers have worked together, they have their own advisory group, . . . and they have come up with kind of a policy of how they're dealing with the kids who fall into that kind of gray zone. And I can't say that every center probably deals with them exactly the same, but they at least discussed it.

Another NBS director articulates similar issues but emphasizes that the transition to NBS identification of "atypical" CF mutations raises issues about whether a certain subset of children should be treated at all. Variants of unknown significance are "certainly very much of an issue relative to CF, with these kind of atypical CFs that they're identifying, or known mutations that we don't know the clinical significance of. And so the kids get monitored by CF center[s], but may or may not need any, you know, much treatment at all."

NBS directors can be well positioned to see how protocols for treating NBS-diagnosed infants unfold in their state. The follow-up system is in many instances connected to the newborn-screening program itself through oversight, monitoring, collaboration, or some combination of these. Once the diagnostic process is over and treatment begins, however, families have little contact with NBS staff—and thus little exposure to their views about uncertainties in clinical care. Parents, then, deal with clinicians when they encounter ambiguities in the diagnosis, prognosis, and treatment of their child's CF.

Questioning What's Answerable

I have already shown how the uncertainty of CF—its maddening, tantalizing, terrifying variability—can powerfully influence the way parents experience the diagnosis itself, as well as their efforts to control the disease. Not surprisingly, CF's unpredictability also affects the experiences parents have with health care professionals. Providers are uniformly decisive in their assertion that early diagnosis of CF, and the prophylactic intervention and close monitoring that follow, means better health for a child than would otherwise be the case. But no matter how persistently parents try, they cannot elicit from their providers a prediction of just how compromised the child's health will actually be.

Some parents regard providers' circumspection about the future as a simple fact of life: accurate forecasting is beyond human capacity, and the unknowability of consequences must just be wrestled with and accepted. This is how Kayla describes her struggle to accept the uncertainty articulated by her son's doctors: "I believe my first question was, 'How long am I going to have my son?' I wanted to know how long he was going to live, and of course they couldn't answer that, and they said that is typically one of the first questions they get, and it is impossible to answer of course, just like it would be impossible to answer how long I am going to live. It doesn't make any difference if you are talking about someone with a disease or a perfectly healthy person; nobody can answer that question, which wasn't the answer I wanted to hear."

Even genetic testing to identify which CFTR mutations her baby has didn't persuade Kayla's provider to hazard a guess about his future. "She told me even when we do know [the] mutation he had, . . . it would still be impossible to tell," says Kayla. "Because that was one of my questions . . . after she spun the genetic side of it. I said, 'With all these thousands of mutations, is one of them known to be more severe than others?' . . . And of course the answer was no. She said you could take one hundred kids with the same mutation and they are all different, so she said there was no way to tell. She said we know what the most common mutation is, but it is no indication of the severity whatsoever. She said, 'One day at a time, that is how you know.'"

Other parents of asymptomatic or only very mildly symptomatic kids, however, are less sanguine about professionals' reluctance to interpret available genetic, medical, or epidemiological evidence and apply it to their newborn-screen diagnosed child. It may not be possible to make precise predictions, sure—but providers' refusal to even speculatively place Bethany or Jim or Tyler somewhere on the well-documented CF spectrum seems disproportionate to the degree of the providers' uncertainty. Other motivations must be behind such watertight circumspection, some parents conclude—and a number offered explanations for what these might be.

One hypothesis articulated by a number of parents is that doctors avoid optimistic predictions about how mild a child's case might be out of a desire to assure strict adherence to the prophylactic regime, combined with a desire to avoid raising parents' expectations too high. "I feel like they don't want to get your hopes up, even if that is essentially what the evidence is suggesting to them," says one father. Selena, who describes her two diagnosed children as "so healthy," puts the issue even more explicitly. Her CF doctor agrees that the kids are in excellent shape, she says, and "he is glad, but he is always afraid that we are maybe going to fall behind, maybe get comfortable where we are and then something is going to go wrong." Selena's sense of the CF clinic's approach is that they are "just trying to cover all their bases at this point," both to make certain she remains vigilant about Jana and Derek's care and to avoid her being "unpleasantly surprised" if symptoms appear.

Another reason for professionals' caution might be the reluctance of experts to acknowledge that they don't have all the relevant answers. Manny worries about this phenomenon as it influences newborn screening in general. "One thing I think that doctors do have trouble with and all experts have trouble with," he says, "is admitting that they don't know. And I think [newborn screening] is a good case of that." Anne is also concerned that doctors will simply avoid questions with which they're not comfortable rather than answering them as best they can. CF is "such a difficult disease because every person's different, so you never know with your child on the whole spectrum of, Are they doing good, are they not doing good? And the doctors don't . . . want to tell you exactly how well they think [your child is doing]. . . . They won't ever say. . . . I mean, they always tell me, 'James is doing great.' And you try and say, 'Well, do you think he has a mild case? Do you think he has a severe case?' They won't [answer]—they dodge that question."

A third reason parents offer for their health care providers' over-caution is the ubiquitous preoccupation with malpractice issues—a concern that in turn can cause parents to "worry about the nature of society . . . having the influence on a medical establishment" with the result that doctors become "afraid to say to you some kids are okay." Ron is one of the parents who see this as a significant issue. When he took his newborn to the CF clinic, the staff there mentioned that just recently a sixty-seven-year-old man had come in for services for the very first time after a full, healthy life with no CF diagnosis. This got Ron thinking: "Okay, maybe there is a lot of this out there, people who have been living normal lives, just because they didn't know." His health care providers had themselves remarked on the major influx of new patients they had experienced now that infants were being identified via newborn screening. Ron notes: "Of course they couldn't say that there were different severities, because it was new to them, . . . but I think they were on the same page with what I was saying." In other words, the providers seemed to tacitly agree with Ron's assertion that perhaps a proportion of NBS-diagnosed infants would be like the sixty-seven-year-old, but "without actually saying it." Why would they hesitate to be more explicit? "Well, I understand how medicine works," says Ron. "I have some family in the medical field, you know, [and] with the whole legal realm today, you have to watch what you say." It's better, safer, for them to be conservative than to be optimistic "and then be completely wrong."

"You Have To Be an Advocate for Your Child": Diverse Pathways to Parental Empowerment

Parents who have lived with and cared for their CF-diagnosed child over a significant period of time understand that they are not only the child's central caregivers but also her best advocates. They need their health care providers, but experience has taught them that, "as a parent, you have to coordinate everything," and that "you have to be a good medical consumer; . . . you have to be an advocate for your child because [the doctors] don't know it all." Parents learn that "in the bureaucratic health care system of changing shifts, multiple personnel, and inconsistent caregivers, the parents are the child's constant protectors" (Taner-Leff and Walizer 1992, 152). Parents have different styles of advocacy. They develop many different ways of working with, relying on, and using health care professionals. But all find over time that it is not only the professional "they" who are keeping the child as healthy as possible, but also the parental "we."

Learning to "Question Things": From Early Diagnosis to Advocacy

For parents who get an early diagnosis, the diagnostic process may be the first sustained contact with health care professionals they experience outside of routine preventive care. "Never having been in the situation," as one mother asks, who could possibly be "comfortable with pushing a doctor, who is someone who's supposed to be knowledgeable in their field?" Only expanded parental confidence, hard-won through experience and experimentation, can change the dynamic and lead parents to conclude that indispensable as professionals may be, "sometimes they don't know everything."

For parents who are just learning their way around the health care system, the sheer number and diversity of providers is bewildering. It takes a while to sort out who does what—who does primary care, for example, and who provides which specialty services related to CF.[5] As Nancy put it: "I didn't know what my rights were as a parent or a patient. Like, can we switch doctors?

I didn't know anything; I had never been through anything like this. I mean, I was unfamiliar with doctors in general. . . . I didn't know anything about the medical field." These parents' crash course, their on-the-job-training in advocacy, thus starts at the time of the diagnosis, when they have little prior knowledge to draw on.

Joan felt completely reliant on professionals at the beginning. "When [our daughter] was diagnosed, . . . we were just so blind going into it," she says. "But the more we lived it every day, the more experience we got, and now we tell the doctors, 'No, we don't agree with that, we think you should do it this way.' So we are more vocal and more advocates for our children, because we know our children and we believe that we are part of the CF team, and their doctors are pretty much in agreement with that [now] too."

Like Joan, Betty—whose daughter had meconium ileus when she was diagnosed shortly after birth—learned as she went. "In the beginning, everything that any doctor ever had to say was gospel. You took that to be the truth, you took that to be the absolute answer. That it was correct, everything and anything that they said, you agreed with. You did not question, that's just the way it was. It took a long time . . . to get an education within myself . . . that I needed to question some of the stuff that was going on with Rose. That I needed to make sure that I was the one who knew everything; everyone else didn't know everything about Rose. . . . *I* needed to advocate for Rose."

With experience, Betty did come to know "everything about Rose," and she certainly no longer takes anyone else's word as gospel when it comes to coordinating, overseeing, and managing Rose's care. "Now I'm not above calling and telling anyone what I think about them or their assessment of my child. And I try to do so as respectfully as possible, but when I obviously disagree with someone, I'm certainly not going to hide it. And if I think that they're not listening to me, I don't stop. . . . I'm not afraid to ask for what I think Rose needs, and I think that I have certainly evolved in that respect."

Leslie also began with much more reliance on her providers and grew to be assertive, to make her own judgments and speak up about them, over time.

I think, you know, we're probably more—we take more care of John's health [than we did in the beginning]. . . . We're more proactive. . . . If something doesn't sound right or if we know there's something that's not quite right with him, we'll push for it and say, "This is the way it's going to be." I mean, we try to play nice but if there's something that we just aren't in agreement with we'll speak up. . . . [If] there's something that's not quite right we'll push a little more. . . . You know, most people, their doctor tells 'em something and they don't question it, and I guess we—we'll question things more.

In some instances, parental advocacy requires not only getting professionals to attend to the child's CF in particular ways or questioning medical opinion but also, at times, giving a higher priority to healthy family life than to elements of the medical orthodoxy. As Cassandra put it:

[My feeling of control] is a lot better; now I feel like when we go if they say something like they don't feel he is gaining enough weight, at first I really took that kind of stuff to heart, and now it is like, Hey, I can only feed him when he is hungry, I can only feed him as much as he is going to eat, it is not my fault. . . . They kept preaching to me that this all had to be done, and I said it is going to get done when it gets done; I am not going to make mealtime a crying affair for everybody. . . . They said you need to work harder, they kept saying you are not steadfast enough [in] your desire in having him eat solids. I said I can't make him open his mouth, we will do the best we can.

For Sally, the food issue was also significant, not just because (as Cassandra discovered) the reality of feeding a young child is radically different from what the CF team envisions, but also because Stephan's overall health seemed ill-served by strict admonitions to deliver calories at any cost.

I think the hardest thing for us is the doctors say feed him a high-fat/high-calorie diet—but that's not nutritious either. And it's hard when a kid goes to school and is around other kids, and everything is telling them fruits and vegetables are nutritious, and here the doctor's telling us . . . instead of giving him an apple, give him candy. Well, I can't go against everything I know about nutrition. . . . They're looking at, we need to put weight on this kid right away. But they're not looking at what a good way to do that is. . . . If I can give him healthy things that have vitamins he needs and if he eats more of it, his body doesn't feel bloated so he'll eat more, then that's more productive than just giving him a couple of things of junk and that gets him the calories. . . . So we have to take what they say with a grain of salt and add what we know is right.

For Paul, the process of becoming an advocate had a lot to do with getting educated about CF on his own, taking charge of the research process himself rather than simply trusting that the doctors were already experts. Over time he developed multiple sources of information and ideas instead of relying solely on his daughter Alexandra's doctors, who may have had general medical expertise but didn't share his passion for every detail about the specifics of his daughter's condition. "From the beginning you, of course . . . you're skeptical, but then you put your trust in [the doctors]. Then we [did] our research, and you feel that you get educated well on some things, and when you ask a doctor maybe about that topic . . . and they just kinda brush that off, . . . you maybe have a negative opinion of the fact that they're not keeping up, maybe they don't know what's going on, maybe *you* know [more than they do]. . . . We can never know how much they truly know, and we also have a different vested interest."

"Hooting and Hollering": Experienced Parents and CF

Parents whose child had symptoms before the diagnosis stand in a significantly different position with respect to the advocacy process than do their counterparts just quoted. These parents have already spent a significant amount of time both caring for an ill child and seeking medical assistance. They have cut their teeth as advocates for their child before the diagnosis and thus enter the postdiagnosis landscape ready and able to assert the value of their own experience, interpretations, and beliefs.

Catherine, who received the CF diagnosis when Joseph was nine months old and already symptomatic, asserted her own knowledge of his condition and needs from the outset of her postdiagnosis interactions with professionals. When medical staff told her they planned to hospitalize her baby after witnessing firsthand a symptom she had managed at home for months, she had no difficulty challenging medical authority and insisting that the baby be tested instead on an outpatient basis.

> The one thing I have learned [from the delayed diagnosis] is that I now fight harder for what I want. I don't stand there and let doctors look at me and think, "Oh, she's crying, she's a mess, she's a first-time mom." After his diagnosis . . . we were at [the clinic] and he had some severe reflux; . . . he threw up all over me, like all over my dress, all over, and it just didn't stop, it kept coming and coming. And they thought he had intussusception, which is when your bowel twists inside your body. And they wanted to hospitalize him and I stood there and said, "No way . . . I'll come back tomorrow for any tests you want. . . . I'll come back, but I'm not staying here. He does this all the time; he's been doing it since he was born. . . . I'll be here at five o'clock AM if you want, but

you're not making me stay here." I was just like, "No way, you've got to
be kidding me. I've been complaining about this since birth and now
finally someone's going to take notice and you're going to admit me?
I don't think so." And he didn't have it; he didn't have intussusception,
he just had severe reflux. Which I had known all along.

Another mother articulated her confidence in her superior knowledge of
her child and his needs—gained over time, and radically different from her
earlier reliance on leadership from her health care providers—this way: "You
can't sit back and let them misdiagnose something when you know it's gonna
be wrong. You know when they're telling me to give a cough suppressant to
him and I know it's gonna be wrong, I can't sit there and go, 'Okay.' I have to
tell them, 'No, you can't give this child a cough suppressant. You need to call
his pulmonologist . . . and you get back to me with the correct answer.'"

Erica, the mother who has three children with CF, two of whom were not
diagnosed until ages six and four, also felt empowered as an advocate from the
time of CF diagnosis. She had a lot to learn and found the adjustment very difficult, but she unflinchingly evaluated her providers on their merits, changing
doctors and pushing for specific kinds of treatment as needed. A third mother
asserts that getting the diagnosis later, after symptoms, "makes you realize that
medical professionals are . . . not always right, and they don't always have all
the answers. And probably I should trust in myself a little bit more." It's not
that the new routines of care and the dynamics of the disease aren't overwhelming; they are, even for the seasoned parent. The difference is that these
parents know right away that when it comes to caretaking and really understanding what's happening with the child, "it's more the parents" than the
health care providers. Diagnosis of a genetic disorder may be no less devastating for parents who find out later, but it is certainly less intimidating. The child
has already been in their care for months or years, and they have already established their own competence. Knowing the child has CF changes many things
for them, but it doesn't change their own baseline of parental experience.

For some mothers, having parented one or more children before the child
with CF comes along also provided a baseline for advocacy and assertiveness
during and after the diagnostic process. Lorraine, the mother whose infant
daughter's diagnosis precipitated the diagnosis of a healthy older brother, is a
case in point.

Well, it was very interesting because I was fortunate in that I was a very
well-established nursing mother when my daughter was born and I was
very comfortable with nursing and I knew I had enough milk output

because my son had done so well. So I pretty much immediately sensed that something [else] was going on [when my daughter failed to thrive]. We were regularly seeing a pediatrician and, you know, I brought her in and he would look concerned but it's really interesting because the immediate thought was there was something wrong with my nursing or my milk rather than something going awry with her digestion. And even in fact my doctor asked us to stop nursing and feed her formula, which for most nursing women would have been the end of their milk production. But I knew enough to and had enough confidence to continue pumping and freezing the milk that I had pumped for basically ten days. She didn't do as well; she lost more weight on the formula than she did on the breast milk. And you know then there were all kinds of theories that my milk didn't have enough fat in it, or that we perhaps weren't actually feeding her. There's all kinds of things that get thrown around in that kind of situation. But we persisted and in the end a friend of mine who's a pediatrician said to me you've gotta get a second opinion.

Cassandra too was an able advocate by the time newborn Jana was diagnosed, but in her case it was experience with an undiagnosed yet symptomatic older child that had seasoned her. "I blame myself for not yelling enough to get the answers I want," she says, speaking about her toddler son whose CF was identified only after his asymptomatic baby sister's positive newborn screen. "I blame myself for that; it could have been caught sooner—when he had been sick I should have hoot and hollered and carried on." She realizes that she didn't do so with Derek because she didn't "know any better" yet, and so "pretty much just listen[ed] to the doctors" without question when they told her he just had asthma. With Jana, diagnosed by newborn screening, things are entirely different. "Boy, I did a 360 turnaround when Jana was born, and I hoot, I holler, I scream, and I yell for the answer I want or I don't leave the office. I say when they hear my name, either the doctors or the hospital, they pretty much cringe."

As care for genetically diagnosed children progresses, many complex factors play into the balance between professional and parental expertise. One factor is the timing of the diagnosis. Is the child not yet born? A newborn? An older child? An eldest child? A younger sibling? Another is the health of the child. At the time of the diagnosis, is she asymptomatic, or has she already been showing signs of the disease? If she is symptomatic, has she been very ill or just bothered by one or two minor problems of uncertain origin? How long has she had symptoms? A third factor is how involved and knowledgeable parents are with respect to the diagnostic process. Did they already know something might be wrong and agree that testing was needed to find out what, or was the screen a surprise to them, a message (from the professional world) that they may not know what dangers lurk for their newborn? Although more research is needed to tease these multiple strands apart authoritatively, parents I spoke to appeared more reliant on professional authority during the period after diagnosis if that diagnosis was made early, and/or for a first child, and/or without their knowledge or consent. They described themselves as less reliant on providers in the post-testing period if their child was older at the time of diagnosis, and/or if the child was a younger sibling, and/or if the diagnosis was the answer to an empirical question about the child's health that the parent herself had raised.

That parents with a later diagnosis were more comfortable acting as advocates for their children from the start of their CF saga by no means implies that these parents had a qualitatively better diagnostic experience. In fact, most of them illustrate in detail how painful the diagnostic odyssey can be. Parents described to me—their rage and frustration still vivid at having been belittled and disbelieved while their child's health suffered—how infuriating it was to have their fears dismissed by professionals, to be told that they were hysterical, uptight, inappropriately "worried about every little thing." Other researchers have concluded that later diagnosis causes significant parental anxiety; increases the chances that parents will consult a lawyer regarding health care concerns; and leads to "a growing sense of fear that their child's deteriorating health [is] the result of their own incompetence" (Boland and Thompson 1990, 1243; CDC 2004; Clayton 1992a; Waisbren et al. 2003). My research certainly corroborates the finding that late diagnosis causes substantial distress, but the interviews I conducted also suggest another aspect of these distressing experiences with health professionals. Looking back at the period before the CF diagnosis, parents with a later diagnosis for a symptomatic child felt a combination of outrage at how they had been treated by professionals, and regret that they had not asserted themselves more effectively on behalf of their child. As Annie put it:

> I am angry about [the delayed diagnosis] to this day, like in my, in myself, that nobody would listen to me. Doing all these things to him, [other tests and treatments] that were totally unnecessary. I mean, I've carried that anger inside of me for a long time because I was like, I knew from the day he was born. You know how frustrating that is? So flipping frustrating. Because I knew from the day he was born and for seven years, and I was intimidated by doctors, you know, and it was like, okay the doctor said no [to testing for CF], so we're not gonna do it. . . . That

day when we found out, I called his pediatrician and I went off on him on the telephone. . . . I had him on that phone for about an hour and a half. I called him every name in the book, and I said, "You know you didn't listen to me. I told you. Mother's instinct knows."

Other mothers also describe how demeaning and infuriating it was to be dismissed and pathologized by the very professionals to whom they were looking for help.

My sister is the head nurse at a hospital and she had gotten us an appointment with this very supposedly renowned pulmonologist. And he examined us and we felt like we were being blown off. [He] jammed a letter in her file and . . . I was reading it through, which I like to do. I was reading the letter and it said: "Doctor observed child, parents are hypochondriacs." As in, it's all the parents, there's nothing wrong with the child. I just remember reading that and, you know, it's something. [Later, my sister] said to him: "You know, you were quick to judge and tell them that they were hypochondriacs. . . . Well, let me tell you something, thanks to you they have two other children [with CF]."

I'd been trying to tell them so long that there's something else [besides what was already diagnosed] that is wrong. And . . . I'm not just a paranoid mom, a first-time mom, you know, it felt like that was the way I was treated, especially with my oldest one. . . . That I'm overreactive, and not to worry, and that kind of thing.

At the doctor's office I . . . would cry every time because he wasn't gaining [weight]. I think they kind of looked at me like this hysterical first-time mother, and the doctor whom I kept going to see kept saying, "Oh, he'll kick in, some babies take a while to kick in." . . . That was really hard, being so powerless. . . . Like if I had to do it over again I would stand on my head in the doctor's office until they did a test. Even if I didn't know what it was called. I'd be like, "You have to do something. I cannot bring this child in here anymore." Like I would have ranted, I would have raved. I would have done something or changed doctors.

I think there were notes all over our chart that we were just overly worried. [The doctor] was convinced it was all reflux and all reflux-related. . . . I had actually found a site where a mom had said you should get your child tested for cystic fibrosis if they have smelly, abnormal diapers, which I thought he did. But again, we had shown them to the doctor at times when we were in the office, and she said they were

normal. But they didn't seem normal to me, because I didn't know any
other parents who said that their infants had smelly diapers before starting solid food. . . . We had been in and out of our doctor's office three
times a week with congestion and kept being told it was normal baby
congestion and it just didn't seem right to us.

In some cases, the confidence and advocacy skills parents have developed
by the time of diagnosis were forged in the course of earlier traumas with
medical professionals. Yes, these parents have already learned to be advocates,
but some of them have done so under the worst of circumstances, motivated
by their child's poor health and their own poor treatment at the hands of
professionals.

It would be preposterous to suggest that empowerment by this damaging
route is preferable to the route taken by parents with an NBS diagnosis—the route
of ceding substantial control to providers, and then gradually struggling for reem-
powerment. But the point here is not to compare the diagnostic odyssey of later
diagnosis with the empowerment odyssey of NBS diagnosis to determine which
is the lesser of two evils. Rather, what seems to me useful about the two kinds of
parental narratives just explored has more to do with what they have in common
than with how they differ. Each demonstrates the problematic nature of power
dynamics between parents and professionals as diagnoses are negotiated and
produced. In both scenarios, the experience of parents is marginalized as a guide
for action once a medical definition of the situation has become dominant—
whether a definition of genetic abnormality in the child (NBS), or one of hysteria
and incompetence in the mother (later diagnosis). In one case, it is the mother's
observation of manifest illness that is devalued and pathologized in the absence
of any scientific verification of real disease. In the other, a system of uniform testing is used in a way that can devalue parents' nascent knowledge and authority
by standardizing care regimens for genetically diagnosed children—regardless of
the true genotype/phenotype correlation for that specific child; regardless of
whether prescribed care routines can plausibly work within the larger household structure; and regardless of whether establishment of complex prophylactic treatments or recommended care routines constitute an emergency priority
in the first few tender weeks of life. Once the child's genotype is revealed,
parental knowledge recedes, replaced with a medically prescribed regimen of
watching, vigilance, and preventive care.

The dangers and costs of delayed diagnosis are significant, as the mothers
I quoted demonstrate. They are also comparatively well documented (see, e.g.,
CDC 2004; Southern 2004; Waisbren et al. 2003). But the impact of mandatory

screening of newborns on parents' sense of competence, and on their relation-ship to professional knowledge, is also significant, and is much less documented. As Dorothy Nelkin and Laurence Tancredi write in their book on the dangers of diagnostics, "testing can transform doctor-patient relationships." In the case of newborn screening, one effect—at least in the beginning—is more reliance by parents on professionals. Nelkin and Tancredi's conclusion that increased focus on diagnostics means "medical professionals are relying more on test results than on the symptoms of the individual" also appears to hold for many families with newborn-screen diagnoses. Identification of CF sets off an imme-diate sequence of care practices and early interventions that are overwhelming to parents, who leave the clinic wondering, as Joan did, how they can possibly "do all this stuff in one day." And yet just as there are standardized procedures for giving the newborn-screen result in each state, there are in most states stan-dardized processes for handling a newly diagnosed infant and getting the baby "into care," whether she is symptomatic and in need of immediate intervention or not. Nelkin and Tancredi observed, with respect to diagnostic testing gener-ally, that "the more physicians rely on tests, the less involved they become with the patient as a person, and the more they distance themselves from the person, the less they are able to assess the implications of professional advice for the life of the individual involved" (Nelkin and Tancredi 1994, 66). I next examine parents' experience with this phenomenon as it unfolds, and is challenged, in the complex system of follow-up services for children with a newborn-screening diagnosis of CF.

Parenting "Up to Code": Professionals Define the Standards

Knowledge of the CF genotype increases parental vigilance and leads parents—particularly those with an early diagnosis—to focus extensive energy on prevent-ing illness in their diagnosed child, as I have shown. Of course the drive to keep the child healthy comes from the parents, from their fierce love, protectiveness, and determination to hold CF at bay. But the tools and strategies for accom-plishing this come to parents largely from the world of professionals. And the same is true, to an appreciable extent, of the standards used to measure the success of their efforts.

The expertise that many parents of sick children acquire on the job, as it were, is awe inspiring. Parents whose children are actively struggling with CF are able to pick up on symptoms immediately and take action. As one mother put it: "I am a firm believer [in] 'Listen to those parents because they know their child better than you do.'" Parents know when the child needs to be seen by a professional, and when it's okay to keep the child at home. They suggest to providers what medications should be tried and adjust levels themselves when necessary. At times, as Andrea describes here, they seem to have a miraculous sixth sense:

> With Bobby, right before he comes down with the respiratory infection, when he was younger his breath would smell sweet, almost syrupy. Now it smells musty. When I smell that, I start right away with the expectorant and I'll call his nurse and say, "Right, I'm adding a couple more albuterol treatments for the next few days because he's starting to smell like he's coming down with an infection." When I first told her that, . . . he was about eighteen months old. I took him in for one of his regular visits and she said, "How's he doing?" I said, "His breath smells sweet, he's coming down with an infection." And she just—she was taken aback by that. I don't know how many other parents recognize that as a symptom. But I can recognize that now.

Many parents exult in their acquired expertise, and a few even playfully lord it over their health care providers. Erica, for example, sometimes likes to "test the doctors." "That's always interesting," she says. "Find out what they would prescribe, . . . you know, would it provide coverage against this or that? And they [the doctors] look at you." Other parents talk with pride about the providers' acknowledgment of their skills. "I have a good enough rapport with my pediatrician," describes one mother. "He says, . . . 'What do you think, you know [your son] better than I do.'" Another mother's doctor told her she "could probably diagnose a child before he could."

These anecdotes illustrate that on one level, power relations between professionals and parents have fluidity. Providers begin with a stacked deck: diagnosticians and treatment specialists have power over parents because of the authority afforded them by their professional status; because they have formal training and codified knowledge that most parents lack; because it is their role to "see [families] as having problems and needing to be fixed" (Conrad and Schneider 1992; Crane 2000, 3; Litt 2000). Yet the messy, difficult, rewarding work of nurturing sick children day by day brings parents an expertise all their own, and sometimes a good deal of decision-making power along with it. A few parents described their relationship with providers now, a long while after diagnosis, as a joint venture on behalf of the child, a satisfying collaboration that's an impressively far cry from the "you guys are the doctors" stance they had at the beginning. As Meredith puts it: "I feel very fortunate to have that outstanding of a team working with me. . . . And I have to say that . . . you really have to work as a team, because, you know, the feedback they get from us and that we get from them is so vital to [my son's] success."

Many parents also learn over time to rely less on the doctors and more on one another, tapping into sources of parental expertise outside the medical context altogether. Despite the infection-control imperatives that impede parents whose children have CF from seeing much of one another in person, many have found ways of connecting with each other via the Internet. Listservs and online support groups were described by a number of mothers in my study as important sources of information and emotional sustenance. Here, parents share tips, experiences, worries, joys, and strategies for coping with medical practitioners. Lorraine notes that she got accurate information about CF in the postdiagnosis period only "when I went to an Internet Web page that hooked me up to other parents." Anne felt the same way, noting wryly that "doctors, they only know how to treat people. They don't know what it's like to actually live with [CF] day to day." Paige says that "get[ting] on an Internet support group" was one of her main "way[s] of fighting the disease."

But with respect to the all-important issue of medical care in clinical settings, the sharing of power between parents and professionals goes only so far. Despite the ingenuity, courage, and aplomb of parents who take charge of their child's care, and who exert their advocacy and their agency in the face of medical authority, structural incongruities remain and were highlighted by parents in several ways.

One issue is that parents continue to perceive professionals as retaining substantial authority to assess how well their children are doing—and how well parents are doing at keeping their children well. Even after time has passed, and all concerned may have come to agree that both parties need to be "part of the CF team," often the balance of power is still weighted toward the professionals. In the language of many parents' accounts lurks an assumption that professionals' expertise gives them the right to mete out praise rather than themselves having to earn it. Some parents talk about how much they trust or distrust their health care providers, but many also talk about how much their providers trust them, about how they have earned the confidence of the professional team. "I am the one who tells them every little thing that goes on," says Kim. And then, laughing a little at the irony but not objecting outright to its implication of who's really in charge, who gets to judge whom, she adds: "They [the doctors and nurses] have told me *they feel safe* that Sarah is with me. I guess that's good for me. The nurse is . . . very confident in my care because I give them so many details" (emphasis added).

Suzanne too is pleased that over time the doctors have come to have confidence in her, that "when Quinn's been sick, *they'll trust me*" to make certain decisions, "you know, *trust you* that you know what's wrong with him and that I live with him to know how he is" (emphasis added). She goes on: "Once you've been in the system for a while . . . they sort of learn to trust you and to know that you're gonna do the right thing by your child. . . . I mean I guess they've had kids where the parents haven't treated their children and what not. But when they know that you do, and that you look after them in the right way, they respect [you] for doing that too, I think."

As this quotation reveals, once the child has a diagnosis of CF, parents' caretaking practices are evaluated against specific standards set by medical and public health professionals. Some of these accord with what anyone would consider humane: taking a child to the hospital in an emergency; administering medicines that alleviate suffering; not intentionally exposing a child to things known to make her sick. But the line between excessive social control and the simple protection of children's rights has never been easy to draw (Donzelot 1997; Katz 1986; Parton 1994). With state-mandated diagnosis of CF at birth, and the concomitant immersion of parents in a world of preventive treatment regimes that may not always be calibrated to accommodate variation in the disease's expression—and that indeed that can be structured one way in state X and another way in state Y—there may be good reason to ask questions about the impact on families of professional expectations regarding the right way to care for these children.

Consider Francesca's experience with the professionals at her CF specialty center in the months and years after the newborn-screening diagnosis for baby Tess. On the first day she brought her (asymptomatic) newborn in to the center, Francesca—like all the parents in my study—was assigned a social worker as part of her treatment team. This is routine, and though Francesca was not looking to any kind of mental health professional for emotional support, she did not object to the intervention per se. "I guess the first time I could understand," she says, "'cause they didn't know where we were going with it, or how we were doing." But the visit with the social worker remains a standard part of every clinic appointment. Now that she's an established mother with substantial experience, Francesca feels second-guessed and criticized both by the social worker's very presence and by her "rude and opinionated" manner.

> To me as a parent . . . I'm not asking for somebody's advice in that area. I'm not, you know, seeking that out. And you can see my child's growing healthy, she's doing fine. I'm coming in for all these routine visits and everything. And I—I've really taken her care into consideration, it's kind of almost like I feel insulted that they're there. . . . She comes in

and she tells you, this is what you're doing, this is what you should do, if you're not doing this you need to do this by next [time]. . . . I mean, I do everything for Tess. I would give my own life if I could to make her CF go away. There's probably a need for parents, you know, that maybe don't get it, or aren't taking as good care, but I've never once missed a clinic. I've never once denied tests for Tess. I always do the best for her. I probably take her in more than I have to sometimes, 'cause I'm paranoid. And then yet the social worker's telling me that it's just maybe not quite good enough yet, . . . You're not doing it this way, so maybe you should try this or that. Or like she'll talk to me all the time about my parenting skills, with treating [Tess's little brother] Gus equally and stuff. [But] he's not lacking in any means. I mean he's developmentally up to code, you know, from a physician's standpoint. He's right on track with kids his age. . . . I don't just neglect Gus and take care of Tess, which is how she kind of makes me feel sometimes.

Francesca holds everything together, working unbelievably hard to take care of both her children. Sometimes the unwanted intervention of the social worker is just too much. Yet she doesn't know if it's possible to say she doesn't want this person's services, or to switch to a different worker. The social worker may be an inevitable part of the package. "We're frustrated," Francesca says. "This is hard enough as a mom to deal with being a parent of a child with cystic fibrosis but then now I have somebody telling me how to parent . . . and step[ping] on my feet. Like I said, I can completely understand if one of my kids wasn't meeting health guidelines or developmentally they just didn't seem to be as sharp as they should be. But my kids are both, you know, tested and go to the dentist and . . . I mean the stuff that she's concerned about we're doing, so it's like why can't you get off my back a little bit?"

Francesca's objections have partly to do with the inappropriate judgments of a professional with poor skills: it is infuriating to be found wanting by some-one who has no idea what the real situation is. Further, for her it is insulting that the social worker is there at all, because it implies that Francesca's parenting needs to be monitored. A number of other parents raised similar issues about social workers and counselors, noting that they resent the presence of these professionals, or—more commonly—that they simply don't need their help. But social workers are by no means the only professionals who make parents feel inappropriately assessed and found wanting, as Sally makes clear:

I start thinking about [being monitored] . . . when the pulmonologist starts giving me the third degree and the riot act about [our son's], you know, weight gain, but we do everything we can, and we try to make sure he eats a good amount of food and healthy and I don't think they should complain too much because we've kept him healthy. He isn't sick like a lot of kids, even a lot of kids who don't have the disease are sicker than him. I think that speaks volumes to the good work that we do as far as keeping him healthy. They don't always say enough, "You managed to make it through a season without an infection." I think a lot of times they tend to look for something negative to say instead of something positive.

To the extent, then, that early diagnosis of CF results in a new kind of governmental and professional intrusion into general parenting styles and psychosocial issues, parents may have a particular bone to pick.[6] Put in sociological terms, they don't want to be subject to paternalistic forms of professional dominance that presume the ignorance or incapacity of the patient, who in this case is not the diagnosed child but the parent herself.

But in my interviews it was not the existence of prescribed rules for parenting that I heard parents objecting to, for the most part: it was the generic, indiscriminate application of systems to monitor and judge compliance with those rules. Suzanne believes that it takes the doctors a while to trust that parents will do the right thing because some parents don't "treat their children" according to medical prescription. Francesca acknowledges that not all parents come faithfully to every clinic, proceed with every test, keep their children "up to code." Sally thinks the pulmonologist has no right to complain—not because her parenting practices are none of his business, but because he's failing to give her adequate credit for how healthy she has kept her son. It is difficult for these parents to feel sympathy with those who don't follow these rules, since they have come to define their own participation in prescribed methods of preventive care, monitoring, and ongoing testing—albeit with perhaps a bit of improvisation around the edges—as the central way they can physically protect their child in the face of the diagnosis. This is a large part of how parents enact their love in the medicalized system set in play by newborn screening; as parents, who among us would not do the same? Despite parents' fervent wishes, they can't make their child's CF go away, even were they to give up their own lives. So they do what the medical system has taught them to do since their child was born. They follow the advice of the day—the professionals' rules—as closely as they can. They go to every clinic, show up for every test, administer every pulmonary treatment (even on Christmas), and hope for the best.

The tacit acceptance of professional codes for parental conduct after an early diagnosis—and indeed the imperative to get an immediate diagnosis in the first place—has its dangers. Screening for CF (and other conditions) at birth is mandatory, and follow-up testing will be overseen by child protective services if necessary. Then—whether the child is symptomatic or not, and whether available medical care is widely accepted as effective in mitigating the disease or not—treatment regimes will be prescribed, with parents again accountable not just for showing up, but for making sure children "meet health guidelines."

Mandatory diagnosis of CF at birth, and the subsequent prescribed regime of clinic visits, follow-up tests, and preventive practices, have created a new code for parents to follow. A new set of expectations, discourses, and regulations now govern the parenting process in these families. That parents accept the code, embrace it even, is not surprising: it is very difficult to do otherwise once the abnormal screening result is reported and its corollary sequence of events ensues. But the automatic testing of infants at birth does more than save the babies. It also provides what researchers of other aspects of the "new public health" call new "norms by which individuals are monitored and classified, and against which individuals may be measured" (Petersen and Lupton 1996, 12). This result may be an unintended consequence of NBS policy. Nonetheless, it is a reality, and one that will exert influence over a growing number of families as testing rapidly expands for CF and other conditions with late onset and/or poor genotype/phenotype correlations.

Becoming a Sorcerer's Apprentice: Warding Off the Unseen

Parents of children who tested positive for CF via newborn screening but are still asymptomatic are the lucky ones in terms of the most important factor: their children's health. But they may also struggle most in their relationships with professionals and have the most difficulty developing confidence in their own ability to manage their child's CF—if ever it were to become manifest— "up to code."

Parents accumulate their impressive knowledge about CF as they encounter symptoms and learn to cope with them, and they develop their advocacy skills as they assert this expertise in health care settings. When the child doesn't have symptoms, parents, ironically, may rely even more on experts than do parents of symptomatic children. Since CF remains a dreaded mystery for most families with asymptomatic children—that other shoe surely just about to drop—where but to the professionals can they turn for reassurance, early identification of incipient problems, and preventive treatments of all kinds? In Paula's words: "[Our daughter's] baseline cough is nothing. She doesn't have one. We're pretty hypervigilant. If she coughs over the span of four hours, we call. So I think we still rely on [the professionals] just because we don't—I don't even know if we know what [CF] looks like yet. . . . That's the harder part—we'll freak out when she gets a cold even though it just could be a kid's cold. We don't know how to differentiate yet."

Sometimes—as I suggested earlier in this chapter—parents do begin to question medical orthodoxy about preventive treatment. However, the promise of healthier outcomes with earlier detection of CF is so compelling that parents' critiques never evolve, never can afford to evolve, into a substantial departure from what has been prescribed. Doubts, criticisms, or resistance to established norms arise for some parents, but always they give way to the conclusion that altering the recommended system of care would just invite trouble—and trouble of any kind for one's child is just too risky, too heartbreaking, to contemplate.

Selena's situation is illustrative. Two of her three children have been diagnosed with CF (the youngest after a positive newborn-screen result, and then an older sibling during follow-up family testing), but both seem healthy. For years, she has implemented prescribed prophylactic routines with precision. She worked closely with her children's CF doctor, even though, as she puts it: "I don't know how I feel about him, he is not very personable, he talks a lot of medical jargon and I am not the smartest duck but I am not the dumbest duck either, so I have trouble sometimes following what he says. I have to ask him to repeat himself and sometimes he seems annoyed with that." Just a few months prior to our interview, though, Selena and her husband had a disturbing experience at the clinic that threatened to turn everything upside down. During one of their visits, the pulmonologist and a medical student who had been working with Selena's family remarked to each other in the exam room that her children are "positive, with no sign of disease." Selena and her husband "look[ed] at each other like, So they don't have CF? . . . Basically to us when he said that, [it] meant they didn't have the disease, that is how we took it. I was like, What have I wasted the last two years for? Am I hurting them by making them take albuterol and all that if they are not really sick? Then I had a hundred million questions when [the doctor] came back in. We questioned him; he goes, 'No, no, that meant positive for CF, but no sign of lung disease.'"

Since the children have both been pancreatically sufficient and also don't have any lung involvement, Selena and her husband tried to probe what it actually means to be "positive for CF." The doctor's response was to reiterate that the sweat test indicated positive status, and thus to "assure us 100 percent" that both have the disease and that all the preventive care is necessary. In the face of such a declaration of diagnostic certainty, and its accompanying assertion about the value of early detection, Selena could not in the end allow her line of questioning about prophylactic routines to result in any change in care, attitude, or expectation. "I said, 'If we take them off and they get sick, I am going to feel awful. Everything is working out the way it is, we should just leave it the way it is.'" She wishes the doctor had taken her concerns about the reality of the disease and potential harms associated with prophylaxis more seriously instead of seeming to laugh about them. Ultimately, however, taking on personal responsibility for risking her children's good health is not a viable option. As Selena sums it up, the doctor "swears they have it . . . and we are just preventing anything from coming up, is pretty much what they keep saying—preventive, preventive, preventive."

These families of asymptomatic children—like their counterparts whose kids manifest illness—have entered a world of intensified vigilance. They have been "urged to turn the medical gaze" upon their children, and to "engage in such technologies . . . as monitoring . . . bodies and health states and taking preventive action in accordance with medical and public health directives" (Lupton 2000, 57). The doctors' report of a genetic abnormality, a lurking disease, leaves parents permanently watchful and unsure—deferring to the knowledge of professionals and then coming over time, despite their doubts, to take their child's continued lack of symptoms as evidence that doing so is the wisest course.

Chapter 5

A House on Fire

How Private Experiences Ignite Public Voices

Newborn screening is clearly changing the lives of parents and children in significant, complex ways. In the public domain, however, these complicated aspects of NBS are rarely discussed or considered. Instead, the relationships parents have with NBS are represented as exquisitely simple, and their attitudes about it are summarized as unambiguously enthusiastic. When questions about the impact of screening are raised at all, it is primarily academic clinicians, social scientists, and bioethicists who articulate them. But commentators, advocates, policymakers, and the media usually depict parents as having uniformly positive experiences with NBS, and negative ones in its absence. Parents are also represented as "almost unanimous" in their enthusiasm for "rapid expansion of newborn screening" (President's Council on Bioethics 2008, 62).[1]

This chapter departs from the preceding three by moving away from a strict focus on the qualitative dimensions of newborn screening and exploring instead why there has been so little space available, in either public consciousness or policy debates, to "take on board" more complex understandings of how NBS touches people's lives (Frank 2006b, 424). Specifically, I examine how a subset of vocal advocates—many of them parents of children with genetic disorders— have shaped a powerful, univocal discourse around NBS that I call the "urgency narrative." This chapter draws on a set of intensive interviews with program administrators in forty-eight of the fifty states (home to 99 percent of the U.S. population), a comprehensive content analysis of NBS media coverage, and additional insights from the parents I interviewed.[2]

Because parent advocates have played a significant role in shaping the public discourse around screening, I spend considerable time here discussing their initiatives. Most often, these are parents whose children have died or become disabled because of a treatable disorder that went undetected. The pain they have endured is enormous beyond quantification or comparison. Their tireless advocacy to spare others such suffering is testament both to their gigantic heart, and to their formidable ingenuity, tenacity, and dedication. Without question many current beneficiaries of NBS are in the debt of these parents, and of parents who had successful screening experiences and then dedicated their energy to the advocacy cause.

The discussion that follows here is in no way intended to diminish either the pain or the good hard work of these parents. Rather, it is offered with the hope that a more careful parsing of the complex issues surrounding the new NBS will help us all better understand the implications of how public discourse about NBS is shaped and reshaped, thereby facilitating more robust and more democratic parental participation in the policy process—an aspiration I explore more fully in chapter 6. I believe this is a goal all advocates must ultimately share, just as they must share a perpetual struggle for influence, legitimation, and voice in a system which structurally disadvantages them (Hoffman 2006; Jewkes and Murcott 1998; Tomes 2006; White 2000). It is also a goal that I think suitably honors the lives of children, both living and deceased.

When a Part Comes to Stand for the Whole

NBS affects every parent, since the very fact of screening exerts an influence—however subtle—over the context of birth and the newborn period. As the new NBS continues to grow and screening shifts more fully away from its original focus, the stakes for every parent will continue to rise. The subset of people who receive news of an abnormal result includes families whose baby was completely false positive, as well as those whose child becomes identified via NBS as a carrier of a genetic disorder. It also includes those for whom abnormal test results do not directly correspond to an identifiable disorder; those who get a diagnosis that has no clinical manifestations; those who get a diagnosis for a condition that has little or no demonstrably effective treatment. And of course it includes the subset of families for whom NBS was originally intended: those whose child has an early-onset, serious condition that can be effectively treated with prompt and accurate diagnosis.

This last group has long been the predominant face—and voice—of parents in debate and decision making about NBS in the United States. Certainly parent advocates are not the only drivers of NBS expansion: other critical factors include the "technological imperative"; interstate competition; the presence of private laboratories; the work of organized advocacy groups; fear of legal vulnerability; and championing by clinicians and other medical experts (Grob, forthcoming).[3] Here, however, because my intent is to examine public representations of parental perspectives on newborn screening, I focus on the influence—both direct and indirect—of parent advocates.

Consumer/community participation in the construction of public discourse and public policy about newborn screening has been dominated by the emotional appeals of parents who hold that their child was, or could have been, saved by the addition of one more condition to the newborn-screening panel. The efficacy of this approach is undeniable: as March of Dimes president Jennifer Howse documents, and as her organization knows from its own work mobilizing parent advocates, "the personal tragedies that families experience as a result of inadequate NBS have often been a key element in winning legislative support for improved screening" (Howse, Weiss, and Green 2006, 282). What's even more striking, perhaps, is that parents' advocacy efforts—both as individuals, and as leaders in formal advocacy organizations—are not limited to demands for inclusion of "their" disease in their state's panel. Instead, they have often argued for the most inclusive possible screening programs, and for policy shifts (as well as normative shifts) that open the door to mandatory screening for conditions that have no proven treatment, that have later onset, or that have ambiguous implications for the child's actual health. At the same time, parents themselves have been strategically enlisted—and their personal stories of tragedy suffered or averted have been extended and leveraged—to support a broad policy platform for expansion that is vigorously championed by other stakeholders, including the media, elected officials, public health professionals, researchers, clinicians, and private laboratories.

Refracted through the lenses of life-or-death drama and parental grief, complex social issues associated with the new NBS are presented and understood in specific ways—ways that can result in simplistic assumptions about how screening can change people's lives. The powerful "saving babies" discourse has impeded rather than facilitated public conversations about what seem to me a series of critical distinctions in the NBS landscape. Among these are the difference between expansion of screening for specific conditions and expansion of screening in general; between screening that can save lives now and screening that can identify people who might benefit from some future treatment; between screening that can reliably result in improved health and screening for conditions that either do not yet have efficacious treatment or have questionable prognostic certainty; between the experiences and preferences of parents whose children have serious genetic disorders and those of all parents.

"Fighter Moms" and "Zealots":
Screaming for Expanded Screening

Over the past thirty years, parent advocates have taken action on a number of health issues affecting their children, pushing hard for research, services, funding, and public attention. Historically, these advocates have produced impressive results through a combination of persistence, effective technique, and searing emotion. For example, in New York City in the early 1980s, parents built coalitions with community and housing groups, children's rights groups, health workers, and others to bring attention to the issue of lead paint poisoning. They successfully used the media and litigation to enforce the housing code, get their children screened, and allocate more resources for lead-poisoning control (Freudenberg and Golub 1987). More recently, parent advocates have been instrumental in increasing services and public education programs for children with fetal alcohol syndrome in Washington State (DeVries and Waller 1997) and in using litigation and public pressure to change public policy for intensive early behavioral intervention for children with autism (Mulick and Butter 2002). Parent advocates also fueled the search for answers about what causes sudden infant death syndrome, and eventually succeeded in obtaining millions of dollars in federal funding for research and in establishing SIDS as a recognized—rather than suspected—cause of death (Hackett 2007).

Parent advocates for newborn screening today—like their predecessors and their contemporaries who have worked for other health-related causes—use both heart-wrenching personal narratives and an array of advocacy techniques to accomplish their goals. As one advocate described it in a presentation to genetic counseling students at Sarah Lawrence College in May 2007: "Anguish is why [an early NBS advocacy organization] began raising awareness among parents, the medical profession and the general public. Because our volunteers were very outspoken, they sometimes described their advocacy work as 'newborn screaming.'" Others talk about themselves as "zealots" (Rubin 2006), or as "fighter moms" who become instant activists and experts because it's therapeutic and makes them feel that they're "working on something, and something is happening" even if they can't directly find a cure (Wynne 2006).

Parent advocacy for NBS is also distinctive in several ways. First, it is driven almost entirely by parents of children with serious, manifest genetic disorders, but its primary policy target is new diagnostic processes, rather than more usual targets such as calling for expanded research, supporting improved services, or creating a support network.[4] Second, the group on whose behalf parents are advocating is the entire population of newborns, all of whose members are theoretically at risk for rare but deadly genetic disorders, and all of whom must therefore be screened no matter how healthy they might appear. Thus, the policy actions of parents with respect to NBS expansion, unlike those of other parent advocates, are aimed primarily not at improving the lives of already-identified patients like their own children but rather at conceptualizing *all* infants as potential patients and making certain that accurate, comprehensive, efficiently implemented testing is conducted so that those with hidden disorders can be identified.[5]

This population-based focus might seem unusual for parent advocacy. As one advocate herself noted: "The advocate's measure of success, to 'make a difference to that *one*,' is almost opposite to that of public health, which measures success by making changes that can be implemented for populations of people" (De Mars Cody 2009, 91). Yet the political logic of this strategy is compelling, for several reasons. First, because NBS screens for rare conditions, the number of infants diagnosed remains small, even when combined across conditions: roughly 6,500 "true positives" annually in the United States estimated for 2006 (CDC 2008). To avoid having the issue dismissed by policymakers and the public as irrelevant, advocates skillfully frame it in terms of risk, and thus as a concern for all parents. Second, describing NBS as affecting all parents also aligns it perfectly with the discourse of the "new public health," which focuses more and more on "analyzing the inner workings of the asymptomatic body" so as to identify and circumvent disease before it is manifest (Lupton 1995, 2001; Nelkin 1996; Nelkin and Tancredi 1994; Petersen and Lupton 1996). Finally, emphasizing that all children are at risk resonates with the contemporary parenting paradigm that gives primacy to risk reduction and to the avoidance— at almost any cost—of potential injury or illness to one's children (Gill 2007; Marano 2008).

NBS advocacy also stands out because it has skillfully avoided much of the competition among groups that has historically characterized disease-targeted advocacy (Armstrong, Carpenter, and Hojnacki 2006; Bazell 1998). In this case, the nature of the MS/MS diagnostic technology created particular incentives and opportunities for parent advocates to work together across disease-specific lines. Because MS/MS makes possible relatively inexpensive testing for tens of disorders all using the same heel blood spot, it (like the DNA-chip technology predicted to supersede it before long) can be regarded as a shared resource across many rare-disease categories. Rather than competing for funding and attention, then, as can often occur in the world of advocacy (Dresser 1999), NBS advocates have endorsed "comprehensive" as well as "universal" screening— that is, implementation of a broad panel of other screening tests in addition to the one that motivated each of them to action in the first place.

The Urgency Narrative

The primary public narrative that has driven parental advocacy for expanded newborn screening—including advocacy for the 2008 federal legislation called the "Save Babies through Screening Act"—has been powerful and straightforward: simple, inexpensive tests at birth save babies. "I want the state to prevent kids from being brain damaged and dying," says one mother, succinctly stating the message of NBS parent advocates and advocacy organizations across the board. "Kids are dying out there. . . . It's about time [the state expanded its panel]" (Somerson 2000). Giving the story its negative iteration, other parents are equally persuasive. "It breaks my heart," says one, "when I hear of a child who died because it happened to have been born in a state run by people who didn't believe its life was worth $20" (Dougherty 2000). Or, in another version of a bereaved parent's heart-wrenching plea to avert further tragedy: "It makes you bitter. . . . They told us if they caught it at birth, there were two procedures that could have been done to save his life, a cord blood transfusion or a bone marrow transplant. And Missouri doesn't have that law yet?" (Taylor 2009).

The message parent advocates deliver—and thus that parents in general are often understood to deliver—has been expertly honed to that streamlined ten-second sound-bite so influential in public discourse. "Imagine your child never realizing their dreams, disabled or dying just because your state doesn't screen your child for more diseases," says one public service announcement developed by advocates. "Newborn screening can change that. Every child, every time, everywhere."[6]

The shifting NBS paradigm and the rapid expansion of panels to include conditions that are not treatable or not well understood, or for which a positive screen may have ambiguous implications, means that an increasing proportion of tests on NBS panels neither save the lives of screened babies nor even improve them in any evident way. A significant number of the fifty-four conditions on the ACMG-recommended panel have no known treatment, or treatment that is likely to benefit only a subset of those identified with a potentially relevant mutation, as mentioned earlier (Baily and Murray 2008; Moyer et al. 2008). Indeed, Jeffrey Botkin, a leading expert on newborn screening, claims that only PKU and perhaps five other conditions on the ACMG-recommended panel have "treatments that are known to work" (Botkin quoted in Kolata 2005)—though the meaning of "work" in this context remains open to debate. Beginning in 2007, some states began adding conditions beyond those recommended by ACMG, such as the highly controversial lysosomal storage diseases (see chapter 1). Expansion of existing pilot testing programs for diseases such as type 1 diabetes and fragile X syndrome (Bailey 2004; Ross 2003), to say nothing of the "radically more expansive approach to genetic screening" (President's Council on Bioethics 2008, 51) many foresee, would further distance newborn screening from its historical legacy of saving lives.

In articulating particular policy recommendations, parent advocates some-times acknowledge that not all screening has immediate lifesaving results. Nonetheless, the message of urgency embedded in the "save babies" narrative—that exhortation to act quickly, through newborn screening, to prevent kids from getting sick and dying—remains a central theme in almost all advocacy, and the dominant one in virtually all public awareness messages. Even when the question is whether states should test for conditions that are not now treat-able, the answer often given—the urgent answer—is, Of course we should save babies' lives. As put by a spokesperson for Save Babies through Screening in a press release entitled "Treatability of Disorders Should Not Be Criterion for Inclusion of Screened Disorders":

> Until we start identifying affected children through screening and giving the doctors an opportunity to intervene early, we won't have treat-ments. . . . In addition, gene defects are quite variable, or can be expressed in different patterns, thus the result is that in any given disorder there is a range of mild to very serious symptoms. Therefore, it can't be said with any certainty that a disorder is 100 percent untreatable. And I have never met a parent that would just let a child die if there was any chance he or she could live a normal, healthy life.[7]

A pamphlet produced by the same organization, entitled "A Simple Test Could Save Your Baby's Life," draws on the urgency narrative to articulate a second important point central to NBS advocacy. Here, the argument is that the tragic experiences of a group of parents whose children had unidentified, treat-able disorders should lead all parents to screen their babies for every detectable disorder. "Almost every family whose child dies or is disabled from a disorder detectable through newborn screening," the pamphlet reads, "and who then learns that their child's death or disability could have been prevented, says, 'If only I had known.' These families urge you to have your baby screened for all detectable disorders."[8]

The Congenital Adrenal Hyperplasia Research Education and Support Foundation (CARES) also moves seamlessly from a focused argument about the need to screen in every state for the emergent and effectively treatable condi-tion congenital adrenal hyperplasia (CAH) to a general endorsement of the broadest possible expansion of NBS. "Because failure to recognize [CAH] at birth has such dire consequences and because treated infants have the potential for a full and productive life," the foundation's website reads, "newborn screening is invaluable." Affected individuals and their families "can truly help fellow sufferers of CAH by getting involved and urging the addition of CAH to newborn screening programs and the importance of comprehensive newborn screening. . . . All children should be screened for all diseases that technology can provide for at this time."[9]

The intent of these advocates is altruistic: to spare others the pain they have suffered. However, use of the urgency narrative to secure universal screening for "all detectable disorders" rather than just for those that are life threatening and treatable obscures the reality: comprehensive NBS leads to positive screen results that change lives but do not necessarily save them. Further, the assumptions embedded in advocacy for comprehensive NBS based on life-and-death experiences with specific NBS tests may prove so faulty as to significantly compromise the advocates' laudable aspiration to help other parents.

The urgency narrative has been used not only to advocate screening for untreatable conditions and for comprehensive NBS, but also to argue for rapidly developing screening tests for additional conditions and then adding these to state panels in order to save lives in the future. Public comments on the ACMG draft report—particularly those that were generated based on a template—are one example of this approach at the national level. The vast majority of those who wrote in urging adoption of the college's recommendations were most passionately interested in expansion for conditions not included on either the primary or the secondary list.[10] The strategy being used here was (as phrased in templates copied by many who wrote) to endorse "the uniform screening panel outlined by the HRSA commissioned ACMG report." At the same time, many of those who wrote told heart-wrenching personal stories about a child who had died, and then emphasized their support for "rapid evaluation and expansion of the screened conditions as new knowledge becomes available" or "development of a procedure for the expansion of core and secondary panels" so as to "give babies and families a chance at life."[11] The urgent argument for adopting a national standard for NBS was thus closely associated from the very beginning with the position that NBS must save lives by continuing to grow, and the associated view (promoted by ACMG and others) that capacity to screen—rather than capacity to treat—must become the benchmark for inclusion.

Ad Hoc Advocates: Just Telling Their Stories?

The urgency narrative's mantra, "Newborn screening saves lives; newborn screening saves lives," has become instantiated in the public domain, and on public record, via several distinct but related advocacy strategies. The first of these, and perhaps the most symbolically powerful, is what I will call here "ad hoc advocacy." Techniques that fall under this umbrella include parents going directly to their state legislators, testifying at state-level hearings about NBS, and pressuring hospitals to make expanded screening panels available directly to parents for a fee through private labs. Ad hoc parent advocates also submit public comment in response to draft reports and policy recommendations; appear at congressional hearings in connection with proposed federal legislation about NBS; and testify before advisory bodies such as the Advisory Committee on Heritable Disorders and Genetic Diseases in Newborns and Children. Not surprisingly, the majority of parents involved in this form of ad hoc advocacy have been those who frame NBS policy deliberations using the urgency narrative.

In some states, ad hoc advocates have had substantial, direct influence over NBS expansion. Over the past decade or so, a number of researchers, journalists, and NBS commentators have noted that parent advocacy has been such an integral, primary component of NBS expansion that the "role of parent advocates in convincing legislators of the importance of NBS reform cannot be [over]estimated" (Howse, Weiss, and Green 2006, 282). A 2001 article in *Science* described a "new grassroots movement . . . raising a ruckus about genetic disease screening—but not for the reasons you might guess. Its leaders want more testing, not less. Specifically, they want every newborn screened for a variety of inherited diseases for which early intervention might prevent disabilities. These activists—many of them parents of affected children—claim that ethicists and public health officials have resisted a new technology that can check thousands of blood samples a day. And health agencies are responding to their campaign" (Marshall 2001, 2272). Another observer states matter-of-factly: "In any particular state, the disorders screened for are directly proportional to the number of proponents for that particular disorder in that . . . state" (Goldberg 2000; see also Clayton 2009a; Paul 2008).

Our survey of state NBS directors provides significant primary data detailing how ad hoc policy advocacy has unfolded in specific states, and how in a number of cases it has relied integrally on the urgency narrative. With the rise in testing capacity made possible by MS/MS and other emerging tools, and the interstate differences created by staggered adoption of new technology, NBS directors described "the whole area of newborn screening" as becoming "much more emotional . . . and dramatic." Plentiful examples of the influence parent advocacy has had were offered by almost a third of the directors we interviewed. One NBS program director described the work of parents with affected children as "absolutely huge and essential for putting the newborn screening

conditions over the top, without a doubt." Another notes that a specific metabolic condition was added in her state because of a parent whose child had
died from the disorder and who was then "very instrumental in getting this
expanded screening bill introduced and . . . ultimately passed." Yet another
describes how NBS expansion that added a number of conditions to the panel
"was really all due to parents" who enlisted a variety of strategies, including
direct work with the media and with legislators.

In most states, expansion of NBS panels is accomplished by amending an
administrative law that governs the state's public health activities—a process
historically initiated and implemented by NBS program staff and (with increasing frequency after the turn of the century) the state's newborn-screening or
genetic services advisory committee. Some of the most powerful parent advocates, however, have taken their story and their plea for action directly to an
influential legislator, bypassing the NBS program and the state's advisory
board. One NBS director, for example, notes that he had never been asked for
any sort of "input on expansion decisions that parents advocated for and acti-
vated the legislature about." Indeed, he was not even asked how much money
should be allocated to initiate screening for a condition not yet screened for
anywhere else in the country—a procedure that his department would oversee
and run. Rather, he would "just be notified that expansion was legislated and
money appropriated."

Another director tells an even more dramatic story, describing in detail
how parental advocacy drove policy in her state, rendering irrelevant the ongoing deliberations about NBS expansion led by program leaders and the newborn-screening advisory committee. "There was a lot of emotion on their part,"
she says of the parent advocates. Also a lot of "anger, and they worked very vigorously on their own." Although the sole existing pathway for adding conditions to the newborn screen in that state had been via a change in administrative
rules, advocates "didn't trust that process, so they went to a legislator, introduced legislation, amended our law, our actual newborn-screening law, to
require us to add these tests." Before the addition of the latest cluster of new,
controversial conditions was written into law, she explained, the NBS program

> kind of went through the gathering information stages where we were
> trying to get together as much information [as possible] to present at these
> legislative committee hearings and tried to utilize the guidances out there,
> the ACMG, and it was basically all dismissed, and it was not even con-
> sidered. . . . They didn't want anyone to hear about that, it was totally
> irrelevant, you know, they just cared about . . . that we were basically

not saving some of these kids. It was very emotional. . . . You don't want to appear to be uncaring, but it was done in a very, you know, emotional way, and they brought these other affected children in for the hearing, and they didn't even really have one of the conditions we'd be testing for, but the perception was that—. . . and they really didn't give it a lot of time to listen to facts, they just really reacted, the committee members, fairly emotionally. So, you know, it was sad for me to see because I felt we were trying to gather as much of the scientific meat as possible and try to show—you know, I'd talked to people at the ACMG and [HRSA], different people, and CDC and tried to just say how we should start on this process . . . and do a pilot. And then, all of a sudden, it kind of took on a life of its own and there was no—. . . there was a lot of anger again and a lot of, it was almost like it was them against us, and that's how it ended up going down, so I think they just felt that we were being resistant and stalling, so that's how it happened.[12]

When celebrities add their voices to a cause, the messages travel far faster and further than those articulated by ordinary citizens (Groopman 2003; Lerner 2006; Smith, Twum, and Gielen 2009). In the case of NBS, former NFL quarterback Jim Kelly has arguably become the country's most visible and effective advocate. Kelly's son, Hunter, suffered and eventually died from Krabbe, a lysosomal storage disease. His parents' belief that Hunter's life might have been saved had he been diagnosed via NBS at birth inspired them to devote much of their lives, as well as their impressive resources, to advocate for expanded NBS. "It's so easy to talk about the wins, whether football games or in business or in any other element of life," said Kelly in a 2008 press release (PR Newswire 2008). "But it's the losses that we learn from—and no loss compares with that of losing a child. That grief is nothing you ever want anyone to go through. That's why newborn screening for 'Every Child, Every Time, Everywhere' is so critical." Kelly's advocacy has been essential to screening expansions or proposed screening expansions in a number of states where he has been active, as well as to passage in 2008 of the federal Newborn Screening Saves Lives Act. In particular, the Kellys and other parent advocates have succeeded in convincing several states to add Krabbe and other lysosomal storage diseases to their panels, despite the highly contested status of research about the efficacy of available experimental treatments and questions about the accuracy of available screening methodologies (Knapp, Kemper, and Perrin 2009; Neergaard 2010). But Jim Kelly's cause is far broader than screening just for the disorder that so tragically shortened his son's life. "Originally, we started out to save the lives of children born with Krabbe and related leukodystrophies," says his organization, Hunter's Hope. "Now our efforts have expanded tremendously: to help save the lives of all children born in America."[13]

Newborn screening's other celebrity proponent to date is actor Scott Baio, along with his wife, Renee. Their baby's newborn screen for the metabolic disorder GA1 came back abnormal and led to follow-up diagnostic procedures that included "an exceedingly painful 7-layer tissue test" and then "the hardest part of all—waiting," Baio said in a 2008 interview. After a period of uncertainty lasting until baby Bailey was ten weeks old, the Baios learned that she is not in fact affected by the disorder, though she may be a carrier. Talking about the trauma of the waiting period, Baio sounds very much like the parents whose experiences I wrote about in chapter 2. "It was the worst time in my life. . . . I don't know how to explain that to you. I don't, other than, every breath that you take, every thought that you have, every moment that you're conscious, it's all you're thinking about. No matter what the conversation is about, what movie you're watching, what you're eating. . . . This disease is the constant thought in your brain. It never leaves you. Ever. You can't breathe."[14]

Bailey is healthy, but the Baios' experience with the false-positive newborn screen alerted them to a range of GA1-related issues, including interstate differences in NBS panels and problems with access to treatment for those who are diagnosed. It also "put everything else in perspective," keeping both parents focused on "what's important" and "thank[ing] God almost every half-hour that [Bailey]'s okay," they said in the same interview. The Baios have since become outspoken advocates for expanded NBS, dedicated—despite the fact that GA1 itself is already screened for in all fifty states—to heightening awareness of NBS issues and to creating, promoting, and facilitating legislation "that will mandate this expanded newborn screening for all fifty states."[15] "The first ten weeks of Bailey's life changed our lives forever," says Renee Baio. "Forever. And we get it. We know we need to be a voice here, and that's what we're trying to do."[16]

In several states, legislators who have a family member afflicted with genetic disease have become outspoken advocates for NBS. As one director notes, tests in her state were often added "through someone in the legislature or someone with a very high visibility that had some influence, . . . often a political-type situation." For example, "when galactosemia was started, there was a legislator that had a grandson with galactosemia. When we added CAH, it was a constituent." Another director says, with humor but also ruefulness, that when trying to argue in favor of expansion, "My joke is, well, we can just hope some legislator's grandchild has it."

Going Professional: Organizational Advocates
Construct a Common Storyline

A second way parents have entered the NBS arena as policy actors is through formal advocacy organizations. These include: (1) parent-driven organizations dedicated solely to expanding NBS (e.g., Save Babies through Screening); (2) parent-driven organizations dedicated to a single disease or a group of diseases, which advocate for expanded NBS, among other things, either through the addition of new screens to state panels or through the development of new screening procedures able to detect additional disorders (e.g., CARES Foundation, FightSMA, Hunter's Hope); and (3) professionally driven organizations that include a focus on newborn screening and utilize parent advocates in their work (e.g., the March of Dimes).

In 2008, a Web-based search and analysis identified roughly six hundred organizations—most of them consumer/parent driven—advocating in the arena of genetic issues under the organizational umbrellas of the Genetic Alliance and the National Organization of Rare Diseases. The same investigation revealed that approximately 27 percent of these six hundred groups include NBS among the issues on which they focus their work. About 7 percent of these, or roughly forty organizations in total, make NBS part of their core mission. In addition, four of the eighteen large, disease-specific advocacy organizations identified in this search—or roughly 22 percent—devote significant attention to, and have multiple mentions of, NBS on their websites. Two of these—the March of Dimes and the Genetic Alliance—have made NBS a central platform in their advocacy campaigns and publicity activities.

Advocacy groups have exerted powerful influence over NBS discourse and policy since NBS's inception in the 1960s (Howse, Weiss, and Green 2006; Paul 2008; Watson 2006). But in the era of MS/MS, the capacity of these groups to push effectively for expansion has arguably reached a new apex. In part, this reflects the fact that many health advocacy organizations have gained traction as they have multiplied and "grown larger, better-funded, and more professional" (Paul 2008, 12), as well as more directly involved in scientific and clinical research (Bazell 1998; Epstein 1995). One trio of commentators documents this trend with respect to what they refer to as "genetic activists," tracing the way "advocacy awareness" is "virtually built into relationships between US scientists, clinicians, and what we might call their genetic constituencies." The advocacy landscape has thus shifted, they continue, in significant ways. "Successful health-advocacy groups may well have begun as 'mom and pop' operations around the kitchen table of a family with a sick child, but if they are to succeed, they eventually 'go national' and 'go professional' as well.

This 'corporatization' of grass-roots voluntary associations represents not merely assimilation into early twenty-first-century capitalist culture, but also a strategic intervention, a move to gain access to resources" (Heath, Rapp, and Taussig 2004, 161).

NBS advocacy groups, both large and small, have been central in the effort to expand NBS in the United States, and in many instances their work has been profoundly shaped by the experiences, convictions, and passion of parent leaders who have transferred their focus from ad hoc to organized advocacy and become leaders of formal organizations. These groups also lean heavily on the urgency narrative, and on the power of individual stories to remind policymakers and the public alike that screening is about "*saving lives*," not about "statistics, politics and government budgets."[17] Most groups also use pictures and videos of healthy, disabled, or deceased children to great effect—on their websites, in social media interventions, and in the form of public service announcements. "The major goal and highest priority" of one such organization, as stated on the Web, "is that through media awareness, every newborn in every state will be tested for every possible disease—saving the lives of thousands of children through the newborn screening program" (PR Newswire 2008). During the period of public comment on the ACMG's seminal 2005 report, eleven advocacy groups wrote in vigorous support of the draft standards. Some of the arguments they advanced were relatively straightforward pleas to adopt the recommendations because of their power to "help *Save Babies* and Families throughout this country," as the Family Support Group for Fatty Oxidation Disorders pled.[18] Others made deft use of the opening provided by the ACMG's own work to extend claims about the necessity to expand NBS screening even when it is not of direct benefit to the individual child, as I indicate later in this chapter.

Once the report was released, key advocacy groups quickly endorsed it, supporting the expansion of state panels to include all fifty-four conditions recommended by ACMG, and additional disorders as technology for screening becomes available. The report's emphasis on screening for twenty-five untreatable disorders, in addition to the twenty-nine it labeled treatable, directly contradicted some advocacy organizations' stated policy of supporting an NBS screen only when there is strong evidence that it is of direct benefit to the child, but I could find no documentation suggesting that any advocacy organization therefore recommended against identifying and reporting the "secondary" group of twenty-five. A case in point is the powerful March of Dimes (MOD), which rightly claims a good deal of credit for expansion of NBS nationwide (Howse, Weiss, and Green 2006). An MOD press release issued on September 2,

2004, explicitly states: "Our policy is to support screening for specific conditions when there is a documented benefit to the child and there is a reliable test that enables early detection from newborn blood spots or other means" (PR Newswire 2004). Several paragraphs later, however, MOD notes their intention to "urge states to provide test results for an additional twenty-five 'reportable' conditions named in the ACMG report for which there are reliable tests but not yet documented treatments." MOD also acknowledged that NBS is a rapidly changing field, and declared its readiness to update its recommendations for what is considered "comprehensive" testing "as medical evidence mounts."

Between 2004 and 2010, it appears that the MOD remained consistent with the public positions stated in the 2004 press release, supporting expansion to all fifty-four conditions but focusing on the "core" twenty-nine and noting in much of its literature that "various organizations have alternate ways of classifying and counting many of these disorders and may have different number totals for these same conditions." Other advocacy organizations, some of which collaborate with MOD on policy initiatives (e.g., Save Babies through Screening, Hunters Hope), are much more explicit and emphatic about promoting universal screening for all fifty-four conditions on the ACMG report and for any other conditions for which testing is possible. Jim Kelly's advocacy organization, Hunter's Hope, provides a compelling example of how the story of one child's tragic death from Krabbe has driven advocacy for NBS expansion in general. Visitors to the Hunter's Hope website are greeted, on the newborn-screening landing page, by a letter from Hunter's grandmother, who begins by offering the "hope and prayer . . . that what you learn on this site will ignite a passion in your heart, a passion so great that you will not rest until every child born in the United States is screened for the most diseases possible; ensuring every newborn in every state has a fair start at life." She asserts that NBS "could have" saved Hunter's life, and that "each year in the United States thousands of children die and many more thousands become permanently disabled because their parents and doctors did not know they had one of over 55 treatable diseases."[19] The public is urged to join Hunter's Hope in pressing for universal screening for all ACMG conditions as well as for the family of lysosomal storage diseases (five, in total) to which Krabbe belongs. A map of the United States traces which states are at, above or below the recommended fifty-five conditions (the ACMG's fifty-four, plus Krabbe), and a Take Action page highlights current state-specific campaigns for inclusion of lysosomal storage diseases.

The direct impact of advocacy organizations on NBS expansion state by state was evident in our survey of NBS directors. Almost half the states identified these groups as having a role in their policy development process—most notably the MOD (twenty states), but also a range of others such as Save Babies through Screening, Hunter's Hope, and "PKU groups." Many states talked about how advocacy groups brought effective pressure to bear in favor of expansion by establishing "report cards" that publicly measure the size of their state's panel against that of other states and against the ACMG's recommended national standard. In the words of one director:

> Well, as soon as the ACMG came out with their report, March of Dimes immediately . . . said that that was their recommendation too, . . . so our [state] chapter immediately contacted us and wanted to know what we were doing and they wanted to be in the media. They set up a whole media outlet or whatever with the governor when he signed the bill, or when we went live and did the pilot testing, they set up the media coverage. And they have been very instrumental every time—every year they would call us and say, Well, are you putting CF, are you adding biotinidase; I mean, they've always been trying to push forward to be comprehensive.

In some cases, NBS directors who themselves had long worked for NBS expansion indicated that advocacy group campaigns influenced legislators to move quickly ahead in ways the program itself is restricted by law, or by norms, from doing. One director told us that in a meeting about NBS program expansion, health department staff told advocates: " 'The only way we ever get things started in [our state] is through legislation. . . . So if you can identify a legislator that, you know, will write legislation . . . that might be a way to do it.' Well, within two weeks, they had an author, and within a few more weeks, they had a bill, and so that's the way it goes." In other cases, advocacy groups—like the ad hoc advocates discussed earlier—pressured states to implement additional screening that NBS directors believed was not justified by the existing evidence base or supportable with available resources. A number of state NBS administrators referred specifically to MOD in this regard, noting that organizational representatives have "been really trying to push" expansion, coming to meetings and saying, "We don't care how you do it, we just want it on board." Another administrator elaborates more specifically on MOD's role in a controversial expansion of the state panel: "Although they didn't want to go on record, saying they were supporting this [lysosomal storage disease] initiative, they were meeting with the [affected] family, . . . they were having a lot of kind of behind-the-scenes meetings encouraging it and really were meeting with our director's office, pushing it, and that kind of thing. . . . They were doing it mainly in the name of, you know, saving babies, not really looking at the science."

Parents as Policy Advisors: Being Called to Represent

A third, more formalized, form of parents' advocacy is through appointment
to state advisory committees. As of 2008, at least thirty-eight of the fifty states
had newborn-screening or genetic services advisory committees charged with
reviewing newborn-screening program performance and making recommendations with respect to the addition of new conditions to the panel.[20] Inclusion of
parents, consumers, or families affected by NBS has been an important recommended element of these committees (Jennings and Bonnicksen 2009; NBS
Task Force 2000; Therrell 2001), in line with growing acceptance of the idea
that "groups affected by policy have a right to a voice and a place at the policy
table" (Jennings and Bonnicksen 2009, 141). As of 2008, of those states with
committees, thirty-four, or roughly 90 percent, have one or more members
specifically identified as a parent or consumer.

Our survey of state newborn-screening directors suggests that on roughly
half these committees, parent members play a notable role in the committee's
work. In some instances parents serve as co-chairs, and thus are positioned to
shape as well as respond to agendas. In other cases, a sufficient number of parent members participate that one or another of them sits on every subcommittee, or they are the largest single group on the committee and thus when it
comes to voting "they swing it." NBS directors are generally grateful for those
"very vocal and interested and astute members who understood the issues and
were very confident in responding." Often a particular task force charged with
recommending whether the state should expand to include a specific condition
will attract activist parents; for example, a father in one state "was very active
for a while, especially as we were . . . discussing whether we should add IRT
technology for cystic fibrosis." In another state, the parent member is described
as "one of the ones who pushed for" inclusion of CF on the NBS panel. In yet
other instances, parent members use their committee involvement as a launch-
ing pad to move toward professional roles in clinical settings, in care coordina-
tion, or in policy work related to NBS—and they remain involved in the life of
the committee or the NBS program from this new vantage point.

But it is not always easy to get parents to participate in NBS development
and deliberation via committee work that is defined by professionals. Ad hoc
advocates and advocacy groups focused on NBS may be working tirelessly on
strategies of their own devising in some states and at the national level, yet
other states "struggle mightily" to recruit, engage, and retain parent representatives for mandatory advisory committees. "We beat the bushes," said one NBS
director. "We tend to . . . beg the support groups that are interested in what it is
we're working on to consider . . . nominating somebody." Another is equally

direct: "It's not like there are a lot of parents who are available" for a job that is uncompensated, and an additional responsibility on top of caring for a sick child at home. Sometimes even when parents do agree to be appointed, they manage to be only "sporadically involved" or hard to retain in the position. "It's very hard for us to keep our parent slots filled on the committee," sums up one director. "They tend to be intimidated and, you know, poor attendees; . . . many of them have disabled children at home." NBS advisory committees thus suffer many of the same challenges other civic organizations face as they strive to involve unpaid members of the public in formalized processes (Church et al. 2002; Lomas 1997; Putnam 2001; White 2000).[21]

Notably, as of 2008, at least thirty-nine of forty-two parent/consumer representatives (more than 90 percent) on state NBS committees had a child with a phenotypically expressed genetic disorder that either was or could have been screened for on the newborn panel.[22] The parents serving on these committees—like those active in unsolicited, uncodified forms of NBS advocacy—thus all bring to their roles the perspective of people coping with symptomatic children who either were or might have been diagnosed by screening. That those making appointments to advisory committees regard this cohort of parents as the appropriate pool from which to draw consumer members is revealing in several ways. First, it suggests that NBS advisory bodies have adopted the assumption that "citizens affected by genetic disease have a special authenticity to contribute to policy making" (Jennings and Bonnicksen 2009, 143), even when the policy making in question is for mandatory, population-wide screening rather than for interventions (such as treatment protocols) specifically targeted to those with genetic disease. Not a single NBS director mentioned, in the context of parent representation on the advisory committees, the tension between a mandated public health program that involves, on the one hand, the entire universe of newborns, and on the other, the statistically tiny subpopulation of infants with screenable, treatable disorders and clear diagnoses.[23] The ability of particular parents to think about NBS expansion beyond its implications for the specific condition suffered by their own child was of concern in a few states, and several directors spoke about the process of carefully recruiting parents of children with "all different kinds of . . . various different birth defects; . . . all of those groups have had somebody on the council at one time or another." By contrast, in no case did NBS directors raise questions about whether parents motivated by the urgency narrative should be the sole eligible representatives on these committees in the first place.

The preponderance on NBS advisory committees of parents who experience the need for expanded newborn screening as a pressing personal cause can also be explained in part on pragmatic grounds. Appointing parents who take the initiative—who get in touch with the committee and ask to be involved—is the easiest way for committees to fulfill the requirement that consumers be included. Self-selection of this kind is not inhibited by any procedural mechanisms, and most advisory committees are not asked to engage in careful deliberation over issues of representation. Consequently, committees in most states are grateful and relieved when they are contacted by parents eager to serve. In the words of one NBS director: "There's just parents who just are really passionate and motivated for a given disorder class and really want to . . . aid and assist and help out. They typically contact us, and they say, 'Hey, you know what, I want to be involved and engaged.' And we're real happy then [and recommend] for strong consideration for the commissioner to make a decision [to appoint]." Another director describes a similar process, facilitated by an advocacy organization. "When we were first contacted by the Save Babies through Screening Organization," he says, "we sat down and talked to them about what was going on and what we thought needed to be done and then, as an outcome of that, and as we moved along further to when we're forming an advisory committee, certainly they were invited to, and did, sit on that advisory committee."

In some cases, having parent members whose children are affected by a particular disorder does raise questions for NBS directors about the ability of these members to move beyond a focus on their own story and circumstance to a broader consideration of pros and cons associated with program expansion to include multiple new disorders. "I think parents may not know a lot about other disorders as much as they know about the one that affects their child," says one director. "Many times, family members have a hard time thinking beyond their specific situation," notes another. This highlights the tension in NBS committee representation between what Bruce Jennings and Andrea Bonnicksen have called a "trustee" model of representation, which implies reliance on one's own "thinking and judgment about what is in the best interest of constituents," and a "delegate" model, which compels active investigation of and advocacy on behalf of the "opinions, preferences and positions" of constituents (2009, 146).

A minority of NBS directors we surveyed, then, raised questions about how capable individual parents are of representing a larger universe of those whose children suffer from screenable (or potentially screenable) conditions. Even fewer, however, went on to reflect on a second important aspect of the representation issue: what does the committee itself do to promote appropriate inclusiveness of multiple perspectives during deliberations and decision making? More specifically, what is the capacity and willingness of the committee as a whole to bridge gaps in knowledge and experience between parent members and professional members, and to address the power dynamics that inevitably exist when groups of people with various kinds of technical expertise strive to incorporate a "consumer" perspective (Hoffman et al. 2011; Jewkes and Murcott 1998; Morone 1990; White 2000)?

Our interview results suggest that explicit approaches to addressing issues of representation that have been developed elsewhere in health policy (Brown et al. 2006; Minkler and Wallerstein 2008) have not gained much traction in the arena of newborn-screening advisory committees. It is indisputable that in many domains "setting up processes for lay participation in research and policy settings is increasingly becoming part of the occupational and professional responsibilities of public health officials and researchers" (Wilcox 2011, 26). But as of 2009, for most NBS programs, the issue of this kind of inclusive practice (or its absence) just didn't register. Only one state described an intentional strategy for revising its procedures because "it seemed that some of the group were sort of just nodding and deferring totally to the medical opinion and not considering some of the other stuff." When NBS expansion was next being considered, this state's solution to this problem was to first conduct a technical review of the evidence with medical experts alone, and then convene "broader, more representative groups" to consider whether each condition met the expansion criteria that had been set.

In several other states—particularly those with strong, cutting-edge NBS programs and a lot of in-state substantive expertise—problems of inclusion were identified, but there seemed to be no sense of obligation to address them. In these instances, NBS is regarded largely as a technical problem legitimately approachable only by experts. "We get parents to come to one or two meetings," says one director,

> and then they don't show up anymore, and in a way I don't blame them, because, you know, our meetings are very technical . . . and the parents plain don't understand, . . . so I think they sort of bail out because they have to commit essentially almost a full day, if they're traveling at all, because our meetings are typically four hours long, so . . . you've shot a whole day, and to come and . . . listen to us and walk away feeling that, you know, I don't have anything to offer; . . . you can see why they don't show up. . . . If you try to bring in a . . . farmer, you know, because his child has PKU, they have no idea—talking about tandem mass spectrometry and this guy knows how to plow fields, . . . they have trouble comprehending, What the heck you talking about?

Given that on most committees there do not appear to be specific norms guiding committee participation, not to mention orientation or training designed to cultivate particular models of representation, it is difficult to imagine that parent members of committees otherwise made up entirely of professionals could possibly do otherwise than draw primarily on their own experiences and those of other parents in their support networks. And parents who might have views about or experiences of the new NBS that are different from those of parents with affected children are not yet represented on these committees at all.

From Voice to Chorus

Ad hoc, advocacy group, and advisory board forms of advocacy are distinguishable, and an accurate understanding of the NBS landscape requires appreciation of the approximate size, shape, and influence of each. But an equally important feature of the topography is that these categories are overlapping, with permeable boundaries, so that the activities of parents in each category have synergistic effects on the others. This synergy is perhaps most evident in the professionalization processes that lead many advocates from ad hoc strategies to participation in or leadership of formal organizations.

The transition from lay person to organizational representative is a salient feature of advocacy in general, as exemplified by high-profile lay-people-turned-leaders such as Fran Visco of the National Breast Cancer Coalition or Sharon Terry of the Genetic Alliance. In the arena of NBS, the nearly flawless harmonization of individual parent voices with the instruments of organized pro-NBS advocacy—conducted and amplified by the media, policymakers, industry, and others—tend to make it difficult for anyone singing a different tune to be heard.[24] The blended chorus can also make it difficult for various audiences to distinguish who is really at the table when policy deliberations occur. For example, state NBS directors in our survey often responded to questions about parent involvement in their state's NBS expansion with answers about the involvement of advocacy organizations. The majority of the 117 comments submitted by parents on the draft ACMG report (59 percent of the 199 comments submitted) were clearly developed based on a template provided by advocacy groups.[25] In public discourse, politicians may refer to vocal advocates such as Jim Kelly and Jill Levy-Fisch at times in their parental roles and at other times in their organizational roles. Finally, the MOD itself seems to credit equally "the sustained efforts of consumers and voluntary health organizations" for their role in NBS expansion, and documents how its own organizational strategies rely heavily on mobilizing "volunteer families" on a state-by-state basis (Howse, Weiss, and Green 2006, 280, 283).

The mutually reinforcing influence of diverse advocacy strategies is certainly not unique to newborn screening. As the twenty-first century rounds the corner of its first decade, there is much truth in the assertion that "decisions about public health are not based primarily on a feasibility study or cost-benefit analysis, but are increasingly influenced by the voices of advocates" (De Mars Cody 2009, 101). Yet the dynamics surrounding NBS advocacy and deployment of the urgency narrative involve many actors and serve many interests. Once they are loosed in the public domain, parents' stories of their children, dead or saved, no longer belong only to them. Rather, they are appropriated for social, economic, political, and policy purposes not necessarily envisioned or endorsed by the parents themselves, either individually or en masse.

Specific examples of parents' stories being used by others for political purposes were not hard to come by in our state survey. Private laboratories, for example, have "trotted out" families as a tactic for pressing states to contract with them for immediate service rather than waiting for the state or regional laboratory to gear up for expanded screening. "I heard horror stories from other states that they [the labs] were picking on a family," says one NBS director. "Or they found a family that had a child that was affected with a disorder that was not being screened for in that state, and they were parading that child in front of the legislature of that state, saying, If we had been there, this child would not be in this wheelchair, this child would not be mentally deficient, this child would, you know, not have all these physical . . . problems, so we knew it was coming, and we just tried to stay one step ahead of them in [our state]."

State NBS directors themselves, or members of state advisory committees, also sometimes strategically enlist parents and parents' stories when pushing for program expansion. Vignettes may be retold by professionals in committee meetings or deliberations, but asking parents known to the program to come and provide firsthand testimony creates the biggest impact (as illustrated in the NBS horror stories recounted earlier). "We had one very vocal member of our advisory committee," recounts one director when describing what factors led to program expansion in her state. This physician member "follows a lot of kids, okay, and . . . he lined up five families with a variety of those metabolic conditions who came and spoke directly to our advisory committee at one of their meetings." The testimony provided by these five families was instrumental in pushing the state to add a number of new conditions. In a second state, the hospital association had voiced objections to NBS expansion because of costs that would be passed on to their member institutions as a result. Before the public hearing about proposed changes, however, the association "representative was lobbied rather heavily, and was told in advance that there [would] be emotional testimony . . . and that if he wanted to stand up in opposition, he'd have to do it right after parents—the tale about their poor dead baby." Fear of "look[ing] like the Grinch" was such a strong disincentive that the association decided not to testify after all. In yet another state, the NBS director notes that nobody spoke out against screening expansion because "it's not a, you know, really good political move to be opposed to screening for an infant." Families new to the world of genetic disorders can also themselves be moved by the stories and strategies of other parents, becoming "quite likely to add their support to groups calling both for universal screening and for increased funding of research to find a cure" (President's Council on Bioethics 2008, 64).

Framing Issues in the Public Domain:
Media Representations and Parents' Voices

The link between health advocacy and media coverage has always been a strong one (Ryan 1991; Themba 1999; Wallack et al. 1993), and NBS advocacy is no exception. In several states we surveyed, program administrators talked about the connection explicitly. "We keep track of a lot of the press reports," says one. "Whenever something might get in the press or [a] parents' magazine or something, we're always—well actually, we can feel the push from the . . . press and the parent groups." In another state, NBS staff described how "the media played a big role" in creating interest on the part of parent activists and legislators. And as I show just below, parents' stories about NBS and media coverage of the issue have been firmly interlocked in a mutually reinforcing cycle across the United States.

Particularly since 2005, as parent NBS advocates have gained increasing traction and visibility in a variety of public arenas, NBS has captured increasing amounts of media attention. In this period, NBS has decisively entered what has been dubbed the "issue attention cycle" created by three mutually reinforcing phenomena: media focus, policymaker response, and public awareness. These cycles follow a consistent pattern: events that had previously been portrayed in the media as poignant individual anecdotes are linked together by a catalyzing event. This event triggers an exponential increase in media coverage, which in turn validates comments by political figures and calls for immediate action to deal with what is characterized as an impending crisis (Downs 1972; Peters and Hogwood 1985).

The intensity of media coverage for NBS fits this pattern, with the ACMG report as one key catalyzing event. Of the 189 newspaper articles on NBS published in major U.S. national, state, and regional papers from 1975 to 2007, fully 55 percent (104 articles) were published in 2006 and 2007. Parents and advocates have a substantial presence in these news stories: parents or advocates are cited as sources of evidence in 50.8 percent of the articles, and they represent almost a third of all the evidence that's cited in all these articles.[26] Parents or advocates are described as drivers of NBS expansion in 28 percent of these articles on newborn screening.[27] A comparison between these 189 media articles and a set of 45 media articles published in the Commonwealth countries during this same time period testifies to the distinctive importance of parental advocacy in the United States. Outside the United States, parents/advocates are used as sources of evidence and cited as policy drivers less than half as frequently—just 14.9 percent and 15.2 percent of the time, respectively.

There is also some powerful evidence of the association between parents and the urgency narrative in the media. We uncovered this association by examining the correlation between parental sources of evidence in a given article and the appearance of the urgency narrative in that same piece. A content analysis of newspaper articles about NBS in the United States between 1970 and 2007 reveals that the more frequently parental anecdotes appear in an article, the more likely that article is to include multiple mentions of NBS's purportedly lifesaving benefits. As table 1 reflects, in pieces with no parental anecdotes, 14 percent have multiple references to lifesaving benefits, whereas in articles with two or more parental anecdotes, 54 percent have multiple references. Similarly, 39 percent of articles without any parental anecdotes portrayed conditions screened through NBS as treatable (presumed so, without presenting any supportive evidence), whereas a full 73 percent of articles that included parental anecdotes implicitly made this assumption.[28]

These newspaper articles also illustrate the persistence of the urgency narrative, despite the increasing distance of NBS programs from the Wilson and Jungner criterion that screening should occur only for conditions with a "well understood natural history." The media continued to portray NBS as lifesaving just as often after the ACMG report as before it. In fact, the proportion of articles

Table 1 **Relationship of Parental Anecdotes in News Articles to Article's Claims for NBS**

Number of parental anecdotes in article	Article's assumptions about NBS	
	Beneficial (%)	Lifesaving (%)
0	38.5	13.9
1	73.2	29.3
2+	73.1	53.9

in which NBS is presumed to be lifesaving remained the same (roughly 32 percent) from 1975 through 2007.

Our media analysis also reflects the movement of parent NBS advocates from ad hoc roles to formal advocacy roles. In the period before 2001, parents' experiences and opinions represented 37.3 percent of all evidence the media cited about NBS; this declines to 19.4 percent from 2001 through 2005, and finally to 15.8 percent from 2006 through 2007. At the same time, advocates are cited as sources of evidence with increasing frequency: from 4.2 percent, to 12.8 percent, and finally to 13.5 percent over these same time periods. Yet while parental sources are cited as evidence less often, there is a concomitant increase in portrayals of both parents and advocates as significant drivers of NBS expansion (from 13.8 percent to 34.2 percent over the same time periods). These simultaneous trends suggest both that parents' effect on the policy process has been increasingly transformed from ad hoc to organized and consolidated avenues of influence, and that narratives recounted directly by parents are quoted less often even while the media's representation of their influence takes on a life of its own.

Spectral Corollaries of the Urgency Narrative

Newborn screening undeniably saves the lives of some infants, and the importance of this reality to those who benefit from it must never be underestimated. However, the claim—whether direct or by implication—that all available screening tests respond to an urgent need, and that all at least point the way to solving an urgent problem, profoundly oversimplifies a range of issues. Commentators with more distance from the urgency narrative agree that these issues must be dealt with if policy is to be made responsibly (see, e.g., Baily and Murray 2008; Botkin et al. 2006; Clayton 1992b; Paul 2008). Further, my qualitative research with parents suggests that the urgency narrative has power to structure parents' NBS experiences even in situations where urgency is questionable—for example, when a child is asymptomatic or only mildly affected—and also that some parents of diagnosed children develop critiques of NBS even as they participate in or comply with its mandates.

To illustrate the complexities inherent in the NBS advocacy process, I examine here various aspects of the argument for expanded screening that borrow lift from the "save babies" narrative. In some instances the urgency narrative's influence permeates more strongly, but in every case its impact is significant—even when the specific argument in question centers around what the ACMG described as "family and community benefit" rather than direct benefit to the screened infant. In this exploration of parents' voices in the public domain,

I again draw from my own interviews with parents of screened babies and from the survey of state NBS administrators that I conducted with Mark Schlesinger.

The Therapeutic Misconception Writ Large

Increasingly, NBS advocates take the position that for all screenable conditions, treatment starts with diagnosis. With respect to conditions (and there are many) with no demonstrated treatment, the argument is that "if we do not ever *try* to save these babies we will never learn *how* to save them" (De Mars Cody 2009, 100), and that no attempt can be made to save them if it is not clear early on—ideally before the onset of symptoms—that they have a genetic disorder. The urgency narrative is thus artfully extended to imply that the research facilitated by at-birth identification of babies with genetic disorders may actually benefit those same babies, and that diagnosis in the newborn period is therefore essential. The term "research," however, is rarely directly employed in NBS advocacy. Instead, the concept of "treatability" is redefined so that effort to treat is the sine qua non, and efficacy of treatment is secondary.

This paradigm shift in advocates' definition of what it means to say something is "treatable" was apparent in comments submitted by advocacy groups and parents in response to the 2005 draft ACMG report, and it has continued to gain currency ever since. As the Genetic Alliance's public comment argued, and many other submissions echoed: "Our community of consumers . . . knows that the medical definition of treatment is more narrow and limited than the one they experience," because "affected families may find treatment essential that is not yet deemed efficacious."[29] These same advocates also directly reject the long-standing Wilson and Jungner principle of screening only for conditions with a "well understood natural history." Instead, they maintain that screening should be universally implemented for conditions in order to understand their natural history. As advocates at Hunter's Hope put it: "We also must highlight our concern over the 'well understood natural history' aspect of the ACMG report as many of the conditions are rare for which there are, and or, will be tests. For conditions like these a well understood natural history would be best achieved with early detection, standardized follow-up and shared data." Clearly, these advocates have deemed it to be in affected children's best interests, "broadly understood, to push their incurable genetic ailments into the column of treatable illnesses, even if no actual treatment is available at the time of their diagnosis," because "an obscure illness for which there is as yet no treatment is more likely to be elucidated and ameliorated or cured if newborn screening gives the medical community an accurate picture of the prevalence of the disorder as well as early access to as many of its sufferers as possible" (President's Council on Bioethics 2008, 60).

Professional advocates articulating their own NBS positions in the professional literature are in some instances explicit about a possible delay in timing between identification of affected children and projected benefit to them or others. Parent advocate De Mars Cody, for example, notes in an essay on NBS advocacy that questions about how treatable or untreatable a condition is "will not be answered unless babies with these conditions are identified and there are potential research participants with whom research treatment protocols may be devised and implemented" (2009, 100). Yet in public discourse and educational material about NBS aimed at families, the heavy emphasis on saving lives remains, even concerning conditions whose treatability is at best uncertain. This brings about an almost guaranteed conflation of possible future benefit for others with immediate benefit to the infant in question. Many advocates whose children are affected by a fatal disease demand "a diagnosis for their child's condition regardless of how proven or unproven the treatment regimens," De Mars Cody notes. However, messages about NBS directed to parents of the "huge number of babies [who] need to be screened" in order to "generate meaningful results on rare conditions" (ibid.)—as well as messages to the public at large—are misleadingly focused on tangible advantages to the infant at hand rather than on the possibility of good for future generations.

The conflation of potential benefit for others with immediate benefit to a research subject is a commonplace one: bioethicists have long pointed to this "therapeutic misconception" as a central concern to be addressed in the protection of human research subjects (Shamoo and Kihn-Maung-Gyi 2002). It is arguable, however, that in the case of mandatory screening for conditions without proven treatment, this misconception is particularly problematic (Moyer et al. 2008). These programs were not created as research protocols at all, but as emergency public health measures, justified as both mandatory and universal precisely on the strength of claims that they serve the state's interest in protecting vulnerable children from death and disability (Botkin 2005, 2009). NBS thus lacks the most basic elements of ethical human-subjects research: education about the protocol, informed consent, and capacity to easily withdraw from participation. As state NBS director Anne Comeau argued in her comment on the draft ACMG report—summarizing concerns voiced by a number of others—confusion about the differences between public health mandates and research protocols is cause for concern at several levels.

I propose that we own up to our national research needs rather than rationalizing decisions to run fishing expeditions. Though we as citizens might be impatient to access services that appear beneficial or that are

beneficial for an as-yet undefined few, we as a nation have yet to determine how the public health service, newborn screening, should be used
to facilitate the generation of data. . . . Nationally, we need to acknowledge
that some of the disorders in the ACMG standardized panel belong in
lists of newborn screening for public health (associated with some abridge-
ment of individual rights) and some belong in lists advertised to citizens
as human subjects research. We need to run our laboratory screening
algorithms in a manner that is true to whether we are screening for
public health or for research.[30]

Why has the new NBS been able to evolve, in most states, without clearly
settling these issues and without adopting broadly accepted standards for ethical research in cases where efficacy of treatment is in question?[31] In substantial
part, I would argue, it is because the potency of the urgency narrative places
NBS in a category of its own. As Jeffrey Botkin was quoted as summarizing:
"In all these cases of newborn screening gone haywire, there is usually some
understandably zealous group of parents of sick kids, patient groups, advocacy
groups saying 'Let's get on with it.' Some ethicists asked for clinical trials,
but these groups said, 'We don't have time to waste'" (Kolata 2005). Survey
responses from state NBS directors in a number of states corroborate that even
when research was not a direct motivator for expansion from the point of view
of the program itself, when new conditions are added they are often touted as
"help[ing to] improve the base of kids that are available for research."[32]

The universal and mandatory nature of NBS distinguishes advocacy for
NBS's expansion for research purposes from advocacy for research on conditions such as HIV/AIDS or breast cancer. Advocacy by affected laypersons in
these latter cases has arguably been as passionate and effective as NBS advocacy. However, these advocates' strategy rests explicitly on the assertion of
patients' autonomy: they argue that terminally ill patients should be able to
take on risks related to experimental procedures at their own discretion. In the
face of fatal disease, HIV/AIDS activists, for example, fought for access to
experimental medications with the "rallying cry, . . . 'We are dying. We will
test the drugs in our bodies'" (Bazell 1998, 114). In that case, what sociologist
Stephen Epstein calls "activist ire" was "directed largely at the FDA, whose
'paternalistic' policies of drug regulation were perceived to rob patients of the
right to assume the risk of an experimental treatment" (1995, 416).

Parents of children with fatal diseases understandably feel a similar des-
peration to obtain any treatment whatsoever, no matter how unproven, for their
sick and dying children. To have done all they could to try and save their child

is essential to them, whether or not the best of what medical science has to offer at the moment is deemed efficacious by scientific standards. But advocating mandatory identification of potential subjects for enrollment in research protocols through population-level screening is very different from gravely ill people advocating for their own right to elect experimental treatment or from parents seeking that right for their own children. The former involves the entire universe of persons screened, rather than, in the latter cases, just the statistically tiny subset of those who would actually participate in the research. Consequently, it is arguably the former group (i.e., parents of all newborns) whose experiences must be understood, and whose approval must be sought, as NBS moves away from its "standard tenet" that only treatable conditions should be screened and toward a model designed in significant part to test preventive interventions (see Alexander and van Dyck 2006; Bailey et al. 2006).

So what is known about parents' perspectives on screening for conditions that have no proven treatment? Not a tremendous amount yet, as far as I can tell. But we do have some information, based on opinion polls, genetic counselors' experience with families, and a small amount of qualitative data (including that presented in this book). And we also know something about how parents' perspectives on these issues have been represented.

Claims that parental attitudes with respect to screening for untreatable conditions are known, and that they are overwhelmingly favorable, have been made not only by NBS advocacy organizations but also in the peer-reviewed literature and by the President's Council on Bioethics. Alexander and van Dyck, for example, asserted in a 2006 *Pediatrics* article: "With the potential of greatly expanded testing and broader understanding of genetic diseases, many have begun to question one standard tenet of newborn screening, i.e., that it is appropriate to screen only for conditions for which an effective treatment already exists" (Alexander and van Dyck, 2006). They then elaborate on this position (for which they offer no citations) in a letter written in response to a critique of their article by a Dr. Wald:

It is the parents who prefer to have a diagnosis early, even for a serious nontreatable disorder, so that they can avoid the long diagnostic odyssey of trying to find an explanation once symptoms begin. It is the parents who want to be able to apply appropriate palliative or ancillary care early rather than late and to have the opportunity to consider enrolling their child in a trial of an experimental therapy before irreversible damage has occurred from disease progression. They are the ones who would like to have information early for family-planning purposes rather than after the birth of a second affected child. They also value having this information early because it allows them to make informed decisions about matters that others may overlook (e.g., the parents would not have bought a 3-story house when their child was 2 years old if they had known at birth that the child had muscular dystrophy that would not become apparent until the age of 3). . . . We urge Dr Wald to talk to parents who have affected children, as we have done, about whether they would have preferred to know even a devastating diagnosis in the newborn period rather than months or years later when symptoms developed. (Alexander and van Dyck 2007, 407)

Alexander and van Dyck draw here on their own knowledge regarding what parents of children with an incurable genetic disorder say they want or would have wanted in the newborn period. They then extrapolate, without acknowledging the potential impact on the larger population of families whose babies are screened, to suggest a mandate for expanding NBS to cover untreatable conditions. They make clear, however, that when they say "parents," they mean "parents with affected children." Not so the President's Council on Bioethics. In their comprehensive 2008 report entitled "The Changing Moral Focus of Newborn Screening," the council quotes Alexander and van Dyck out of context as claiming "an 'almost unanimous preference of parents for knowing the diagnosis in the newborn period'" without the requisite qualification specifying which parents purportedly have such a preference (2008, 62).

The council then offers misleading evidence in support of their claim that "many American parents seem increasingly willing, if not eager, to learn whatever they can about their children's health, including any genetic abnormalities that can be detected at birth" (63). Citing a report summarizing public-opinion survey research conducted in 2007, they note that "fifty-four percent of adults endorsed genetic testing of children even if no effective treatment is available"; the actual finding (published in full in 2009) was just over a third (Tarini et al. 2009, e435). The council's assertion that the subset of parents with affected children "believe that they have a *right to know* whether their child has a genetic disorder, even if it is untreatable, and they believe such knowledge is good" is also misleadingly documented in the report. Citing a 1998 survey, the council reports the finding that 71 percent of parents in this cohort said they would want NBS for a condition for which there is "*sometimes* no treatment" so as to "find out if your next child would have a genetic condition" (President's Council on Bioethics 2008, 63). They neglect to note, however, that only 24 percent of parents indicated support of NBS for a condition represented as entirely untreatable (Wertz and Fletcher 2004, 70). In short, a fair reading of the evidence suggests that though some parents with affected children would want to know about the condition regardless of treatability, even among parents with affected children this does not translate into majority support for mandated NBS of such conditions. And this is a long way from the claim that all parents embrace NBS for untreatable conditions.

Other research (my own included) suggests caution about using survey data of this sort, even when accurately presented, as evidence that "the parents have spoken" in a coherent manner. Conventional attitudinal surveys may be problematic in several ways, especially in light of the still-cogent power of the urgency narrative. One issue involves the documented discrepancy between hypothetical preferences and actual uptake of predictive tests. For example, about three-quarters of surveyed families at known risk for Huntington's disease indicated they would want to be tested for the condition despite the fact that no effective treatment exists (Kessler et al. 1987). However, only about 10 percent or fewer actually come forward to be tested, and of these, a significant number may be using the test to confirm their own suspicion that they are beginning to have symptoms or to confirm their sense that they are free of the gene because they are past the usual age of first onset (Richards 1993). More recent studies outside the United States found predicted uptake for testing between 50 percent and 80 percent, yet the percentage of adults who actually requested testing when approached by testing centers "varied from less than 4 percent in Germany, Austria and Switzerland to 24 percent in the Netherlands" (Tibbena 2007, 165) and 13–15 percent in Victoria, Australia (Tassicker et al. 2009, 66). Similarly, a study of parents who receive CF diagnosis through NBS found that the way parents thought they would use prenatal screening in a subsequent pregnancy and what they actually did when they became pregnant correlated only about half of the time (Sawyer et al. 2006). As Sally Macintyre concludes: "Asking a global hypothetical question about whether people want screening may be neither helpful nor predictive of what people actually do, and . . . what people actually do is extremely context-dependent" (1995, 227).

Another difficulty with the representation of parents as willing participants in NBS regardless of treatability is that parents are prone to presume, even when explicitly told otherwise, that if conditions can be identified through medical technology, technology must also be able to treat those same conditions (Campbell and Ross 2003; Leiberman and Chaiken 1992). In other words, the therapeutic misconception may persist even among those who have been directly informed about lack of treatment because "many parents [are] unwilling to accept that no preventive measures could help" (Campbell and Ross 2003, 211). This is not so surprising. In these contexts, parents are asked to imagine having a child at risk for a life-threatening condition. Which of us would not long, under these circumstances, for the hopeful notion that what medicine is able to detect, it ought also to be able to treat?

Of course, the vast majority of parents are not well informed about newborn screening; in most states, if parents know about NBS at all, they understand it in the context of the urgency narrative that structures virtually all public representations of the program (media coverage, policymakers' pronouncements, public service announcements, and health department brochures). When children are screened for conditions that fall outside the Wilson and Jungner criteria for treatability, or for conditions with broad genotype/phenotype variability, their families most likely have no concept that the program may discover disorders with unpredictable courses, mutations that will never cause symptoms, or diseases without proven treatment. Most families therefore do not even have the opportunity to develop a therapeutic misconception in the context of individual decision making about NBS. This is both because they do not apprehend NBS as including conditions for which identification of potential research subjects is a primary motivation, and because their informed consent for screening is never sought.[33] As Wald summarized in his critique of the Alexander and van Dyck article, being presented with the opportunity to enroll in experimental protocols is "not what most people expect from screening. They expect a personal benefit, not to be a potential candidate for a research study. If screening were to be performed for the latter reason, it should be made clear at the time that screening is offered, and screening should then be restricted to areas in which there is a reasonable expectation that such research will be conducted instead of recommending screening generally" (Wald 2007, 406). The misconception under which families labor, then, is writ large at a generalized social level, where NBS programs continue to be broadly understood as lifesaving and health giving even now that most states have begun testing for at least some conditions for which traditional treatability criteria have not been met.

Not surprisingly, there appears to be no published research exploring the actual (rather than anticipated) experience of NBS for parents with children who were identified through screening as having genetic abnormality, but to whom only experimental treatment, or not even that, could be offered. As noted during a 2009 meeting of the Advisory Committee on Heritable Disorders in Newborns and Children: "Evidence on family functioning in the kids who screened positive but stayed asymptomatic"—a large subgroup of those who may benefit least and be most at risk for harm from NBS—is "relatively uncommon" despite the fact that it would be "very helpful" to know more about the impact of NBS on their "family functioning, beliefs, quality of life, et cetera"

(2009, 32). This is a hard group of people to locate, though as the new NBS continues to roll out it will likely come to represent an increasingly large proportion of the entire screen-positive population.[34] This is also a hard group for social science researchers to gain access to, given the current politics of institutional review boards in the NBS arena (Au 2009).[35]

Genetic counselors are the group most likely to interact with this cohort of parents regularly, since it is often their job to describe the results of diagnostic tests and to interpret their meaning. Counselors whose experiences have been captured in the published literature discuss how challenging ambiguity can be in cases where affixed disease labels do not clearly correspond to any particular form of understood clinical problems or known treatment. In her testimony before the Secretary's Advisory Committee, Michelle Fox from the National Society of Genetic Counselors comments about how difficult it is "to call out newborn screening results . . . when we really don't know what the answer is. We don't know what the prognosis is, and we don't know what the diagnosis means. My metabolic nurse tells me, 'Tell everybody relax, reassure, and retest.' But that's easy to say and hard to do" (Fox 2009, 40).

A study that includes interviews with fourteen genetic counselors reports that though these professionals have a good deal of faith in the overall utility of molecular genetics, they are also "witness to some of the paradoxical challenges of new diagnostic capacity" as applied in NBS and other settings. Genetic counselors understand that the "clinical needs of their patients" are not necessarily met by merely providing molecular details about their disorders, particularly in cases where there is a good deal of uncertainty. As one counselor in this study elaborates: "That's a really difficult concept for people to understand, that if you have the gene, when do you actually have the disease?" And from another, who uses the example of the disorder CMT-1 to illustrate the problems caused by unclear diagnostic information from the perspective of patients:

> At the end of the day, what patients are most concerned about is, "What's going on with me?" and, "How can you help me?" And for a disease that has 15 or 16 sub-types and every form of inheritance pattern, for a patient to get a diagnosis . . . it may not necessarily mean anything besides the fact that, "Oh, each of my kids has a 50 percent chance," and that's it. But besides that, "You can't tell me when I'm going to be affected with CMT, even if you can find the change in my genes or how old my kids are going to be when they're affected with CMT. You can't tell me how severely I'm going to be affected with CMT . . ." And those are the things that are most important, I think, to a patient. (Miller et al. 2005, 2539)

Data from my own research with parents of children whose positive newborn-screen tests did not easily lead to definitive, stable, or useful disease diagnoses, suggest that Comeau's concern, noted earlier, that NBS should "own up to our national research needs rather than rationalizing decisions to run fishing expeditions" is shared by at least some parents most at risk of harm as a result of NBS's research agenda.

One mother whose child's initial CF diagnosis was later rescinded by her doctors notes: "I don't think she'll ever have any health issues with cystic fibrosis" and observes that "therefore it's like, Okay, so the tears and the worrying, what have I gotten for it?" She understands that as NBS proceeds and "data is more pinpointed," the criteria will likely shift and that "five years from now maybe we wouldn't have been marked . . . because they would've then put us below, and we wouldn't be put in the grey area anymore, we would be below." This parent is adamant that genetic counseling and other services must be in place for parents around the NBS experience, yet she remains fairly sanguine about the research agenda of the NBS program. "Look at all those people who would never have been tested who are finding out, who have a much harsher case," she said. "You know, if you're gonna test, there's always gonna be someone on the low end of the spectrum. . . . Somebody's gotta be the guinea pig, and it just happens to be us."

Other parents urge much stronger caution, centered on several distinct but overlapping themes. The first is a conviction that the NBS program's literature must be continuously updated so that it reflects the realities of the actual panel of screens being administered and does not focus so insistently on the urgency-narrative version of treatability that other possible outcomes are omitted entirely.

> Info sheets for the screenings are written in terms of if you turn up something then you need to get treated for it. Not that "sometimes you are in this gray area where you take [the child] in, he keeps showing up with something [on the test] but nobody knows what it is, he doesn't have any other symptoms, we don't really understand why it is that way." . . . I feel that they need to go back and look over their info sheets again as they expand these programs because I think a lot of the assumptions being made in these sheets don't hold true anymore, especially about . . . having treatment for things which affect certain populations in which the sort of biological basis is well understood. It seems that is not the case anymore.

These parents want to be told explicitly where the existing evidence base is strong, and where it is not. They are concerned about the consequences for families of screening for little-understood genetic abnormalities. The same parent says: "They are screening for all types of things and we have absolutely no idea what to do about them, and that is very dangerous, I think. Essentially what you are telling somebody is, We have noted this, we don't really understand it, and we don't know what you can do about it. Good luck with that."

Lived experience of the new NBS has brought these parents to questions akin to those raised by the NBS directors I quote in chapter 1, and to those voiced in the published literature by bioethicists and other professionals. "I think this is the case where the technology has gotten out in front of . . . the ethics, or something like that," says one director we interviewed. "Because they certainly have this way of running these multiple battery of tests all in one screening so they are only taking blood once and they can do all these different things at the same time. I don't think anybody considers kind of the ramifications of doing that."

Scanty though it is, preliminary testimony about a prominent example of new NBS—New York State's pioneering screening program for Krabbe—indicates that the experimental nature of that endeavor has been highly problematic from the point of view of parents whose infants are identified as at highest risk for the fatal, early-onset form of the disease. Of the seven infants in this category, as noted in chapter 1, two have been referred for experimental cord blood transplantation at Duke University: one died shortly after the operation, and the other is reportedly doing fairly well. A physician treating at least one of these families and familiar with Krabbe services overall testified, two years into the new initiative, that "this level of prognostic uncertainty, of how well our clinical risk levels actually work in practice, . . . has made following these children and counseling these families very difficult." For the family with whom he had been working directly, the blurred boundaries between research and treatment were evident and disturbing.

> My understanding of the best information available at the time that I met with this family was that this patient was very likely to have early onset disease. When I met with the family, she was three and a half weeks of age, and I outlined our protocol of investigation and referral to Duke University. She also met with our geneticist, as well as our own center's bone marrow transplant team, as well as the electrophysiology team and the anesthesiologist. The family continues to be followed by me, but they are not followed per protocol. They were very upset at the diagnosis, as you can imagine. It's a heart-wrenching and horrifying diagnosis. Furthermore, the fact that they would go through this very invasive suite

of testing in order to be categorized as possibly being eligible for a treatment that they felt was experimental and highly risky was very offensive to them. They were lost to follow-up for some time because, as they told their pediatrician, they were convinced that they were part of someone's research experiment, and they were uncomfortable in following up with us. Their pediatrician was able to smooth things over to allow them to at least follow up with me. (Advisory Committee on Heritable Disorders 2009, 38)

Krabbe is one current example of parental experiences on the expanding edge of NBS. Though we know little about it as yet, what we do know suggests that issues with the therapeutic misconception may merit substantial public attention as the new NBS continues to unfold.

Rare Genetic Disorders: Foremost Threat to Infants' Health and Well-Being?

Most conditions screened by NBS are extremely rare: they range from approximately one in 1,856 births to as few as one in 384,142 births.[36] However, the drama of the "screening saves lives" story—complete with its showcasing of technological innovation on the one hand and elegantly simple dietary treatments on the other—is so compelling that it can easily claim status as a central plank in the overall campaign to give babies the start in life that they deserve. Political support for NBS-related legislation is skillfully framed by advocates as "an investment in the health and the future of our children" deserving of gratitude to legislators from "families in every community across the country" (States News Service 2008b). Expanded screening for some conditions is good for children, but the public relations benefits it garners are likely to be disproportionate to its actual impact given how rare conditions fitting the original NBS paradigm are. Also, quite often the legislators to whom families ostensibly owe gratitude for NBS-related legislation have a dismal overall track record on other child health issues.

This disproportionately high-profile status for NBS relative to its numerical impact—and relative too to the status accorded other rare diseases (Marcus, forthcoming)—is aided by two factors that combine with technological innovations in NBS to create a perfect storm for elected officials who use NBS as a political calling card more powerful than other programs that might yield more widespread benefits to children. The first of these two factors is a health-care–policy environment disposed to high-tech diagnosis and treatment and indisposed to addressing the social determinants of health (Schlesinger, forthcoming). Here the "NBS saves lives" narrative perfectly bolsters the more general tendency of messages about diagnostic technologies to "exploit [parents'] hope of controlling frightening conditions, [and] of predicting and eradicating risk" (Nelkin 1996, 546). The media further bolsters this tendency by framing stories episodically—that is, in terms of dramatic individual stories rather than of systemic causes or effects.

The second factor is the fierce interstate competition that has undergirded NBS expansion for at least the last decade, leading advocates to chastise or praise the size of their own state's screening panel relative to that of others at every opportunity.[37] An *Atlanta Journal-Constitution* article reflecting these intersecting biases notes: "Mississippi, the state that's perennially at the bottom of health status charts, leads the nation when it comes to sparing children from the ravages of rare genetic diseases." Despite this opening reference to the possible ways Mississippi may not be best positioned in the nation with respect to general health and child health indicators, the article quotes the March of Dimes president as asserting: "If you're a baby born in the United States, Mississippi is your best bet. . . . Georgia has more work to do if it wants to catch up" (Guthrie 2005).

That the infant mortality rate in Mississippi during 2005 was 11.4 per thousand births compared to a national average of just 6.9 (Eckholm 2007) is neatly obscured by the representation of newborn screening as an easily implemented plan for saving lives, and by a history of glaring differences in the number of conditions screened for from state to state. Further, advocates' assertion that "due to disparities in state newborn screening programs, a healthy start and a healthy life is not a guarantee for all newborns" (Urban 2007) is difficult to counter with the statistics and complex proposals for addressing structural underpinnings of health disparities—disparities that have fallen largely on deaf ears for decades. A dead baby on one side of the state border, and a living one on the other—what more compelling evidence of an unacceptable disparity can there be? As Baily and Murray of the Hastings Center for Bioethics point out, when it comes to comparing return on the investment of resources in helping children across child health programs (e.g., asthma management, home visits, prenatal care, newborn screening) rather than within a single program across states (e.g., NBS in Mississippi versus NBS in Georgia), we just "do not know which of these programs would produce the greatest benefits for children—but that ignorance is itself a major problem" (2008, 24). Further, it is difficult to make the complex point that discrepancies in the number of conditions screened for from one state to the next are sometimes less dramatic than they appear because they are in part a byproduct of whether states elect to list conditions singly or to group them.

Many state NBS directors are quite aware of how screening can be used to boost a state's political image. As one respondent from a poor region noted, her state is "last in most all health statuses," but NBS is "one area that we could move to the forefront and be one of the leaders of the country and not one of the lag-behinds." Further, this strategy is a relatively easy win because "it was something that . . . the behavior doesn't have to be altered to do it, such as smoking and obesity and things." Other administrators highlight NBS not as the silver lining in an otherwise less-than-stellar track record in child health, but as an investment with clear opportunity costs. As one interviewee put it, some directors would "rather see every family get a carseat, you know." They believe "there's things that are more important, and . . . I think there are states that would rather spend their money elsewhere than do this but . . . once the federal government gets behind it, you know, and in turn the March of Dimes, . . . you're really out on a limb if you're going against recommendations."

Comprehensive, Universal Screening: The Antidote to "Newborn Roulette"?

NBS advocates have used interstate competition as leverage not only by suggesting that states owe it to newborns to expand screening panels but also by declaring that the failure of all states to test for as many conditions as the state with the broadest panel constitutes a violation of equal rights. As one parent advocate put it: "In one state you can live and lead a normal life, and in another state, you can die or be mentally retarded. . . . It's like newborn roulette" (Miller and Guthrie 2003). This point is emphasized by advocates in media interviews, in official testimony before legislators and national advisory committees, and in public comment on the 2005 ACMG report. "The life of my Stephen," one advocate argued, "should not be so devalued in a society where our constitutional rights are supposed to promise us equality. . . . States are left to their own means and only 18 have decided that children's lives are worth the effort and cost."[38] Another advocate asserts that "Each newborn in the United States should have an equal chance for a healthy, productive life. Not because they live in Illinois, but because they live in the United States of America."[39]

For some advocates, pressuring a particular state to add any given condition under consideration in that state is part of a long-range strategy for gradually assuring that all screenable conditions are added, including whichever one is of greatest personal importance to them.[40] Once any given state panel reaches the upper limit of what available (but ever-changing) technology can produce, the next strategy for some is to pressure other states to expand their panels to at least equal breadth. By linking the argument that comprehensive newborn screening (CNBS) saves babies with the argument that all babies should have equal access to screening, advocates of expansion effectively set the bar for laggard states at the highest possible number of disorders screened for anywhere in the country. The result is a cascade effect whereby inclusion of a new condition in any state immediately triggers pressures for other states to follow suit. An NBS advocacy brochure available online pushes this agenda: "Imagine your child's life cut short or devastated by disability, just because they were born in the wrong state. Universal Newborn Screening seeks to provide necessary newborn testing for every child in every state. All it takes is one heel prick—one test—and together, we can save lives."[41] And in the era of new NBS, "necessary newborn testing" is most often defined as screening for all conditions detectable with current technology.

Equity arguments often have trouble gaining significant traction in the United States. Many health advocates (motivated, like NBS advocates, by the conviction that "each newborn in the United States should have an equal chance for a healthy, productive life") work passionately on such issues as poverty, environmental toxins, and the availability of essential health and social services—but despite their efforts children's access to basic benefits such as the Women, Infants, and Children nutrition program or high-quality public education continue to vary wildly from state to state.[42] Yet in the case of NBS, where a thriving baby on one side of a state border can be contrasted with a disabled or deceased one on the other, efforts to move toward a national norm have been hugely successful (PR Newswire 2009).

State NBS directors have much to say about this issue; more than half of them identify interstate competition as a major driver of expansion, and many elaborate in substantial detail. "We wanted children in our state to have the same benefits and to have opportunities to have the same services [as] in surrounding states," say program directors from one state. "We want . . . an even playing field with other states to the degree possible." Other directors explicitly emphasize real or potential bad publicity relative to other states as a motivator for adding new conditions. During the period of rapid expansion that followed the ACMG report's release, says one respondent:

Newborn screening was very much in the news . . . and [our state] got a lot of bad publicity about being so slow to jump on board. . . . "Stop dragging your feet"—that kind of thing. . . . Like I said, my advisory was not 100 percent behind the ACMG, so I think it was peer pressure, you know, from what other states were doing. . . . We work very closely with our neighboring states and we have very short panels, and everybody else all around us, you know—a baby born in [our state] was being screened for, say, six, or I mean ten, conditions, but if that baby was born one mile south, . . . that baby would have been screened for thirty conditions, you know?

Or from another director, succinctly: "The extreme where [competition] would be influential was . . . 'Mississippi is screening—that makes us look really bad.'"

Some NBS program administrators view interstate competition as a powerful driver not just of the recent past and the present, but also of the future as the new NBS continues to roll out. As one of them put it: "Unfortunately . . . we're no longer looking at our criteria that we used to use in order to select a disorder," because now, "there is a lot of pressure, you know, they shame the states that aren't doing as many disorders or at least the full twenty-nine panel. So . . . it's going to be peer pressure, absolutely. It doesn't matter what the disorder is, whether it's diabetes or fragile X . . . , it's going to be peer pressure."

Interstate competition fueled by advocacy efforts is also a significant influence for states as they cope with how to handle ACMG's so-called secondary conditions. Although some states may still appear to screen for only the twenty-nine core conditions while others screen for all fifty-four on the larger list (or more), there is more variation in what states publicly declare themselves to be screening for than in what they actually screen for. Why? Directors described, and the NBS literature corroborates, at least two reasons. The first has to do with the politics of nomenclature. There is no consensus about how to refer to various conditions, so some states use the name of the analyte deficiency, some the name of the disorder, and some the name of the screening analytes (Sweetman et al. 2006, S309). Further, "counting disorders creates even more confusion, because multiple variations of a disorder sometimes are counted in different ways or are not counted at all" (ibid.). In the colorful words of one state director:

> Right, so there's "lumpers" and there's "splitters," and in [my state], we're lumpers, so we say "hemoglobinopathies," you know. And another state will list out . . . eight different hemoglobinopathies. I get a lot of calls because people look on the website of the National Newborn Screening and Genetics Resource Center and it'll just say how many conditions each state screens for, and I had to give them the lumpers and splitters thing, because they'll say, "Well, we only screen for twenty-nine conditions and they screen for eighty-six," you know. And so, there really is, even if you look, some of those states aren't actually screening for more than the others, it's just a different way of expressing it.

Another reason why there is greater perceived than actual interstate variation has to do with the relationship between following up on identified analytes associated with secondary conditions, and actually declaring that screening is available for the disorders of which these analytes may be indicators. Some states set their MS/MS equipment to detect secondary conditions, and they communicate about all abnormal results to pediatricians, specialists, and parents. However, they decide against publicly announcing some or all of these disorders as part of their panel, for reasons specific to their state's policy deliberations and its criteria for what constitutes appropriate NBS. Such reasons include that the disorders are extremely rare; that they have a little-understood natural history; that they violate state-level criteria specifying that screening be done only for treatable conditions. Maintaining this commitment not to advertise inclusion of conditions that don't fit the state's own screening paradigm can be tough, though, say many NBS directors, when advocates send out "report cards on how states are doing," making it "somewhat of a political issue about, you know, [our state]'s got a screen for one more than [the state next door], to make ourselves look good." Thus, the focus on interstate competition and pressure for all states to announce screening for as many conditions as possible can result, NBS administrators say, in states "bow[ing] to the political environment" and "revis[ing] our literature to include all of the disorders that we can detect both on the core panel and those on the secondary"—even though this may go against the NBS director's own convictions.

Saving Lives by Preventing Births?

There is another strand—a complicating one—in the argument of those who advocate screening for every detectable condition: the claim that screening saves lives in the future by allowing families to "choose to avoid having more children after having a child diagnosed with an untreatable inherited disorder," or at least to make "educated family planning decisions."[43] In this framing, "urgency" does not involve safeguarding an infant who is at risk of a medical crisis if left undiagnosed and untreated. Rather, it's the rush to be sure the diagnosis of an existing child is made before the conception of a subsequent child. This critical distinction, however, is easily lost when buried in the metanarrative of saving lives.

The importance of preventing deaths of children not yet conceived via NBS is most urgently articulated in connection with one particular strand of the new NBS: fatal, early-onset, untreatable diseases. Here the tragedy of losing one child turns seamlessly into a plea to be spared—or at least to have the option to spare oneself—yet more heartbreak. As one NBS advocate put it, in her ACMG public comment:

> Affected children are born anyway, with or without newborn screening. Losing one child is bad. Losing subsequent children is worse. Maximum benefit from newborn screening includes being given knowledge that will lead in most cases to the prevention of a second death. By the time a correct postmortem diagnosis is made, the mother can already be pregnant with a subsequent affected child, and/or a subsequent affected child can already be born. In cases of "no treatment," families still gain maximum benefit from newborn screening in that the families can use family planning options available to them for future children, thus preventing subsequent deaths.[44]

This argument may seem to contradict the exhortation to save babies by testing for these conditions in the first place, but its heartfelt urgency makes it almost irrefutably persuasive; of course the possibility of sparing additional loss to parents who have already suffered tragedy is an unmitigated good. However, here as so often in NBS discourse the urgency narrative threatens to inaccurately imply that the experience of a small number of families in a very particular kind of situation can be generalized to all families that receive screening.

For the vast majority of families, NBS's impact with respect to future pregnancies will not be the opportunity to avoid the future conception or birth of fetuses consigned to death during infancy or early childhood. Rather, as coined in NBS parlance, most families will derive only a more generalized "family benefit": optimal "choices" for "future reproductive planning." Importantly, the timing of NBS means the reproduction-related information it provides can be used to prevent future pregnancies rather than to terminate existing ones, thus circumventing—at least in part—the contentious abortion debates that inevitably mediate the politics of prenatal testing (Rothman 1986). However, that voluntary genetic testing for many NBS-screened conditions is offered to most women during or before pregnancy is rarely, if ever, explicitly addressed in public discourse about NBS and reproductive choice. Despite the fact that not all pregnant women consent to all such tests even in the face of significant pressure to do so (Rapp 2000; Rothman 1986), and despite a lack of definitive research demonstrating strong and consistent public opinion in favor of the new NBS as a mechanism for informing future childbearing (Whitehead, Brown, and Layton 2010, 10–14), reproductive risk information delivered by mandatory newborn screening is often implied—when connected to the urgency narrative—to be universally good and highly desired.[45]

Surveys of families indicate that a substantial proportion of them view information related to reproduction as a valuable aspect of NBS (Campbell and Ross 2003; Götz and Götz 2006; Poppelaars et al. 2004; Sawyer et al. 2006). My own research with parents of NBS-diagnosed children, however, reflects a more complicated view. Not a single parent described better-informed future reproductive decision making as a benefit, per se, of their NBS experience. Further, only one mother indicated that, though she wouldn't have wanted a prenatal diagnosis for her NBS-diagnosed baby, she would like to know the CF status of any future fetus just so "we know what to expect and we can start right away." The remainder voiced concern of various kinds about the idea of CF encroaching on pregnancy, both past and future—or were in the throes of difficult decisions about having more children in light of positive NBS screens with uncertain health consequences.

Nearly all parents I interviewed whose children were diagnosed at birth or later were grateful to have been spared foreknowledge about the NBS-diagnosed child. They did not know prenatally, and they are glad they did not—with one or two exceptions. For many, remaining free of a diagnosis until birth was important because they imagine knowledge of the disease would have destroyed their enjoyment of the pregnancy, without any compensatory benefits—would have "spoiled the pregnancy" (Rothman 2000). Lilly, for example, notes that fetal diagnosis would have just been "more worrying and 'what if.'" And from Francesca: "I just think it would have taken away from my pregnancy with her. . . . I was so happy pregnant, . . . I wouldn't want that to [be] taken away." Kayla says that knowing about CF while pregnant would have changed the experience "in a more negative way," since "you are already miserable enough when you are pregnant—I was, anyway. And you are already an emotional wreck, so maybe it is better not to tell people while they are pregnant—we are wacky enough." For Anthony, the main point is whether or not a diagnosis during pregnancy could improve the health of the baby. "[Since] there's no course of treatment that could happen in utero," he says, "then I don't think that I would need to know beforehand in any way."

Parents whose older child was diagnosed with CF after the younger one was identified via NBS were grateful they hadn't had an earlier diagnosis for that older child: otherwise, they are quite certain their younger children would never have been born, and who could wish for that? For Cassandra, prenatal testing and making "that choice to end the pregnancy if I found out" would not have been an option. At the same time, "having one child with a chronic illness would have been enough," had she known about CF with the first affected sibling. Thus, her son Neil would never have been conceived if her daughter

Vera's CF had been identified by NBS—an unthinkable situation now that Neil is here. Maddy is grateful about the identical situation for her family: "I guess in a way I have to be thankful for the way things turned out, because if things had turned out differently we probably would not have had a third child. I guess I have to be thankful that my guardian angel was at least awake—wasn't doing her job but at least she was awake. [If we had known about Derek's CF], we would not have had Jana. We already discussed that; we know that for a fact, that if he had been diagnosed at birth . . . she would not be here." Roxanne, whose older children are not affected, also expresses relief that it was her youngest who got diagnosed, because if the child with CF "would've been our first . . . , I don't know that we would've had any more children."

A few of the many families I interviewed who were glad about not having a prenatal diagnosis for their NBS-diagnosed baby did in fact get CF testing during a subsequent pregnancy. Others I interviewed may still do so. But regardless of what they do if they are again pregnant, the choice to conceive without having to decide about CF testing (for what will now inevitably be considered an at-risk fetus) is no longer available.

Having been spared an explicit decision about prenatal CF testing for their NBS-diagnosed child—and thus spared the corollary choice that arises for many parents about continuing or terminating the pregnancy—was in retrospect a huge relief for a number of mothers. As Lara put it, comparing her situation when pregnant with the predicament of a couple in her family who have now both been identified as CF carriers:

> They're in a very unique position of knowing ahead of time that they both carry this. And if [my husband] and I had known that, it would be much more difficult to make decisions. . . . I had people ask me when word got out that [my family member had] been tested and was a carrier—I had people ask me, What would you have done? And I don't know. . . . I tell people their decision is so much more difficult than anything we've gone through emotionally. Because it was thrust upon us, but they have to decide to take it on.

For a subsequent pregnancy, Lara too would have this "much more difficult" decision to make. The same is true for Paige, who could not be more clear about the relief of not having faced a prenatal diagnosis and the ensuing negotiation with the baby's father. "Do I wish that I would have had a prenatal diagnosis?" she asks. "Absolutely not. I think if I would have gotten a prenatal diagnosis, although I didn't believe in abortion, I think I would have been incredibly overwhelmed. I think my husband would have wanted an abortion. I think it

probably would have ended up an abortion, and something I would have regret-
ted for the rest of my life, so I'm glad I did not have a prenatal diagnosis."

Parents who know that they are at elevated risk of conceiving a child with
genetic disease are not obligated to proceed with prenatal testing. Choice still
exists, but its context is changed by the additional information, and it may
become much harder for women to refuse such testing in clinical settings (and
familial contexts) where consent is often expected. As Ruth Hubbard put it,
when "'choices' become available, they all too rapidly become compulsions to
'choose' the socially-endorsed alternative" (1982, 210). In the case of prenatal
testing, what is generally endorsed is "having all the information" so as to
"be prepared, act rationally, not bury your head in the sand" (Katz Rothman
1986, 84). Once a woman knows she's at high risk for a child with problems,
the pressure to find out whatever testing can reveal may become even more
intense (Baughcum et al. 2005).

Parents I interviewed who were in the midst of deciding whether to have
another child provide perhaps the most poignant insight of all about the
complicated, life-changing repercussions of NBS for future childbearing. "It's
definitely changed things in figuring out if we're going to have a third child,"
says Paula.

> We don't know if we can handle another. We've seen so many [families]
> with more than one CF child, and it's a lot of work and it's scary, and the
> possibility of losing two children and then having—putting another
> child through [the preventive treatments]. Because she does not always
> enjoy it. . . . I'm hoping by the time she gets old enough to understand,
> there will be many more treatments and possibly even close to a cure,
> but the possibility is that she may have to be a twelve-year-old child who
> knows she may not live as long as her friends. Or, you know, just have to
> do their treatments twice a day when they want to go out hanging, or
> hang out with their friends. It's so much a part of their day, it's going to
> affect her forever. So we're thinking about putting another child through
> it, is that fair? It's going to change things. . . . And [our oldest, unaffected
> child] Z. has also lost—I think he loses some of our attention because of
> it. And that's, you know, if we had another one, who could possibly
> require more care, would he lose out more too? It's not fair to him.
> So there's lots of things to consider.

For Paula, the question of whether it is possible, right, and fair to have a
third child looms large. For Abby, the same question is even more preoccupy-
ing. Her first child's diagnosis (and thus prognosis) has remained ambiguous in

the fifteen months since his abnormal newborn screen. As she and her partner begin to contemplate a second child, it is unclear to them how to proceed. "Honestly," she says, "I think about this all the time." The information they have about her existing child, now a toddler, is "incredibly imperfect," so "do you assume you might have another asymptomatic child? And what is the likelihood of that, and who knows?" Abby elaborates:

> Which is worse, the pain of trying to decide whether or not to go ahead with a pregnancy that you have gotten amnio results that you have another possibly affected child and either going ahead with that, and then having a child that dies or is very, very sick—the impact that that has on our son or our extended family; or the pain in having to make a decision yourselves and the dice are just too risky to roll, and see if we have an asymptomatic child or not, so we are going to terminate this pregnancy? And then how many times do you do that, in the hopes of having a child that is just a carrier, when [what we have already] is an asymptomatic child who is perfect in every other way. . . . To choose to [go through the odyssey of ambiguous diagnosis after a positive NBS] more than once, I can't even imagine the strain that would place on my marriage. I can't imagine the strain of having a child and losing that child for my whole family. So it is easier to say, Well we have got a kid, and what else are we going to do? We would probably have to adopt, which is crazy, or maybe go down the road of pre-implantation genetic diagnosis, maybe. I don't know what we are going to do, it is just like this huge can of worms. . . . We are going to have to make some very tough decisions about having other biological children.

The urgency narrative is enormously compelling. Its role in pressuring states across the country to initiate lifesaving screening for serious, early-onset, treatable conditions cannot be underestimated and should not be undervalued. However, its deployment in the service of broad NBS expansion, and the resulting impassioned policy activism for expanded NBS now burning hotly all around us, arguably represent what John McDonough has characterized as "the misuse of anecdote" in policy making—that is, the development of large-scale policies in response to individual narratives that may or may not accurately characterize the experience of a larger group (McDonough 2001). In the case of the new NBS, the larger group of relevance is all parents whose lives are touched by screening, not just those whose babies were or could have been saved from death or disability by a timely diagnosis. As the likelihood of a shift from newborn screening to newborn profiling becomes more and more probable, the group of stakeholders expands even further, to include all of us whose future will be touched by the increasingly prominent role of genetic information in individual, family, and community contexts. Nonetheless, as I have shown here, stories about newborn screening's heroic properties tend to take up all the available narrative space in the public domain. Similarly, the dynamics of parental advocacy around NBS have made it very difficult to achieve polyvocal, broadly participatory advocacy.

Political historian Diane Paul points out that some of these dynamics have inhered in newborn screening from the beginning. "Then as now," she writes, NBS debates "pitted those with an immediate stake in the outcome, who were emotionally involved and easily organized, against those speaking on behalf of hypothetical patients who might either be spared future harm or receive future benefits from research—unorganized and, for all practical purposes, unorganizable constituencies that rarely count as 'stakeholders'" (2008, 10). Earlier chapters of this book made audible the stories of some of those parents who have not typically been heard. These are not hypothetical people, but very real ones. Their perspectives deserve to be given voice in the policy-making process, along with those of other currently silent constituencies.

Chapter 6

Brave New Worlds

Visible in a Single Drop of Blood?

The world around us is changing very quickly. While we're not looking, while we're working at our jobs or washing the dishes, the context in which we live is continuously transformed. The new NBS is part of that rapid transformation, and its impact on infancy and early parenting deserves notice.

This book has focused on the NBS-related experiences of parents whose children were diagnosed at birth with a relatively rare genetic disorder, but all signs point to a future in which newborn screening programs touch the lives of many others as well. More and more parents will now be getting news of abnormal screens at birth—results that signal a true positive, or that the test was faulty, or that the baby carries a genetic disorder, or that the screen turned up ambiguous findings with unclear consequences. As NBS expands yet further and becomes more publicly prominent, an increasing proportion of the families who welcome a new baby each year will come to see screening as part of the newborn period, just as expectant parents have come to understand prenatal testing as a routine aspect of pregnancy and to redefine their relationship with the fetus accordingly (Rothman 1986).

Perhaps most significantly, parents like those whose stories appear in these pages belong to the vanguard of what Deborah Heath and her colleagues have termed "genetic citizenship" in the "Genes R Us" era when genetic attributes and limits are gaining increasing influence over identity and participation in the public sphere (Heath, Rapp, and Taussig 2004, 159, 166). "To the extent that the widespread and chronic diseases of 'advanced civilization' are increasingly understood to have a genetic basis," they write, "we all have 'screenable futures'" (159). The coalescence and rapid growth of the politically influential

Genetic Alliance, an umbrella group for disease-specific organizations, illustrates this point perfectly. By emphasizing genetic identity as a unifying
element across a broad array of disorders and susceptibilities, the alliance has
built a far-reaching coalition. Its leader, Sharon Terry, described it in 2004
as 600 organizations "representing" fourteen million people (though relatively
few of these individuals have a formal affiliation with either the Genetic
Alliance or its member organizations). By 2008, these numbers had swelled to
650 organizations "representing" twenty-five million people.[1]

Technology-enabled genetic profiling of newborns would of course mean a
much more heavily screened future, beginning at birth, for each infant in the
United States. Within the decade, a *New York Times* article reported in 2009,
"every baby born" is predicted to "have its genetic code mapped at birth"
(Henderson 2009). And this is precisely what most NBS administrators also
envision—with apprehension, excitement, or some combination of the two.
As one of them suggests, echoing the predictions of many commentators, innovations in testing methodologies will mean "there's going to be an explosion of
disorders that we will . . . begin testing, and, I mean, you kind of have to look
at the big picture, you know, when a baby is born, do you want to know everything about that baby? . . . Newborn screening is going to play a bigger role, and
I believe that in ten, twenty, thirty years . . . when you bring your baby home
from the hospital, you're going to have a printout of their genes. . . . I absolutely
believe that that's the way newborn screening is going." In the words of another
administrator: "Where this field is going in general [is], . . . Why don't we just
screen for it because we can screen, not because we can treat."

The screenable future is predicted to mean many things: better health and
improved longevity (Alexander and Hanson 2006); an acceleration in existing
eugenic tendencies (Rothman 1998); and "new forms of democratic participation," as coalitions continue to form around genetic identity (Heath, Rapp, and
Taussig 2004, 152)—to name just a few. It will also mean more widespread
changes in parenting and in early childhood, like those described in this book.
In this final chapter, I reflect on some of the persistent dilemmas that accelerated testing creates. I also suggest how the nuanced view of NBS's consequences that I have tried to develop here can point toward a clearer articulation
of how screening changes lives, toward some concrete improvements in NBS
practice, and toward more robust deliberation about the future of NBS policies.

Doing Some Sociology

In a *New York Times* interview published several years back, sociologist Troy
Duster asserted: "By looking at what's in the blood, [geneticists] avoid the

messy stuff that happens when humans interact with each other. It's easier to look inside the body because genes, proteins, and SNP patterns are far more measurable than the complex dynamics of society. . . . But few of these basic processes happen outside a social context. . . . You can't . . . [do] biomedical research . . . without also doing some sociology" (Dreifus 2005).

Duster was referring here to genetic research based on race, but the insight applies equally to the new NBS. When we mandate testing of a newborn's blood for expanded numbers of disorders, we do so in a specific context. Furthermore, the implications of this action are far messier than most people realize: the new NBS is not just an isolated laboratory practice that leads to life-saving interventions for the few who are diagnosed with a treatable disorder. It is, rather, a particular form of social practice made possible, in its present form, by a number of converging factors: technological innovation; compelling advocacy; state power as enacted through the modern public health apparatus; the rise of the genetic paradigm; a laudable commitment to child health that is heavily influenced by some less-than-benign ideas about safeguarding children from risk at all costs. The cycle of expansion created by these forces is then reinforced by NBS itself as screening fuels an even higher perception of risk, a heroic view of technology, and a compelling underdog narrative about parental advocacy. We cannot continue to understand newborn screening only as a medical intervention with quantitatively measured effects on health and longevity. We must apprehend it also as a phenomenon that both reflects and influences how individuals interact with each other; how they relate to social institutions (such as public health programs and medical clinics); and how they conduct themselves—consciously, and also unconsciously—within a specific historical and cultural context.

Risky Business

When we "do some sociology" to understand the new NBS, it's easy to see how aspects of it exemplify larger trends within what Alan Petersen and Deborah Lupton have dubbed "the new public health" (1996). In both arenas, constant awareness and calculation of risk are primary strategies for selecting certain dangers as worthy of energy and attention while relegating others to the margins of public consciousness. In much mainstream discourse, as I have shown, the risks of failing to know, from birth, what genetic disorders may threaten one's baby are represented as disastrous, while the risks of finding out everything screening technology can reveal about that child when she is just a few days old are represented as minimal (if they are noticed at all). But when we set aside for a moment the research paradigm that compares risks according to quantitative measures of cost and benefit, the possibility of illuminating other aspects of how risk is constructed via the new NBS suddenly opens up. Now we can ask a different set of questions, like those Lupton raises in her work on risk. "What statements are used to construct certain kinds of knowledge about risk at a particular historical moment and sociocultural setting? What rules prescribe certain ways of talking about risk and exclude other ways? What types of subject are constructed through risk discourses? How does knowledge about risk acquire authority, a sense of embodying the 'truth' about it? What practices are used in institutions and by individuals for dealing with the subjects of risk discourses?" (Lupton 1999, 33).

From within the risk paradigm of the "new public health," molecular signs detected by genetic tests are often treated as "more important than behavioral or physical expressions" (Nelkin 1996, 539). Newborn screening, by intensifying the search for genetic explanations of human health, draws attention away from an examination of other significant determinants, particularly those that are environmental and therefore more integrally connected to social structure than to biological endowment. "Geneticization," as this process is sometimes called, thus results in the selection of genetic disorders as a critical target for risk reduction, while at the same time relegating other risks—like poverty, racism, social isolation, poor access to primary health care, to name just a few— to the margins of public consciousness.

Individual health conditions should be diagnosed and treated with the best solutions medicine has to offer. But particularly as the old NBS paradigm gives way to the new, it is also important to heed Lupton's admonition to look carefully at "how knowledge about risk acquires authority," and at what "rules" encourage certain ways of talking about risk while discouraging others. As we confront the likelihood of further growth in screening programs, we must try to be clear about when it is sensible to safeguard our infants from risk by looking for additional disorders at birth, and when more tests cannot realistically mitigate danger despite our heightened worry about genetic risks and our desire to spare our children. As emerging forms of genetic citizenship are rapidly uniting "diverse genetic constituencies" (Heath, Rapp, and Taussig 2004, 159) in potent political and organizational coalitions, developing a public discourse that assesses one by one the consequences of screening for each specific condition will not be an easy task—but it will be a necessary one. Screening for Krabbe disease is not the same as screening for PKU, and we need a language for describing NBS—not just in the bioethics literature but in the public domain broadly writ—that acknowledges these differences instead of summarizing them under the "saving lives" banner.

Equally important is to assure that the authoritative risk discourse associated with NBS—its promise to spare our babies from genetically induced danger—does not prevent or distract us from asking larger questions about the range of child health issues that deserve public attention, and how these should be prioritized. The dedication advocates and policymakers have brought to the task of narrowing interstate screening inequities since the ACMG report has been impressive. But—we need to ask—what would it take to transfer this political commitment to other child health domains where risk rhetoric is less heated, but where the stakes are at least as high? And what would it take to focus public debate on the fact that a skewed allocation of public resources may mean children get more and more diagnoses and genetic information at birth, yet lack the basic necessities that we know foster healthy development—such as access to high-quality primary care or a safe outdoor space in which to play? What would it take, in other words, to loosen the NBS success story from a narrow genetics frame and view it instead as one element in a broad call to action for children's health?

A few states have already begun to answer these questions by interpreting the mission of the newborn-screening program to include a long-term commitment to at least monitor the well-being of children who have been identified via NBS. It might be possible next to envision, champion, and fund an equally long-term commitment to the services those children will need to cope with their genetic condition as successfully as possible. To date, however, I know of no state that has actually taken even this next step, much less developed a more comprehensive approach to addressing persistent child health issues.

The Two-Way Street Connecting Risk and Disease

As this book has illustrated, once genetic information is identified, it can quickly be used to predict problems, monitor health, and structure preventive care regimes. When it comes to early NBS diagnosis for complex, often later-onset conditions like CF, one result of this approach seems to be what social historian Robert Aronowitz calls a "convergence" of "the experience of being at risk for disease . . . with the experience of the disease itself" (2009, 417). His description of how this works in adulthood for a number of chronic diseases also compellingly captures what is happening to a subset of families coping with NBS-diagnosed disorders.

"For many patients," Aronowitz writes, "the experience of chronic disease is not dominated by symptoms of the pathological processes but by reading the body for signs of future problems, negotiating different secondary prevention measures, and making decisions about the future." Thus "asymptomatic does not mean no experience of disease." Parents, like adult patients, "understand that [their children] are at higher risk . . . and will need to be screened aggressively. . . . They are [also] likely to pay special attention to any [symptoms]" (432). Sounds exactly like parents' caretaking practices after an NBS diagnosis, doesn't it?

As additional later-onset conditions such as fragile X syndrome and type 1 diabetes are proposed for mandatory NBS, we must acknowledge that shifts in family relationships and experience like those described in chapters 3 and 4 of this book will become an increasingly prominent part of "what happens when medical technology, for the sake of prevention, [continues to] make otherwise hidden bodily processes visible" (Baughcum et al. 2005; Reventlow, Hvas, and Malterud 2006, 2721). The cumulative impact on infancy and early childhood of an increased focus on genetic risks and differences—and the attendant convergence of early disease diagnosis and early parenting—will not, I believe, be a trivial thing. Accordingly, policymakers should make this impact part of the equation when they make decisions about new screening tests—and particularly when they consider whether screening for nonurgent conditions should take place with consent in the pediatric setting rather than on a mandatory basis at birth (see, e.g., Clayton 2009b). If a child is symptomatic as a newborn, or if an infant's health is imperiled beginning at birth by a treatable and early-onset condition, there can be no question of separating the moment of diagnosis from the postpartum period; the disease must be dealt with immediately. But it is possible to separate these two events for asymptomatic children with nonemergent conditions—and if NBS expands as predicted, a majority of those receiving true-positive newborn screens will soon be in this situation.

Unexpected and unsolicited genetic information has enormous implications for families. As I have shown, when the diagnosis of an asymptomatic infant is made immediately after birth, that diagnosis—not the disease, but the diagnosis itself—significantly defines the early relationship between parents and their newborn, coming as it does when they have "no other dimensions of [the baby's] identity to counterbalance this early signifier of disability" (Rosner 2004, 20). There has been no public outcry about how radically the newborn period is transformed when an immediate diagnosis is imposed on it, and policymakers have thus not been forced to make it an issue of central concern. But lack of public discussion on this issue may be due at least in part to the fact that nobody has ever asked parents to describe in detail the impact newborn screening has had on their lives. Without serious consideration of how optional genetic screening might be incorporated into pediatric care rather than mandated at birth, and without rigorous research about whether later diagnosis for each screened or potentially screened condition might compromise an infant's health, we should not accept an increased focus on risk and disease during the newborn period—and also should not accept newborn genetic profiling—as an unavoidable consequence of doing well by our children's health. When diagnosis of a given condition at birth is not substantially more beneficial to the infant than later diagnosis, screening conducted in primary care rather than in hospital settings should be considered a viable alternative. If policymakers made pediatric care cost-free during, say, the first year of life (following a principle enunciated in the Patient Protection and Affordable Care Act of 2010), perhaps oft-cited barriers to reaching parents in clinical settings would become less significant. As a result, the exigent need to front-load the postbirth hospital stay with screening and other services would recede.

The High Risk of Doubt

When a parent raises a child in the shadow of cystic fibrosis beginning at birth, it is clear that the promise of improved health via NBS diagnosis and subsequent treatment will powerfully structure their experience of risk and later their opinions about newborn screening. As Botkin notes, when NBS-identified children remain healthy, it is assumed that screening has successfully lowered the risk of deleterious health outcomes and led "to improved survival rates . . . compared with historical control subjects." However, continued good health for screened children is at least partly "because screening identifies a subset of asymptomatic children who would have fared well anyway" (2005, 865). Even for CF, where gold-standard randomized controlled trials indicate some aggregate improvements for children identified via NBS over children identified clinically, it is clear that children who would have remained asymptomatic even without any preventive care are also being identified and treated. But how can any single parent be certain if this would have been the case for her own child? And in the absence of knowing definitively whether one's diagnosed son or daughter will be helped or not, what option does any particular parent have but to minimize potential harm by believing wholeheartedly in the promise of NBS and committing herself absolutely to the preventive regime that follows in its wake? For most parents, the risk of doubting the efficacy of this explanatory model is prohibitively high.

Parents do not always view getting information about genetic disease at the earliest possible moment as desirable. For example, as I have shown, not all parents want information about genetic disease before birth. When knowing about the disorder earlier won't lead to improved health for the child (as is most often the case when it comes to prenatal diagnosis), parents may not feel that the benefit of "being prepared" outweighs the risk of helpless anxiety and a "spoiled pregnancy" (Rothman 1999). With NBS diagnoses, however, the promise of direct benefit to the child makes it almost impossible for most parents to even ask themselves (much less ask their health care providers) similar questions about the pros and cons of genetic knowledge. As Marta put it, reflecting on her decision not to pursue prenatal diagnosis even after both she and her husband had been identified as CF carriers: "When I had [my daughter], at least I felt I could do something to try and help her, because even if I had the amnio there is nothing in utero you can do."

Several of the parents I interviewed know, in the abstract, that NBS is identifying kids who would remain asymptomatic for decades, or forever, even without diagnosis or treatment; they told me, without prompting, that this is the case. Some also have questions about the efficacy of the prophylactic regime. But, with the exception of the mother who was told that her daughter's CF diagnosis would be "declassified," the possibility that their own child might not be benefiting substantially from early diagnosis is not imaginable: the "rules" operative in NBS discourse, which "prescribe certain ways of talking about risk and exclude others," don't permit it.

Listen, for example, to Ron. When he took his child to the CF clinic for the first time, a technician there told him "how a few weeks before, there was a patient who had come in, sixty-seven years old, his entire life was treated for asthma, and just on a whim they had him come do the test and found out he was positive for CF." This, "coupled with the knowledge that they had only just started newborn screening for CF, . . . put thoughts" in Ron's head. He realized that until recently NBS clinics had "only been seeing the severe side of CF." But if there was one relatively healthy undiagnosed sixty-seven-year-old, similar cases must exist. "Maybe there is a lot of this out there," he says. "People who have been living normal lives, just because they didn't know." Yet when it comes to his own five-year-old child, who is generally healthy and "only . . . different from any other child" because he takes vitamins and digestive enzymes, Ron is happy for the diagnosis immediately after birth because it made them "able to get him moving in a direction that was good for his health."

In Cora's case, her child's CF mutation is known to be very mild. The baby tested as "borderline" on the sweat test; he is entirely asymptomatic at two years of age; his diagnosis was so unusual that the health care institution where he is treated changed its protocols so as to "rule in" as CF a formerly "ruled-out" genotype. In other states or at other CF centers, this child would not have been considered to have the disorder at all. Nonetheless, Cora too remains very grateful for the early diagnosis, and unfailingly faithful to every aspect of the prophylactic regime. "Even though he's asymptomatic in all this stuff," she says, "he still is doing every treatment. . . . We try to be as incredibly conscientious as we can."

CF NBS's early-intervention mantra—"prevention, prevention, prevention"— also gains potency for parents because its target is their children rather than themselves. As I have suggested, coping with risk ourselves is one thing. If we make a bad call, fail to follow the most conservative path, sustain illness or injury that might have been avoided—well, so be it. We have only ourselves to blame. But when we're making decisions for someone else, for our child, the level of acceptable risk is likely to be much lower (Dickie and Messman 2004). As Clayton notes, parents "repeatedly say that they want to know what is going on with their children," and "these sentiments underlie the current assault on the 'consensus' that children should not be tested for adult onset disorders, even though many adults continue to avoid genetic tests themselves, especially for untreatable disorders" (2009b, 203). The same sentiment was evident in my research. Evelyn, for example, describes herself as "the au naturel person generally"—someone who favors natural childbirth, is committed to breast-feeding, seeks approaches to health problems outside of as well as within the paradigm of Western allopathic medicine. When it comes to managing her child's CF diagnosis, though, she is "totally there with the doctors . . . using the pulmonologist and the team, . . . like, 'Take care of it and do everything you can.'"

The risk of doubt significantly influences attitudes toward screening for the majority of parents—but not for all. Among those I interviewed, there emerged at least two subgroups who approached early genetic testing from a slightly different perspective: mothers of CF-diagnosed children who again become pregnant, and families whose abnormal newborn-screen results led to follow-up testing that was inconclusive with respect to diagnosis.

Members of the first subgroup, like most parents, say that as a matter of policy, they think newborn screening is a good and important thing. Yet mothers of CF-diagnosed children sometimes choose—when choice is an option—to wait a while before pursuing testing for a subsequent child. Nine mothers in my study went on to have another baby after CF was a known genetic risk in the family. None of them had any intention to abort, and all of them knew there would be no diagnostic odyssey, as the risk of CF was clearly established. Three got fetal diagnoses (one affected, two unaffected). Four mothers did not seek prenatal tests but knew that NBS for CF was mandatory in their state and that they would learn about the new baby's CF status that way. The remaining two mothers lived in states where CF NBS was not yet mandatory. Neither of these mothers opted for prenatal testing, and neither sought testing for her infant immediately at birth. Both were anxious, very anxious, about whether the child was affected. But they waited to do the actual test until they had known the child for a number of months (four in one case, and approximately eight in the other). And by the time the test was done, each had a clear sense based on observation and experience of what the result would be.

Meredith and her partner refused prenatal testing for baby Jim, whose older brother Steve was diagnosed with CF at birth because he had meconium ileus, reasoning that it would not "have made any difference on whether we continued through the pregnancy or not." Once Jim was born, though, Meredith watched him nervously, looking for any first indication of a problem or symptom. "I don't know how many times [my boyfriend] said, 'Meredith, will you just relax, he's fine.' [But] it's just that whole not knowing. I have to say that did just totally encompass me, the not knowing, the wondering, Okay, so could this be a sign of that, or could this be a sign of that?" For Meredith, those early months were full of stress, of "watching every move he made and then wondering." Yet she held off on getting Jim tested until he was about eight months old.[2] "I think it was fear of possibly getting the diagnosis was why we didn't," she says. "With Jim, it was just more of a wanting to know but being afraid to, I think is the best way to put it." By the time the test was done, it served mostly to confirm her sense that he did not have CF, yet it was still nerve-wracking. "It was more, I really don't think he does, but let's be positive. Let's not wait till he is two years old and begins having symptoms and then say, 'Oh yeah, he had CF too.' . . . It's just that reassurance, that proof. . . . So we were pretty positive that it was gonna be negative, but still that fear was there of, Okay, what happens if he's just a very moderate [case], you know, very, very mild?"

Erica, whose two older children had been diagnosed with CF, originally thought she might test her third child at birth, but her doctor suggested delaying a bit. Even though she didn't feel that this physician "was someone who had my best interest at heart," she decided she "wanted to wait." Rather than labeling the baby right away—something she is wary about—she decided to just watch for and treat the symptoms, to "treat how he presents." As it turned out, he was symptomatic for CF very soon. Like Meredith, Erica used the test to confirm what she already knew, what she had learned little by little from parenting her child. And she was very glad that she got the confirmatory news later rather than right after birth.

Many people embrace diagnostic technology and use it to gather information, to make decisions, to prepare psychologically for what will be coming next. But some people choose to find things out in other ways. They learn by observation and experience, and want to protect themselves from the blunt reality of a test. A black-and-white indicator of yes or no is too harsh for some. When newborn testing is mandated, parents may be grateful that the decision has been made for them. But as a matter of volition, immediate testing even for children known to be at risk for CF may not be a universal norm. Some parents will prefer instead to "see how the baby presents" before subjecting her to the test.

The second subgroup of families who seem to have a different relationship to NBS's discourse of risk comprises those with abnormal newborn-screen results that led to follow-up testing which was inconclusive with respect to diagnosis. Although my sample included only two parents in this category, the contrast between them and the rest of those I interviewed is striking. Instead of hopeful promise for health improvement through preventive care, these parents are left with endless diagnostic procedures and no clear sense of whether symptoms of any kind will ever emerge in a seemingly healthy child. Not surprisingly, once it becomes evident how tenuous the relationship between firm diagnosis and direct health benefit to the child may actually be in the face of so little medical knowledge, even the prospect of arriving at a specific disease label can lose its appeal. "The metabolic specialists are really, really focused on pinpointing [our son] has something and we are going to label it," says Abby.

> They want to pin it down and I understand that's how they are trained, but it is very much like getting down to the bottom of it and doing test after test. We actually skipped a couple of appointments with our old doctor because she was just so focused on testing and testing and testing, with the tests not getting us anywhere and her in some cases not able to tell us what she was trying to accomplish, so we just stopped going. Focus on a diagnosis versus on, like, is there actually anything going on. It wasn't until we went to our new doctor that he gave us [something useful], an ER protocol letter, so if you want to go to the hospital, give them this. . . . We don't need his blood to be taken for the seventeenth time just to show you the same elevation it had last time. I understand it is important and they need to see that those things are still there and if there is anything else, but at the same time to just walk in the door, to be told the same thing over again. . . . Just because they are trying to find a different diagnosis on its face is not particularly helpful. . . . It is definitely medicalized; it is very much medicalized and not so much health care.

In the face of enormous uncertainty, what this mother most wants from her child's doctors is candor. She wants them to be honest enough to "throw up their hands" and say, "'We don't know what this is. We are going to monitor you, and we are going to make you feel like you know what to do, and we are going to work with you.' Because [my husband and I] understand that there may not be an answer, and the problem with our other doctor was that she was just always trying, or seemed to push him into different categories even if they really didn't seem to fit."

Manny expresses a similar perspective, describing how it feels to confront medical uncertainty as he and his wife try to decide how risky it would be to conceive a second child.

> Here is what I am afraid of. I am afraid that you are going to go in and talk to the genetics counselor, you are going to talk to the metabolic special-ist and you are going to ask them those questions, and they are going to give you answers but they are not going to know, they are not really going to know. So they are going to try and tell you something because they don't want to admit they are [not] going to know, and that is almost worse in some sense, instead of if they said, "You know what? We can't really give you an answer, we don't have any other instances with this happening, or we don't have any other instances of mildly affected chil-dren and what their siblings are going to be like, there is just no evidence of that." So, it is hard, because I don't know if we are going to get a straight answer or not, to some extent. I am hoping that our current specialist is at least willing to say, "I have zero certainty in this answer but I can tell you what my gut feeling is," or "There is one documented case" and the sibling was much more severely affected or was not at all severely affected. All you can really go on is the case studies.

Meanwhile, as his child's diagnostic odyssey stretched into a second year, Manny began to lose patience with some doctors' view of him as "a ticking time bomb," when "good empirical evidence sort of seems to suggest otherwise."

This father's critique of medical expertise is trenchant, and he has no trouble describing at the intellectual level how vast the uncertainties associated with genetic screening can be. Like Ron and others, Manny knows that once you start screening an entire healthy population, you may find that mutations believed "relatively rare" actually aren't "all that rare," and that "there are going to be a lot of people who just happen to have one of the many different kinds of things [screened for] but they are asymptomatic." When it comes to Manny's role as a parent, however, these analyses are very little help. The unusual test results first identified on Ben's newborn screen changed everything, catapulting Manny abruptly yet seemingly permanently from the domain of normal parenthood into the no-man's-land of ambiguity.

> I think the key thing with an asymptomatic child to me was that you are constantly [walking] the tension between saying, I am in denial about this, because you don't feel like anything is wrong, and feeling like you have to acknowledge it mentally, or the gods of irony, or the gods of poetic justice will make something actually wrong with your child. It is like when you get on a plane, you have to acknowledge plane flying is dangerous or the plane will crash. . . . He is growing well, he is meeting all his physical and developmental milestones and so on and so forth, but you still don't know what to tell people because you don't fit into any of the groups. You don't fit into the "something is really wrong with my child" group, but you don't fit into [the] "my child is perfectly healthy" group, so there is, like, there isn't any place for you.

As it was for Abby, Manny, and others in their situation, the risk of doubt experienced by most parents of asymptomatic children who get NBS results can be transformed, over time, into doubt about NBS's risk discourse itself. "It is so complicated," says Abby. "And yet they say with the number of children that they are screening now that they are getting so many more hits." As those hits include more and more children in her son's situation—identified as abnormal on screening tests but undiagnosed and perhaps undiagnosable—Abby believes there will "come a point . . . where somebody realizes that there is a problem. Like somebody beyond us." But "usually what it takes," she adds—invoking in the name of caution precisely the same dynamic that has worked so well for expansion—"is that it happens to some congressman's kid. And then they care."

If a congressperson's baby did in fact have an abnormal newborn screen followed by an ongoing diagnostic odyssey that profoundly restructured family life without any apparent health benefit to the infant, as has been the case for Abby and for Manny—perhaps then the NBS debate would shift. But for the moment, doubt about NBS can be as risky for policymakers as it is for most parents. Newborn screening saves lives; it is popular with families; it is relatively low cost; it has few, if any, detractors; and to dig below the urgency narrative's structuring story is a time-consuming and complex task. Under such circumstances, policymakers have little incentive to pause and ask if the deliberative process has been sufficiently inclusive and well rounded, or if the new NBS calls for different approaches to policy development than did earlier NBS, unless they are specifically persuaded that it is necessary to do so.

There "Must, Must Be a Safety Net" for Parents:
The Practice of Newborn Screening

The narratives that parents entrusted to me reveal a lot about how newborn-screening programs feel to those they touch. NBS practice at the ground level profoundly affects parents' lives, and many of those I interviewed had a lot to say about how it ought to be done. Qualitative research about health care should "feed into the improvement of . . . planning, organization, or delivery" (Murphy and Dingwall 2003, 3). Here, I present some insights parents shared in our interviews about NBS. I hope readers will take these up, debate them, and even perhaps use them as a template for how laypeople's perspectives on important issues can be sought and used to improve health care and health policy.[3]

Better Education about NBS

Providers should take the need for education about newborn screening as seriously as they would if informed consent were required. Parents whose infants have had abnormal screens hold complex views about how much information it is optimal to have before screening.

Many parents I interviewed fervently wish they had known more from the beginning about the test and what might happen. "I would have wanted to know exactly what they were testing for and why and what exactly it was," says one mother. "Like, where do we go from here if it is positive? I mean, it just seemed like such a whirlwind at the time. They were like, we think she has CF, we're not going to tell you what it is, you have to go here and do this. And those people were like, well, we did the test, and it looks like it's positive but we're not sure. You have to go here and do this. And we just felt that we were running in circles, just not knowing."

Other parents, however, are cautious about how much more information would have been optimal. They say that a plethora of details about the conditions being screened for might have given them "too much to worry about" between when the heel prick was done and when the results came back, and would have caused excessive "aggravation and worry."[4] "I'm kind of torn," one of these mothers said, but "I know what it is to be a first-time mom. With my daughter, if they'd have explained to me these are the ten or fifteen diseases that we check for and if you get a positive hit on any of them, this is what we're gonna do, I think that would have just made me worry more. So I guess, kind of, no [I wouldn't have wanted more information ahead of time]. I think I would have gotten myself into a real state by the time they called me."

Regardless of whether parents would want to know everything, however, all those I interviewed feel they needed more information than they had. When a routine hospital procedure turns out to be a life-changing event, it is unaccept-able for parents to be left "digging for anything they can find" among the papers and forms they may have carted home, or to be desperately calling family and friends in an attempt to get more information. As one mother put it: "I would have wanted more information, [since] I didn't know anything, . . . maybe just a bit more educating as to what's on it so . . . maybe it would trigger something, or maybe a more comprehensive list of things that could be found through genetic testing, just to make people a little more aware of what they're testing for."

Treating NBS education as if it were mandatory would likely assure that parents begin getting what they most want and need before screening takes place—even while practical, legal, and ethical issues related to informed con-sent continue to be vigorously debated (see, e.g., Clayton 2005; Downie and Wildeman 2001; Tarini et al. 2008). Given how large and complicated NBS pan-els already are, and how diverse parents' desire for detailed information is, the education process should provide a baseline of information about the nature, purposes, risks, and benefits of screening—and then allow parents to choose whether they want to learn more right away or to learn more later (if they have a more pressing need for additional details). And as NBS continues to evolve toward the new NBS, educational material designed for parents needs to be kept up to date.

Parents also feel that education about newborn screening should happen during prenatal care. Since the time of birth is obviously not optimal for learn-ing about NBS, the best option is to incorporate it into obstetrical/midwifery care. As one mother articulates the point:

> I guess if they could give you more information during your last trimester about the newborn screening in your state, and, "Here's what we test for, do you have any questions, and do you want any more infor-mation on it?" that would be so much [better]. Maybe it's just because I've had an experience now with the screening where something came back positive, maybe I'd be different if I never did; . . . but just to me now looking back that would have been a time where at least I was thinking about it. . . . I would have [heard] the word before. You know, even like, CF, that's right, they told me about that they were gonna test for it in the newborn screen. And I maybe wouldn't have been so panicky about it earlier . . . , maybe I wouldn't have been such a basket case over a word I'd never heard before.

Recommendations to provide NBS education during the prenatal period have already been made by commentators and professional associations (Clayton 2005).

However, implementation remains spotty at best, in part because obstetricians view NBS as the province of pediatricians and have therefore been reluctant to address it (Faulkner et al. 2006).

Help for Parents Trying to Make Sense of NBS Results

Parents want to be contacted with screening results at a time and in a way that allows them to ask questions and absorb information—and it should be possible to design flexible ways of doing so when the abnormal result does not signal an immediate potential health emergency for the child (as PKU and other metabolic conditions do). Being face-to-face with a provider makes it easier for parents to ask more questions, to get more information, and to receive appropriate reassurance. If providers do have to tell parents about a positive screening result by telephone, they should call at a time when it won't be necessary for the provider to rush off the line or be otherwise unavailable for questions and follow-up communication. As one mother put it, when parents are told their baby screened positive for a disorder, "they need to be counseled appropriately. . . . There has to be a person on hand to provide that link" to follow-up testing, information, and services.

It is also important to families that professionals coordinate their messages about the differences between screening and diagnosis. It is very difficult for families when providers give conflicting information about the complex and anxiety-producing diagnostic process. For example, if DNA analysis has been conducted as part of the newborn-screening process, then pediatricians, those who administer the sweat test, and other CF clinic staff should all communicate consistently with parents about whether the screen is considered diagnostic in nature, and what the purpose of follow-up testing is. Otherwise, parents can arrive for what they believe is confirmatory testing, only to be greeted by providers who view the infant as already definitively diagnosed and are therefore moving straight into treatment mode. Avoiding this "confusing and overwhelming" situation is important to parents, who are otherwise left asking clinic staff, "Why are you doing this" treatment-related intervention when the confirmatory test is "not even positive yet?"

Individualized Timing of Education and Treatment

When the diagnosis does not constitute a true medical emergency, it is best for parents if providers work flexibly with them to design an individualized schedule for getting their child into care and for learning about the disease. Receiving the abnormal screen result, and then a diagnosis, can be overwhelming for families. Some parents' anxiety is eased by having a comprehensive

CF-clinic visit—complete with education about treatment regimens—on the same day as the sweat test. In other cases, though, it's simply too much, and a separation of days or weeks between the diagnosis and the first clinic visit would work much better. As one mother explains: "At first when we got the diagnosis, and, like I said, it happened to be clinic day, so they introduced everybody to us, so we ended up being there for three hours, and we were just devastated, and then they are introducing all these people to us, and it was too much. . . . I wish they would have just sent us home with the written information, gave us the basic, 'This is what we need to do now, and then this is what is going to happen in the future,' cutting some of the information, and have us come back the next week."

Similarly, in the case of conditions with highly variable outcomes and little exigent danger during infancy for identified children, health-care providers need to emphasize normalcy over disease, especially during the tender newborn period. One mother's description of her interactions with CF-center staff could serve as a model:

> I said to the nurse, "I only had a healthy baby for two days," . . . [but] she was able to say to me, "You know, your kid isn't sick." I was able to learn from there that she's not sick. . . . I think a lot of people aren't, a lot of parents aren't taught that your kid is okay, and I think that . . . if there's anything to take out of this, that's the part that's really lacking for these families. . . . Hopefully in the future . . . parents will eventually all get the same methods and the treatment, but, you know, . . . when your kid is sick, your kid is sick, but the rest of the time when they're not in the hospital, and . . . they don't have a cold, they're not sick, they're just kids like any other kid. I think that that's not really being relayed to the parents.

Especially during the exhausting, exhilarating, and complex period immediately following birth, parents want to be asked how much information they want at any given time, and they want providers to respect the pace of learning that they set, as well as the methods by which they choose to educate themselves. Parents have highly variable needs for information, and they process it at different rates. When the infant's health is not in immediate peril, it would be optimal for providers to individualize teaching about the disorder, checking in with parents along the way about how they are doing with what they are learning, what they would like to know next, and whether they need some time to process the information between consultations.

More Support and Services for Families

Many parents who have just received a newborn-screening diagnosis would welcome optional home-visiting programs. Here is one parent's description of why this would be useful, and what the home visitor might do:

> A lot of . . . parents . . . find out these results, either at the doctor's office or by phone, and then they go home and they know nothing. . . . They were handed a book that says, "Cystic Fibrosis for the Patient and Family." Now I don't know how they feel, but when my daughter was first diagnosed, I wasn't really up to reading a 150-page book. . . . I was just a little bit on overload, and what I did read didn't really stick. [What I wanted was] somebody who could, you know, come in my house, sit down with me, look at my baby with me, tell me what would be normal or what would be abnormal, . . . show me, tell me, maybe let me cry, maybe hold my hand, maybe just look in my eyes and hear what I'm saying.

Parents also want providers to be up front about uncertainty if information from the NBS is inconclusive or if its meaning is otherwise unclear. Parents appreciate honesty and often yearn for providers to just say: "We don't want to give you any false hope or false fears. This could be very serious. It could be nothing. You need to [get] more information before deciding anything."

It is essential that there be appropriate resources reliably available to help parents who have just received an abnormal screen result cope with both the long- and short-range implications of the information they are getting. As one mother implored: "If [newborn] testing is gonna be done, there must, *must* be a net in place to catch people." There was such a net in her state—a system that put her in touch immediately with genetic counselors who held her hand through every step of the process. But she knows that in other states "they don't have anything set up. So if it's positive, what are [they] going to tell these people to do?" Another mother emphasized that being informed of a positive newborn screen "could be devastating" for parents unless good genetic counseling is in place as a standard protocol.

> The counseling provide[s] information for parents about a particular disorder, but it also provides an avenue for where you go from . . . the screening results, to the diagnostic testing and results, to connection to whoever they need to be connected to. . . . You can't just get a letter in the mail saying your kid's screened positive for CF or whatever. . . . That is the scary part. What are you [as a parent] going to do with this

information? ... There has to be some protocol; ... there has to be established [a] qualified person who can explain.

Finally, parents desperately want to know about NBS's insurance and cost ramifications. Newborn-screening results, and subsequent testing of other children in the family, may have implications for future insurance coverage; despite passage of the Genetic Information Nondiscrimination Act in 2008, many parents remain concerned about this issue. Similarly, costs associated with treatment of problems identified via NBS may create significant financial burdens for families. Being informed about these issues from the get-go would be helpful to many parents. As one of them put it: "One of the things I wish they would put on the genetic sheets and info screening sheets is this may result in significant financial costs for you. If you turn up positive, even if you have insurance, it is not free, you still have to pay for the doctors, ... all kinds of stuff. ... I think it is a hidden cost, because it is not like some benefactor swoops down after your child has been diagnosed. The state doesn't come in and [pay for you]."

Presentation and Representation:
From a Parent's Voice to Parents' Voices

Preventable death and disability are tragedies. Not a single life is expendable, and no unnecessary death should pass without notice, without mourning, and without action by all who can usefully participate in change designed to protect other people from suffering a similar fate. If systems need to be shaken up, if parents need to be "fighters" and "zealots," if they need to be "screamers" to make others pay attention, so be it. In *The Brothers Karamazov*, Dostoevsky's character Ivan describes to his brother Alyosha the response of a mother who witnesses her child's death: "I don't want harmony. From love for humanity I don't want it" (Dostoevsky [1880] 1957, 226).

Our health care system badly needs patients (including parents of patients or of future patients) to be part of creating and transforming policy—even when their inclusion results in messiness of various kinds. It must be responsive to those who have the courage to sacrifice harmony and give voice to their experiences and their convictions. However, full inclusion of patients in policy making on critical issues like NBS involves such high stakes that more must be done than simply to make room at the proverbial table for those who spontaneously transform themselves from service recipient or citizen to policy activist. Indeed, we must move beyond mere responsiveness to proactive solicitation of broad and democratic participation. Put another way, those with the most power to shape health policy have a duty not only to listen to what they are being told but also to ask, in various ways, for the perspective of people who may not voluntarily stand up and speak.

The narratives I have shared in this book demonstrate that when it comes to newborn screening, parents' experiences and parents' perspectives—even with respect to true-positive test results—are not all the same. Rather, parents are polyvocal and defy easy categorization or straightforward policy response. As is true for so many areas of health policy, what is needed as we address the challenges of the new NBS is an approach to democratic participation that acknowledges this heterogeneity.

One potentially effective tool for moving toward more participatory policy making has been quietly embedded in NBS programs from the beginning. Among Wilson and Jungner's central criteria for evaluating proposed screening tests is that they should be "acceptable to the population" (1968, 31–32). The implication of this principle is that "the *introduction, design* and possible *expansion* of (newborn) screening programmes are essentially collective decisions" (Wieser 2010, 928). This principle has received almost no attention in NBS debates in the United States over the last forty years; now, in light of the high-stakes policy decisions facing us, it is time to reaffirm and implement it.

In her work examining the ideal process by which public participation in policy decisions can be fostered, ethicist Rebecca Dresser notes it should include: fair distribution among interest groups of opportunities to participate; an inclusive perspective on the part of advocates about how best to serve the public; and provision of information from public health officials and others that would "assist public participants to understand and debate the values and trade-offs that are at stake in these decisions" (Dresser 1999, 259). The urgency of the life-and-death narrative in NBS is so compelling, however, and the activism it ignites is so powerful, that with few exceptions these safeguards are not in place.[5] Thus very little attention is paid to either the values or "the processes by which patients' interests are defined, measured, and protected" (Tomes 2007, 698). Policymakers and NBS program bureaucrats hear only from the "usual suspect" parents and believe that, as a colleague of mine in public health commented to me in October 2005 while I was working on this book: "The parents have spoken, and the government has listened. Parents want to know their diagnoses no matter what."

We need to move beyond simplistic ideas about "the parents" as a representative entity, and to muster what it takes to promote more democratic mechanisms. What's required here is more than *pro forma* acquiescence on the part of policymakers to concepts of lay participation. They must grant entree not only to those who speak loudest, but to the quieter voices as well. What will be needed is commitment not only to specific new NBS policies that address problems of representation in existing practices, but also to a set of principles for enhancing patients' (and parents') engagement in policy development that can be flexibly implemented over time as NBS continues to evolve (Grob and Schlesinger, forthcoming).

What would such principles look like? When it comes to newborn screening, where parent advocates with a particular set of experiences have been almost the only lay representatives in the policy process, an explicit commitment to representing diverse parental experiences may be most crucial. As the history of NBS advocacy so clearly demonstrates, both individual advocates and advocacy groups can fail to be adequately representative for a variety of reasons: exigent situations (for example, the tragedy of losing a child) lend themselves to the formation of groups more easily than other circumstances do; some issues and frames (for example, the urgency narrative) muster resources and attract policymakers' attention more readily than others; individuals purporting to represent a group (for example, a parent member on an NBS advisory committee) may fail to apprehend, understand, or articulate issues that have little significance to him or herself, but that do matter to others. Given these vulnerabilities, NBS policymakers should actively elicit experiences from a representative cross-section of parents who neither come to the fore voluntarily nor belong to advocacy groups active in the policy process.[6]

Qualitative social science research designed to solicit nuanced voices that might not otherwise be heard is one useful mechanism for this important work. When we make a commitment to learning in depth about parents' diverse experiences with and perspectives on newborn screening, and thus to expanding our collective understanding of what it means, public discourse can become much richer and decision making much more informed. Narratives such as those recounted to me by the parents I interviewed are seldom included, as yet, in legislative hearings, in NBS advisory committees, or in media coverage. Generating, publishing, and discussing qualitative research findings about NBS can, I believe, contribute to changing that.

Another way we can promote more robust participation in NBS-related deliberation is to carefully revisit operating guidelines and procedures governing parent/patient participation in formal committee structures—both with respect to who is qualified to be a member, and with respect to how representation of a class of people is defined, encouraged, supported, and evaluated (see chapter 5). As the new NBS increasingly confronts us with questions about the line between newborn health promotion and newborn genetic profiling, it becomes more important than ever to ensure that parents and other lay persons on these committees reflect a range of perspectives. Further, those with authority over these policy-making bodies must deliberately move away from what Jennings and Bonnicksen have called a "consumer orientation" that defines representation according to "the private interests of individuals or groups," and toward a "civic orientation" that firmly places common good for the entire community of affected persons at the center of concern (2009, 147).

Civic engagement around issues in genetics via mechanisms such as community-based participatory research (Minkler et al. 2003) and deliberative policy making (Jennings 2003) is another promising avenue. These approaches can function to democratize decision making and to demystify common conceptions about who has the expertise to weigh in on questions involving science, technology, and medicine. As Harry Collins and Trevor Pinch put it, the public needs to understand that "even a dubious hypothesis can be maintained almost indefinitely and against almost any evidence if its proponent is determined enough." Further, people "need to know how to weight antiestablishment scientific opinions and discriminate between kinds of scientist. To understand this, they need to know, not more science, but more *about* science" (2005, 202). If more people understood, for example, the degree to which the multiplex capacity of MS/MS has driven the rapid uptick in number of screened conditions across the United States, prevailing views about NBS might be altered. Such knowledge will not provide straightforward answers to complex questions—but it may function as just the sort of "input to judgment" (ibid.) required for more robust public deliberation on questions of general concern.

Models of decision making about NBS from other countries can offer some additional perspectives on U.S. policy dilemmas. Bernhard Wieser, for example, highlights how the public sector influences acceptance of NBS through the knowledge-making process by comparing how two European countries structure the "institutionalized practices by which members of a given society test and deploy knowledge claims used as a basis for making collective choices" (Jasanoff 2005, 255, quoted in Wieser 2010, 928). In Austria, he explains, governmentally appointed institutions are responsible for assessing knowledge claims. "There are no public demonstrations, nor is the objectivity of the underlying knowledge tested in public. The experts involved are not known to the public and they do not speak or report (directly) to the public. The decisions made are not publicly justified. In essence, the process behind newborn screening is for the most part invisible and, therefore, not available to public assessment of a collectively shared knowledge basis." In the United Kingdom, on the other hand, there is in Wieser's view a "very substantial effort to account publicly for the way in which [the] screening programme is designed. This is done mainly by the extensive display of scientific facts produced by empirical studies" (Weiser 2010, 929).

In the United States, there is now in place a transparent federal process for soliciting from the public nominations of candidate conditions for NBS, and for assessing the appropriateness of such conditions, through a new Secretary's Advisory Committee on Heritable Disorders in Newborns and Children in the Department of Health and Human Services. The committee's recommendations are not binding on the states, but they do offer a process at the federal level well beyond what existed prior to the ACMG's 2005 report (albeit far short of the national model in the United Kingdom). The committee's meetings are open to members of the public, who are invited not only to listen but also (by prior arrangement) to comment. Its evidence reviews are conducted by a contracted third-party research group, whose findings and rationale are also publicly posted. Individual states might be able to create more robustly participatory NBS policy making by reviewing and selectively adopting elements of this federal process.

This federal commitment to an evidence-based and open policy process in the United States suggests some movement toward the kind of model embraced in the United Kingdom over the past decade and evident sporadically elsewhere (Borowski, Brehaut, and Hailey 2007; Potter, Avard, and Wilson 2008; Wieser 2010). However, numerous impediments remain. For one thing, U.S. states continue to set their own NBS policies and to be heavily influenced by ad hoc and organizational advocates working hard for inclusion of conditions (such as Krabbe and the other lysosomal storage diseases) that were specifically designated by the Secretary's Advisory Committee on Heritable Disorders in Infants and Children as unready for screening due to insufficient evidence. For another, the committee does not actively solicit input from affected parties; rather, it tends to rely on and to attract mostly the same advocates and NBS champions who have been active at the state level. Further, the committee itself has not yet developed a process for dealing with the complex interpretive elements inevitably associated with evidence review. As a large group of authors integrally involved with the committee notes: "Despite creating a rigorously standardized method for evaluating the evidence, how the weight of evidence is interpreted by Advisory Committee members—and others—may vary depending on differing values and perspectives. Variation in interpretation is inherent in any group decision-making process and may be more pronounced when evidence is limited to nonrandomized experience with screening or intervention" (Calonge et al. 2010, 158).

Finally, we should not underestimate the impact of the urgency narrative on U.S. policy making, and on fledgling efforts to move toward more participatory policy making. I have shown how this narrative has evolved from a heartfelt solo sung by those for whom it has personal meaning to a powerful chorus chanted by an ever-expanding group of people whose motivations and experiences are not directly shaped by the death or disability of a loved one. In the process, the powerful threat of tragedy and the promise of averting it have been extended from specific situations where they have clear or arguable merit to a general analogy that no longer accurately captures the complex consequences of policy for affected groups. Indeed, since about 2004, the tide of NBS expansion has begun to turn and parent advocates encounter less and less resistance. As I have already suggested, their policy interests have come to coincide more and more closely with those of an array of other actors pursuing their own ends in shaping newborn-screening policies and practices: private companies, pushing to sell screening technology and lab services; states, coping with pressure to save money by purportedly preventing future births of disabled children; the media, looking for compelling stories; the research establishment, anxious to translate genetic bench science into clinical practice. Advocacy for NBS expansion also speaks eloquently to politicians, who can see political advantage in "saving lives through screening"—especially since screening costs are cheap and funding for follow-up services is not necessarily on the public radar (Baily and Murray 2008).

Though the urgency narrative had its origin in the experiences of parents who suffered or averted crises related to their children's screenable, treatable genetic disorders, policymakers, private industry (Paul 2008), and the media have all appropriated it to a significant extent, making it difficult to formulate questions about NBS in any other terms. This tendency is visible in the rhetoric of federal legislators in several ways. National NBS legislation—signed into law in 2008—is named, in full resonance with the urgency narrative, the Newborn Screening Saves Lives Act. Not surprisingly, the powerful prospect of death or disability from a preventable disorder—and emphasis on the risk that one's baby might be among the statistically tiny cohort of those who could benefit most from expanded NBS—dominated both congressional testimony and public discourse as the legislation worked its way to the president's desk. As described by Sen. Christopher Dodd, one of the act's primary sponsors: "In the most direct sense, newborn screening saves lives. . . . Although the disorders that are tested for are quite rare, there is a chance that any one newborn can be affected, a sort of morbid lottery, if you will. In that sense, this is an issue that has a direct impact on the lives of every single family."[7] When the act passed in 2008, Dodd and his cosponsor, Sen. Orrin Hatch, issued a joint release quoting Hatch's statement that "health screenings for newborns can mean life or death for infants" (States News Service 2008).

A 2008 press release also illustrates the persistence of this "risk society" framing over time. "The lives of 500,000 newborns hang in the balance because they still are not being screened for the 29 core conditions," U.S. Rep. Lucille Roybal-Allard's release declared, attributing the figures to the March of Dimes, as the Newborn Screening Saves Lives Act gained passage and promised another "major step towards correcting . . . disparities" in the scope of NBS panels across states. The release goes on to note: "The tragic result is that hundreds of infants suffer lifelong disabling consequences or even death from otherwise treatable disorders."[8] However, the overall impression created by this strategic ordering and framing of the data might well be that it is half a million babies (that is, the entire newborn population each year who are being screened for somewhat fewer than the twenty-nine core ACMG conditions), rather than a few hundred (that is, the number who might be identified as true positives for as-yet-unscreened conditions that may or may not be treatable), whose lives are in any way affected.

It is our shared responsibility to protect the integrity both of the original solo and of the chorus that has swelled in its wake, by ensuring that as newborn-screening policy evolves, its changing implications and expanding scope of influence are mirrored by changes in who and what is included in policy discussions. To make this aspiration a reality will require both an active campaign for more balanced media coverage, and concerted education for reporters about NBS's complexity. It will also require that we think through the role of parents and of parental voice with significantly more analytic nuance and imagination than has been evidenced to date.

Newborn screening's urgency narrative tends to bolster conventional perceptions of professional expertise and to lionize heroic medicine. But ironically, over time, the high degree of uncertainty associated with many aspects of the new NBS may begin to have a different impact. If made public, test results with unclear implications, for example, could catalyze reconsideration of common ideas both about who is considered to possess expertise, and about the predictive power of genetic screening. As one parent in my study observed in his extended meditation on how NBS changed his own life, the difference between experts and other people no longer seems as clear-cut as once it did. "I don't want to walk in and tell somebody how to do their job," he says, "or act like I know more than I actually do. I am very respectful of experts." But being treated like an amateur by "experts" who have been able to do little to safeguard his child's health has had a profound impact on this parent, triggering new perceptions about the way he himself enacts the role of professional in his own line of work.

> I have actually tried to take that into sort of my job function, and, say, when somebody comes to me, they can say the piece of software that I wrote for them or that my company built for them isn't working and here is the reason why. I feel like I used to be much more dismissive of that than I am now, where I say, "You know what, I am actually going to listen to you because what you have to say you don't really understand, but maybe what you are telling me is telling me a lot more than I would have otherwise heard." And I think experts can sort of learn something from that.

Perhaps as the new NBS continues to grow, all those involved in constructing its discourse would do well to learn from this kind of willingness to use an encounter with uncertainty as a catalyst for more democratic forms of knowledge production.

In Closing

More than twenty years ago, Barbara Katz Rothman concluded her study about the impact of amniocentesis on mothers by observing that with prenatal testing and selective abortion, "we ask mothers to decide just what kind of child they choose to mother" (1986, 243). In so doing, we alter motherhood, putting at risk what Michael Sandel, in an article entitled "The Case Against Perfection," describes as the ability to "appreciate children as gifts . . . [and] accept them as they come, not as objects of our design or products of our will or instruments of our ambition." Parenthood is and must remain, Sandel asserts, "a school for humility . . . in a world that prizes mastery and control." The "openness to the unbidden" we embrace by having children in the first place "invites us to abide the unexpected, to live with dissonance, to rein in the impulse to control." It teaches us to keep in balance what the theologian William F. May describes as "*accepting* love [that] affirms the being of the child," and "*transforming* love [that] seeks the well-being of the child," assuring that "each aspect corrects the excesses of the other" (Sandel 2004, 55, 57, 60, emphasis added).

   With ever-expanded newborn screening, a different but related change in parenting looms large. In addition to asking mothers to decide what kind of child they want to mother, we are now beginning to tell mothers right from their baby's birth what kind of child they have in fact given birth to. Of course, as parents discover over time, the diagnosed abnormality is just one aspect of who that baby will become. But because the newborn is still so little known at the time of diagnosis, it is difficult—as it is during pregnancy—to separate the disorder (or the possibility of a disorder) from the child's overall identity. As we screen for more and more conditions, and as awareness grows that such testing is a routine aspect of newborn care, I worry that parents might become hesitant to happily announce the birth of their baby until the results come back, and that the screening process might displace parents' attention from the baby to the test. I worry that the tentative pregnancy created by prenatal tests might be replaced by as tentative parenting, as the next diagnostic battery—the mandatory one we do at birth—runs its course. I worry, ultimately, that tests designed to rule out, diagnose, or predict genetic disorders will become instead tests that babies must pass, a bar they must meet, before they gain full entry into their families and communities. Let's think very carefully, and with broad participation, about what it is we want to ask of them at such a young age.

Notes

Chapter 1 — Saving Babies, Changing Lives

1. Save Babies through Screening Foundation, Inc., http://savebabies.org/stories/fod/ben.pdf, accessed May 2010.
2. Although most NBS tests are still biochemical rather than molecular or DNA analyses, NBS is considered genetic testing because all conditions for which screening is conducted except two (congenital hypothyroidism and hearing loss) are inherited disorders (Grosse and Gwinn 2001).
3. My adoption of the term "new NBS" was sparked for me by Peterson and Lupton's term "new public health" (1996).
4. U.S. GAO 2003; National Newborn Screening and Genetics Resource Center, http://genes-r-us.uthscsa.edu, accessed May 31, 2007 (hereafter NNS).
5. I am using the term "chip" here as shorthand for a variety of emerging multiplex technologies that can be used to test DNA for many hundreds of thousands of variations that may (or may not) have clinical significance and may (or may not) lead to increasing accuracy in predicting individual risk of disease.
6. The ACMG's report (ACMG 2005) describes its own criteria and methodology, of course, in detail. For critiques of its approach, see Botkin et al. 2006; Baily and Murray 2008; Moyer et al. 2008; President's Council on Bioethics 2008.
7. The ACMG's overall methodology has also been criticized on a number of grounds. Doubts have been raised, for example, about who participated in the process, since the group that was assembled was made up entirely of newborn screening "insiders" and thus did not include anyone with an "outsider" perspective. ACMG was also criticized for releasing its recommendations to the public before publishing its report, and for failing to make public in a timely way some aspects of its methodology.
8. As I explore further in chapter 5, the notion of testing preventive treatments and asserting, at the same time, that they are effective exemplifies one of the potentially problematic features of new NBS.
9. Hoff and Hoyt 2005; National Newborn Screening and Genetics Resource Center, http://genes-r-us.uthscsa.edu/.
10. March of Dimes press release, February 18, 2009, http://www.prnewswire.com/news-releases/national-standard-for-newborn-screening-is-announced-94627034.html.
11. These figures are aggregated from statistics for 2008 on the National Newborn Screening and Genetic Resource Center website (http://www.genes-r-us.org).
12. There are a number of other published examples along these lines. See, e.g., Botkin 2005; Cunningham 2002; Kaye 2006, E936.
13. See, e.g., *Minnesota Lawyer* Staff 2009; Neergaard 2010; Roser 2009; Stein 2009.
14. See, e.g., Edelson 2003; Hehmeyer 2001; Nawn 2005; Oliver 2002; www.savebabies.org/familystories, accessed February 2010.
15. Associated Press, www.intelihealth.com, accessed October 31, 2004.
16. March of Dimes, www.marchofdimes.com; Greenville News (Greenville, S.C.); www.greenvilleonline.com, January 16, 2003; WPTZ, Burlington, Vt., www.TheChamplainChannel.com, September 27, 2003.

17. For an excellent analysis of how the press treats issues of science and technology in general, as well as genetics in particular, see Nelkin 1995.

18. More recently, evidence has begun to mount that in some instances even one copy of a mutated gene can have consequences for human health (Miller et al. 2010)—a finding with potentially vast and as yet relatively little-examined consequences for NBS.

19. More recent studies suggest that increased parental stress may not in fact lead to perceptions of child vulnerability and thus to increased health care utilization (Lipstein et al. 2009).

20. Bridget Wilcken (2003, S64) seems to dismiss the data reported in Al-Jader et al. 1990 when she asserts that "studies of patients correctly diagnosed with a disorder have not shown early diagnosis to affect adversely the parent-child interaction"; however, she offers no citations to back up this statement.

21. The sociological literature in these areas is rich. Examples include Ariès 1962; Condit 1999; Conrad 2001; Conrad and Schneider 1992; Cunningham-Burley and Bouton 2000; Duster 2003; Ehrenreich and English 1978; Hays 1997; Hochschild 1997; Hubbard and Lewontin 1996; Hubbard and Wald 1999; Hulbert 2003; Kerr and Shakespeare 2002; Lupton 2000; Marteau and Richards 1996; Petersen and Bunton 2002; Peterson and Lupton 1996; Popenoe 1988; Rapp 2000; Rieff 1966; Rothman 1998; Stearns 2003; Szasz 1961.

22. When clinicians have no reliable way of knowing which cases will be severe and which mild, they are most likely to intervene aggressively, thereby guarding against the risk of not doing enough for a highly symptomatic child. Treating a mild case too intensively doesn't evoke the same anxiety or the same legal risks (see chapters 3 and 4).

23. However, traditional definitions of carrier status are increasingly coming into question as paradigms in genetic science shift. With respect to CF, research now suggests that even a single mutated gene may lead to increased probability of asthma and other problems (Dougherty 2010).

24. Cystic Fibrosis Foundation, www.cff.org, accessed May 25, 2010.

25. People with cystic fibrosis who live into adulthood are beginning to tell their own stories about their experience of CF, either by autobiographical work or by participating in qualitative research studies. See, e.g., Rothenberg 2003; Schubert and Murphy 2005.

26. For a critique of how CF has been framed in racial terms, see Wailoo and Pemberton 2006.

27. "Cystic Fibrosis Carrier Screening-2," Handbook of Genetic Counseling, July 13, 2010. http://en.wikibooks.org/wiki/Handbook_of_Genetic_Counseling/Cystic_Fibrosis_Carrier_Screening-2. Accessed January 2011.

28. In the United States, when CF was diagnosed clinically, twenty-four mutations accounted for 80 percent of all identified CF cases; the remaining 20 percent of affected persons had much less common alleles.

29. There is also a declining overall prevalence of CF, linked to increased rates of newborn screening as well as more "carrier screening" (i.e., testing of women before or during pregnancy) and subsequent prenatal testing (to see if the actual fetus has two mutations). See Dupuis et al. 2005; Hale, Parad, and Corneau 2008; Massie et al. 2010.

30. For a sense of how this controversy unfolded, and of what researchers asserted about the quality and meaning of evidence gathered in CF research, see Bonham,

Downing, and Dalton 2003; Farrell and Farrell 2003; Farrell et al. 2001; Wilfond, Parad, and Fost 2005. See also the CDC cystic fibrosis meeting, criteria for newborn screening, www.cdc.gov/ncbddd/cf/day1/8–10am/criteriaNBS.htm.

Chapter 2 — Diagnostic Odysseys, Old and New

1. Cystic Fibrosis Foundation, http://www.cff.org/aboutcf/faqs/, accessed February 5, 2010.
2. The 2004 median age of 14.5 months for CF diagnosis could drop rapidly with the expansion of CF NBS to all fifty states as of 2009. Or, because pediatricians will assume that CF would have been picked up on newborn screen and may be decreasingly likely to suspect it as the cause of symptoms in children not identified with the disease at birth, the time it takes for symptomatic children to be diagnosed could lengthen and the median age could rise.
3. Cystic Fibrosis Foundation, http://www.cff.org/aboutcf/; accessed June 18, 2005.
4. New Jersey, for example, in 2007 looked for only the DeltaF508 mutation. All other states used larger screening panels, which as of the end of 2007 ranged from twenty-three to forty-six mutations (Janson 2007).
5. In eighteen of these twenty-two states, even if no mutations were identified, a sufficiently high IRT by that state's standard resulted in parental notification of a positive screen. This is because mutation analysis detects only a fraction of the possible mutations of the CFTR gene, and some states consider that an extremely elevated IRT may indicate the presence of a mutation not included among those for which the analysis tests. This fail-safe threshold also varied considerably among states in 2007; its modal value was 170 ng/ml, with a range from 130 ng/ml, to 270 ng/ml (Janson 2007).
6. At the end of 2007, values for these second screens ranged from 70 to 80 ng/ml; if the first two IRT screens were inconsistent, three states required a third screen. It is striking what a perfect example this is of how microprocesses structure scientific definitions of disease. In this case, it is also striking how widely these processes, and therefore the resulting definition of disease, can vary, even within the United States. For a fascinating examination of how "genetic explanations play a role in the reclassification of Cystic Fibrosis" at the more general level, see Hedgecoe's argument that the availability of genetic tests for CFTR mutations played a critical role in constructing male infertility as a form of CF and his conclusion that "the CF classification system has settled down to include certain cases of male infertility where mutations in the CFTR gene have been detected." But this outcome "should not obscure the socially constructed, contingent nature of this (and any other) classification system. CABVD [i.e., male infertility where the CFTR gene is implicated] does not *have* to be classed as a mild form of Cystic Fibrosis" (Hedgecoe 1993, 59).
7. Widespread lack of parental knowledge about and understanding of NBS is well documented. See, e.g., Duff and Brownlee 2008; Tluczek et al. 2005.
8. Duff and Brownlee make this point in their review of psychosocial aspects of CF testing. Audrey Tluczek and her colleagues make this point as well, noting that the way parents react to CF NBS is connected to their prior knowledge of screening processes as well as what they know about the disease itself (2005).
9. When Erica subsequently tested her younger children to confirm her sense that they too had CF, however, she asked for and got the results over the phone. In those cases, she says, "I liked the phone thing better . . . because I knew already [that the test would be positive], and I think it was also, for me, it is more private. . . . And I was able to just hang up the phone and cry."

10. Receiving the news even of false-positive results by phone can be problematic. Waisbren et al. found that mothers receiving repeat screening results after a false-positive newborn screening test were considerably less stressed when they received these results in person rather than by phone or mail (2003, 2570).

11. Many parents I interviewed offered heart-wrenching vignettes about the insensitive or even callous treatment they received at the hands of various health care workers. Others described great and unexpected kindness. I have not included many of these narratives here, however, because unique though the experience is for the individual, stories about how personality and communication techniques affect care experiences already abound in both the clinical and the sociological literature (see, e.g., Fisher 1986; Helft and Petronio 2007; Makoul 2001; Salander 2002). I focus instead on aspects of getting bad news that are particular to the institutional and structural arrangements that characterize NBS.

12. When I use the term "NBS diagnosis," I intend it as shorthand for a diagnosis established by follow-up testing after an abnormal newborn screen.

13. One other parent was advised by the doctors to have her child put on weight between the suspected diagnosis and the sweat test, but this was a planned delay and one she did not seem to find objectionable.

14. Distress associated with the NBS waiting period is documented via other research as well; see, e.g., Tluczek et al. 2005. Data from a study of 104 parents in Wisconsin indicated that while waiting for sweat testing after a positive newborn screen they felt concerned (96 percent), depressed (77 percent), and shocked (76 percent) (CDC 2004, 24).

15. A parent's disposition can also be a significant factor in determining how much information they want about their child's disorder at any given time. One group of researchers found in their focus groups that "individual personality affected whether participants would choose testing. Self-described planners wanted as much information as possible for long-term decision making. . . . Those who did not want the information did not want to mar time with their child with prior knowledge of the child's diagnosis before he or she developed symptoms" (Whitehead, Brown, and Layton 2010, 25). I examine a similar phenomenon in chapter 4 with respect to how much information parents want about CF right after the diagnosis.

16. My research did not include any parents who adopted a child with CF. However, the issue of how adoptive parents get and respond to diagnosis is little documented and would be useful to take up in future research.

17. Although this is by no means a universal truth, it is a generalization that holds for the group of families I interviewed in connection with this research.

18. The fact that identification of genetic disorders in one family member influences not just that individual but the entire family is well documented in the genetics literature (see, e.g., Kerr and Shakespeare 2002; Marteau and Richards 1996; Parsons and Bradley 2003). Disclosure of positive test results is a complex process for all involved, because others besides the diagnosed person can suddenly understand themselves to be at risk as a result. One mother I interviewed recounted: "When you start telling [family members] it's genetic, well then some people can kind of get a little freaked because it's like, what do you mean, that means I could have it or they could have it, you know. . . . People are really shocked when you tell them that like one in twenty-eight people's a carrier because that's a really high number." Another mother talked about how hurtful it was to deal with family members whose primary response to the diagnosis seems to be "How's this gonna affect me?"

Chapter 3 — Specters in the Room

1. Cystic Fibrosis.com, http://www.cysticfibrosis.com/forums/messageview.cfm?catid= 2964&threadid=31325&enterthread=y, accessed February 5, 2010.
2. The literature on the impact of serious childhood illness on the parents and family is substantial. For some illustrative perspectives, including particular issues related to CF, see Berge and Patterson 2004; Feldman and Eidelman 2007; Quittner et al. 1998.
3. Wadsworth Center, New York State Department of Health, http://www.wadsworth .org/newborn/babhealth.htm.

Chapter 4 — Encounters with Expertise

1. I found no data about the percentage of families with a diagnosed child that are not connected to consistent medical care for CF. Researchers estimate that 80 percent of diagnosed children are seen at one of 115 accredited CF specialty centers nation-wide, but it is not clear what proportion of the remaining 20 percent are treated in other settings, and what proportion are not receiving medical care of any kind. I have also not found any data about what proportion of families might be using some form of alternative or complementary health care instead of or in addition to allo-pathic medicine. I did not ask specifically about this issue during my interviews, but none of the parents in my study noted making use of any form of care for CF outside the allopathic norm during our extensive conversations about the professionals and the treatment routines in their lives.
2. Not all professionals—especially primary-care practitioners—have substantial knowl-edge about genetic disorders, but even a poorly informed provider likely has more information about CF than a parent who has just received an unexpected diagnosis.
3. At least one state administrator we interviewed for our state survey has taken a different approach. They follow asymptomatic babies in clinic but don't prescribe respiratory treatments unless symptoms emerge.
4. Occasionally there is a lag time, either because the state NBS program is able to delay implementation of new tests while it attempts to prepare, or because a given condition is so rare that no infants screen positive for it during the first months or even years of testing.
5. The relationships of parents to each of these groups of professionals, as well as the connections among providers themselves, are complex and multidimensional. Parents did talk in my interviews about some issues relating to differences between primary and specialty care, and what was helpful or problematic for them in each arena. In future research, it would be useful to gather data on this issue more sys-tematically. However, for the purpose of the overview in this chapter, I have lumped providers together.
6. See Katz 1986, chap. 5, for an excellent review of historical examples of this phenomenon.

Chapter 5 — A House on Fire

1. The primary exception to this generalization is the emerging critique not of NBS per se but of current methods of collection, storage, and use of blood spots, which some (including libertarian and other antigovernment groups) see as an invasion of privacy. Some parents have also begun to publicly voice objections to having their child's DNA collected, stored, and potentially used for research purposes without consent or privacy protections (see chapter 1).

2. I conducted the semi-structured survey of state NBS program administrators in partnership with Mark Schlesinger between September 2008 and March 2010. We examined how each state grapples with newborn-screening policy questions, and how various actors influence the process (parents, legislators, advocacy groups, NBS administrators, industry, media, clinicians, researchers, advisory board members). In particular, we explored how decision makers value and apply criteria for adding new conditions to NBS programs, and how technological assessment capacity and political institutions in each state shape these choices. Respondents were asked to describe particular episodes in which the scope of the program was expanded—both before and after the influential ACMG report was issued in 2005 (see chapter 1). We identified appropriate respondents in each state NBS program with the assistance of the National Newborn Screening and Genetic Resource Center. Our telephone interviews lasted an average of forty-five to sixty minutes. They were conducted by me, by Dr. Mark Schlesinger, or by our research associate Barbara Robb. Interviews were recorded and then transcribed verbatim. The transcripts were then coded using the same grounded-theory methodology I used with the parent interviews. Several states requested that the interviews not be recorded. In these cases, the interviewer took comprehensive notes, and these notes were then included in the content analysis.

3. For thoughtful documentation and analysis regarding private laboratories, see Clayton 2009a; Paul 2008.

4. Many *organizations* advocating for NBS—including Save Babies through Screening and CARES Foundation—work diligently on these issues as well. Also, as I show later in this chapter, the boundaries between diagnosis and research have become increasingly blurred since the advent of the new NBS.

5. Use of NBS as a mechanism for identifying research subjects also can facilitate progress toward effective treatment for all those living with a given condition, as we will see.

6. YouTube, http://www.youtube.com/watch?v=KhYugh9Ii-o&feature=player, accessed February 26, 2010.

7. Save Babies through Screening Foundation, Inc., http://www.savebabies.org/pressreleases/release1–20–02.php, accessed May 25, 2007.

8. Save Babies through Screening Foundation, Inc., http://www.savebabies.org/, accessed February 2010. Author files.

9. CARES Foundation, http://caresfoundation.org/nbs.html, accessed May 28, 2007.

10. Of the 117 comments submitted by family members of children with genetic disorders, fully 100 were from persons whose loved one had either severe combined immune deficiency syndrome (SCID) (N = 78) or Krabbe disease (N = 22). Neither of these was recommended at that time for inclusion in the ACMG-endorsed list.

11. The first quote appears in at least six comments sent by family members of children with SCID to HRSA in response to the draft report. The second appeared in all twenty-two comments submitted by family members and friends of children who had died of or were suffering from Krabbe. The third quote is from an ACMG comment dated April 28, 2005. Public comments on the ACMG report are available through the Genetic Services Branch of the Health Resources and Services Administration of the U.S. Government Department of Health and Human Services, http://mchb.hrsa.gov/screening/.

12. Diane Paul's historical account of advocacy around PKU in the 1960s and 1970s suggests that some of these NBS policy dynamics date back to the program's inception. "Although PKU directly impacted very few lives," Paul writes, "those touched were

highly motivated and politically engaged. The medical societies' arguments, on the other hand, could be dismissed as self-serving, while researchers' worries about evidence seemed petty and abstract" (2008, 10).

13. J. Kelly, comment on "Newborn Screening: Toward a Uniform Screening Panel and System" (ACMG 2005), May 8, 2005. Public comments on the ACMG report are available through the Genetic Services Branch of the Health Resources and Services Administration of the U.S. Government Department of Health and Human Services, http://mchb.hrsa.gov/screening/.

14. Moms and Babies, Celebrity Baby Blog, http://celebrity-babies.com/2008/06/16/scott-and-ren-1/, accessed February 26, 2010.

15. Bailey Baio Angel Foundation, http://www.baileybaioangelfoundation.com/, accessed February 26, 2010.

16. Moms and Babies, Celebrity Baby Blog.

17. Save Babies through Screening Foundation, Inc., http://www.savebabies.org/family_stories.html, accessed March 6, 2010.

18. Comment on "Newborn Screening: Toward a Uniform Screening Panel and System" (ACMG 2005), March 21, 2005. Public comments on the ACMG report are available through the Genetic Services Branch of the Health Resources and Services Administration of the U.S. Government Department of Health and Human Services, http://mchb.hrsa.gov/screening/.

19. Hunter's Hope, http://www.huntershope.org/site/PageServer?pagename=unbs_landing, accessed March 5, 2010. The formulation "could have" is masterfully employed here, since it leaves ambiguous whether the writer's intention is to claim that early diagnosis *would* have saved Hunter's life, or that early diagnosis *might* have saved him.

20. Six states reported that they do not have such a committee, and another six—Arizona, California, Kentucky, New Mexico, Rhode Island, and Tennessee—did not respond to our survey, so it is unconfirmed if they have or don't have such committees. Ten of the states with committees (29 percent of total committees) mandate, by law, that there be a consumer member. According to a GAO report published in 2003, thirty-five of forty-five advisory committees, or 78 percent, included parent representatives.

21. The difficulty some states have recruiting and retaining parent members suggests that many of the parents most dedicated to NBS advocacy find ad hoc and advocacy group work of their own design more effective or rewarding than service in formalized advocacy roles. Several hypotheses about why this may be seem promising, though I have not verified them. The first is simple: geographic distribution. Passionate lay advocates who are inspired rather than invited to public action about NBS are not evenly spread across the states. Their impact, both as individuals and as leaders of advocacy organizations, surely extends beyond their own jurisdictions. But it does so via strategies such as media and public relations campaigns, a push for federal legislation, or targeted interventions in other states. When it comes to membership on state advisory committees, however, often only parents who are residents qualify, so the pool of eligible members is severely restricted. In some cases, representatives of national advocacy organizations with local chapters (such as the March of Dimes) are appointed either in addition to, or as proxies for, local parents/consumers. But when the mandated slot is for unaffiliated members of the lay public, the available pool is limited to in-state parents. Another factor that might explain enthusiastic participation and active voice by parents on advisory committees in

one state, and difficulty finding parents willing and able to participate at all in other states, is how effective any given advisory board is—or is perceived to be—as a vehicle for advocacy. As I have just shown, some parents with passion in the belly about NBS issues choose to bypass their state committee altogether, judging that expansion can be more quickly and effectively accomplished through direct legislative action. And as I illustrate later, the technical focus and deliberative style of many committees can make them less than optimal targets for the interventions of NBS activists.

22. It was not possible to ascertain whether or not the remaining three parent representatives had a child or children with a genetic disorder.

23. In contrast, the NBS advisory committee in at least one Canadian province is actively deliberating about *which* of the multiple groups of parents affected by NBS should have representation on their committee.

24. Again, publicly expressed concern about storage and use of the newborn-screening blood spots does not, for the most part, extend to any sort of critique of screening itself.

25. Diane Paul also makes this point (2008, 12).

26. Other forms of evidence in newspaper stories include interviews with experts, expert reports, and vignettes regarding the symptoms associated with the condition in question. These are cited, respectively, in 50.8 percent, 21.2 percent, and 22.7 percent of all articles on NBS.

27. Other drivers of policy expansion that are cited in the mass media include expert testimony and experts' reports (mentioned in 27 percent of all articles on NBS), and changing technology (mentioned in 21.7 percent of all articles).

28. To be certain this effect is real, we also looked at the overall ratio of represented costs and benefits of screening in these articles, and discovered that these are roughly constant.

29. Genetic Alliance comment on "Newborn Screening: Toward a Uniform Screening Panel and System" (ACMG 2005), May 9, 2005. Public comments on the ACMG report are available through the Genetic Services Branch of the Health Resources and Services Administration of the U.S. Government Department of Health and Human Service, http://mchb.hrsa.gov/screening/. See also Bailey et al. 2006.

30. Comeau also criticizes the ACMG for the circularity of its logic in recommending that screening for conditions for which there is not sufficient evidence to justify screening should go forward because "data collection and surveillance through newborn screening for these disorders will generate the evidence base upon which to make decisions about newborn screening." This argument is flawed, she goes on, "because it ignores other options by which we can collect data in order to make decisions about the public health service." A. Comeau, comment on "Newborn Screening: Toward a Uniform Screening Panel and System" (ACMG 2005), May 9, 2005. Public comments on the ACMG report are available through the Genetic Services Branch of the Health Resources and Services Administration of the U.S. Government Department of Health and Human Services, http://mchb.hrsa.gov/screening/.

31. As noted in chapter 1, a number of states have in fact implemented pilot programs in the form of research protocols to test the efficacy and impact of screening for new conditions. Massachusetts, for example, ran an extended and well-evaluated program over a number of years. As already noted, Wisconsin ran a randomized clinical trial for CF for many years and is conducting research about the efficacy of NBS

for SCID. California implemented MS/MS as a research protocol for a couple of years but had difficulty with implementation. Montana ran a research-oriented pilot program starting in 1999 for the hemoglobinopathies. There are other examples as well.

32. Seven states reported that pressure for research was actually very (N = 1) or somewhat (N = 6) influential in screening expansion decisions.

33. As noted, informed consent for NBS is sought in Maryland, the District of Columbia, and Montana.

34. In 2010, sociologist Stephen Timmermans and his colleagues were poised to release their study of the impact of newborn screening on families when the screened baby's diagnosis remained ambiguous.

35. Researchers are required to receive approval of their proposed projects from institutional review boards before implementing any study involving human or animal subjects.

36. Newborn Screening in New York State, A Guide for Health Professionals, www .wadsworth.org/newborn/phyguidelines.pdf, accessed May 31, 2007.

37. See, e.g., "Diseases Added to Infant Testing Cost of Screening Increases to $89.25," *Arkansas Democrat-Gazette*, November 3, 2007; *Connecticut Post Online*, November 14, 2007, http://www.ctpost.com/, accessed November 2007.

38. Jana Monaco, comment to the Advisory Committee on Heritable Disorders and Genetic Diseases in Newborns and Children, http://www.hrsa.gov/heritabledisorders committee/meetings/2004june/Monaco.htm, accessed May 28, 2007.

39. Tess Rhodes, comment on "Newborn Screening: Toward a Uniform Screening Panel and System" (ACMG 2005), March 10, 2005. Public comments on the ACMG report are available through the Genetic Services Branch of the Health Resources and Services Administration of the U.S. Government Department of Health and Human Services, http://mchb.hrsa.gov/screening/.

40. Parent interview with author, Association of Public Health Laboratories, Newborn Screening and Genetic Testing Symposium, Minneapolis, May 7, 2007.

41. Hunter's Hope, http://www.huntershope.org/site/DocServer/HH_Newborn_Screening_ Brochure_031109.pdf?docID=1321, accessed March 26, 2010.

42. As Diane Paul notes, NBS advocates' claim that "'A child's chances for life shouldn't be dependent on where he or she is born' would seem. . . . to have broad implications for a federal system of government since many policies affecting children's life chances vary significantly by state" (2008, 11).

43. Save Babies through Screening Foundation, Inc., http://www.savebabies.org/ pressreleases/release1–20–02.php, accessed May 26, 2007.

44. Wendy Nawn, comment on "Newborn Screening: Toward a Uniform Screening Panel and System" (ACMG 2005), March 30, 2005; A. Comeau, comment on "Newborn Screening: Toward a Uniform Screening Panel and System" (ACMG 2005). Public comments on the ACMG report are available through the Genetic Services Branch of the Health Resources and Services Administration of the U.S. Government Department of Health and Human Services, http://mchb.hrsa.gov/ screening/.

45. Here, I am focused on how advocates have argued for the value of information related to reproductive planning gleaned from NBS diagnosis. A related set of debates, which I do not address here, centers on the utility and ethics of reporting to parents on the carrier status of their newborns after NBS determines that the disorder (as defined by two copies of a mutated gene or other measures) is not actually present. For a provocative discussion of this issue, see Miller, Robert, and Hayeems 2009.

Chapter 6 — Brave New Worlds

1. Genetic Alliance, http://www.geneticalliance.org.

2. Meredith could not recall exactly how old Jim was when the CF test was done, but thinks he was eight months old or younger.

3. A number of the suggestions parents have made to me mirror recommendations now appearing in the published NBS literature and initiatives now being developed by Regional Genetics Collaboratives and other organizations (both public and private) around the country.

4. This reticence on the part of some parents to know more about newborn screening in advance may signal a form of self-protection from the endless warnings and calculations about risk that now mark everyday life more generally. As medical and public health practices focus more and more on analyzing the inner workings of the asymptomatic body so as to identify and circumvent disease before it is manifest (Lupton 1995, 2001; Nelkin 1996; Petersen and Lupton 1996), some parents may want to avoid introducing this discourse of danger into the newborn period in such a prominent and explicit form. Perhaps they have had enough of this risk assessment and testing in the prenatal setting, where it is already an inescapable standard of care. When providers "explain about ten or fifteen diseases"—or, a few years later, about seventy or eighty of them—and say that the baby must be tested for each, they actively label the baby as at risk, and "to be labeled as being 'at risk' means entering a state in which an apparently healthy body moves into a sphere of danger" (Petersen and Lupton 1996, 48).

   It is understandable that some parents would like to avoid knowing about this particular "sphere of danger" ahead of time, and thus to avoid adding worry about the tests to the list of anxieties already flooding the newborn period. It is also reasonable that for others, it is critical to know everything that is happening to their child, and to avoid being blind-sided by a devastating test result. Does this mean we must choose between medical paternalism on the one hand, and increased submission to the discourse of risk prevention and danger on the other? Or is it time, instead, to redefine the terms of NBS debates over informed consent in some of the insightful ways suggested by several of the minority statements in the recent report by the President's Council on Bioethics (2008)—including a consideration of an "opt in" rule or an "opt out" rule as most appropriate and beneficial in the era of new NBS.

5. One example of NBS policy making appears close to (though not perhaps precisely an exemplar of) Dresser's ideal type: the Massachusetts experience (Atkinson et al. 2001; Grosse and Gwinn 2001). In 1997 the Massachusetts Department of Health developed a pilot program to add twenty conditions to the state's newborn-screening tests after a private company offered the use of its tandem mass spectrometry technology. An advisory committee was brought together that solicited the opinions of professionals and parents of children who had rare metabolic disorders. The committee developed a consensus on such prickly issues as criteria for mandated screening, disorders to be screened, a research protocol, and informed consent. The committee concluded that screening for more conditions was not necessarily better, and that there needed to be a balance between providing information to parents and the condition's treatability, prevalence, and test accuracy (Atkinson et al. 2001). This process of inviting and valuing the consumer's opinion is described in the cited sources as a recommended alternative to the more "extemporaneous" model of policy development characteristic of most NBS policy processes.

6. Elsewhere, Mark Schlesinger and I take up in more detail the question of how advocacy groups themselves might be asked to adopt practices that would make their voice more representative (Grob and Schlesinger, forthcoming).

7. U.S. Senate Committee on Health, Education, Labor, and Pensions, *Newborn Screening: Increasing Options and Awareness, Hearing before the Subcommittee on Children and Families*, 107th Cong., 2d sess., June 14, 2002.

8. Congresswoman Lucille Roybal-Allard, https://roybal-allard.house.gov/News/DocumentSingle.aspx?DocumentID=126763.

References

Advisory Committee on Heritable Disorders in Newborns and Children. 2009. Transcript of nineteenth meeting. Department of Health and Human Services, Health Resources and Services Administration. September 25, Bethesda, Md.

Albrecht, G. L., and P. J. Devlieger. 1999. "The Disability Paradox: A High Quality of Life against All Odds." *Social Science and Medicine* 48:977–988.

Alexander, D., and J. Hanson. 2006. "NICHD Research Initiative in Newborn Screening." *Mental Retardation and Developmental Disabilities Research Review* 12:301–304.

Alexander, D., and P. van Dyck. 2006. "A Vision of the Future of Newborn Screening." *Pediatrics* 117:S350–S354.

———. 2007. "Neonatal Screening: Old Dogma or Sound Principle?: In Reply." *Pediatrics* 119:407.

Alford, R. R. 1998. *The Craft of Inquiry: Theories, Methods, Evidence.* New York: Oxford University Press.

Al-Jader, L. N., M. C. Goodchild, H. C. Ryley, and P. S. Harper. 1990. "Attitudes of Parents of Cystic Fibrosis Children towards Neonatal Screening and Antenatal Diagnosis." *Clinical Genetics* 38:460–465.

American Academy of Pediatrics [AAP]. 2000. "Serving the Family from Birth to the Medical Home: Newborn Screening; A Blueprint for the Future. A Call for a National Agenda on State Newborn Screening Programs." *Pediatrics* 106:389–427.

American College of Medical Genetics [ACMG]. 2005. "Newborn Screening: Toward a Uniform Screening Panel and System." *Federal Register* 70 (44). Maternal and Child Health Bureau, http://mchb.hrsa.gov/screening/.

American College of Medical Genetics/American Society of Human Genetics Test and Technology Transfer Committee Working Group [ACMG/ASHG]. 2000. "Tandem Mass Spectrometry in Newborn Screening." *Genetics* 2:267–269.

American College of Obstetricians and Gynecologists [ACOG]. 2003. "ACOG Committee Opinion Number 287, October 2003: Newborn Screening." *Obstetrics and Gynecology* 102:887–889.

———. 2005. "ACOG Committee Opinion Number 325, December 2005: Update on Carrier Screening for Cystic Fibrosis." *Obstetrics and Gynecology* 106:1465–1468.

American Society of Human Genetics and American College of Medical Genetics [ASHG/ACMG]. 1995. "Points to Consider: Ethical, Legal, and Psychosocial Implications of Genetic Testing in Children and Adolescents." *American Journal of Human Genetics* 57:1233–1241.

———. 2005. "Points to Consider: Ethical, Legal, and Psychosocial Implications of Genetic Testing in Children and Adolescents." *American Journal of Human Genetics* 57:1233–1241.

Andrews, L. B., J. E. Fullerton, N. A. Hotzman, and A. Motolsky. 1994. *Assessing Genetic Risks: Implications for Health and Social Policy.* Washington, D.C.: National Academy Press.

Annas, G. 1982. "Mandatory PKU Screening: The Other Side of the Looking Glass." *American Journal of Public Health* 72:137–160.

Ariès, P. 1962. *Centuries of Childhood: A Social History of Family Life.* New York: Knopf.

Armstrong, E., D. Carpenter, and M. Hojnacki. 2006. "Whose Deaths Matter? Mortality, Advocacy, and Attention to Disease in the Mass Media." *Journal of Health Politics, Policy, and Law* 31:729–772.

Arn, P. 2007. "Newborn Screening: Current Status." *Health Affairs* 26:559–566.

Aronowitz, R. 2009. "The Converged Experience of Risk and Disease." *Milbank Quarterly* 87:417–442.

Atkinson, K., B. Zuckerman, J. Sharfstein, D. Levin, R. Blatt, and H. Koh. 2001. "A Public Health Response to Emerging Technology: Expansion of the Massachusetts Newborn Screening Program." *Public Health Report* 116:122–131.

Au, S. 2009. "Equal Access: Providing Genetic Services to Families Living away from Urban Centers." www.geneticalliance.org/conference09-symposia-services.

Baile, W. F., R. Buckman, R. Lenzi, G. Glober, E. A. Beale, and A. P. Kudelka. 2000. "SPIKES—A Six-Step Protocol for Delivering Bad News: Application to the Patient with Cancer." *Oncologist* 5:302–311.

Bailey, D. B., Jr. 2004. "Newborn Screening for Fragile X Syndrome." *Mental Retardation and Developmental Disabilities Research Reviews* 10:3–10.

Bailey, D. B., Jr., L. M. Beskow, A. M. Davis, and D. Skinner. 2006. "Changing Perspectives on the Benefits of Newborn Screening." *Mental Retardation and Developmental Disabilities Research Reviews* 12:270–279.

Bailey, D. B., D. Skinner, and S. F. Warren. 2005. "Newborn Screening for Developmental Disabilities: Reframing Presumptive Benefit." *American Journal of Public Health* 95:1889–1893.

Baily, M. A., and T. Murray. 2008. "Ethics, Evidence, and Cost in Newborn Screening." *Hastings Center Report* 38:23–31.

Baughcum, A. E., S. B. Johnson, S. K. Carmichael, A. B. Lewin, J. X. She, and D. A. Schatz. 2005. "Maternal Efforts to Prevent Type 1 Diabetes in At-Risk Children." *Diabetes Care* 28:916–921.

Bazell, R. 1998. *Her 2: The Making of Herceptin, a Revolutionary Treatment for Breast Cancer.* New York: Random House.

Berge, J. M., and J. M. Patterson. 2004. "Cystic Fibrosis and the Family: A Review and Critique of the Literature." *Families, Systems, and Health* 22:74–100.

Berger, P., and T. Luckmann. 1966. *The Social Construction of Reality: A Treatise in the Sociology of Knowledge.* New York: Doubleday.

Bluebond-Langer, M., J. B. Belasco, A. Goldman, and C. Belasco. 2007. "Understanding Parents' Approaches to Care and Treatment of Children with Cancer when Standard Therapy Has Failed." *Journal of Clinical Oncology* 25:2414–2419.

Boland, C., and N. L. Thompson. 1990. "Effects of Newborn Screening of Cystic Fibrosis on Reported Maternal Behaviour." *Archives of Disease in Childhood* 65:1240–1244.

Bonham, J., M. Downing, and A. Dalton. 2003. "Screening for Cystic Fibrosis: The Practice and the Debate." *European Journal of Pediatrics* 162:S42–S45.

Borowski, H. Z., J. Brehaut, and D. Hailey. 2007. "Linking Evidence from Health Technology Assessments to Policy and Decision Making: The Alberta Model." *International Journal of Technology Assessment in Health Care* 232:155–161.

Bosk, C. L. 2001. "Irony, Ethnography, and Informed Consent." In *Bioethics in Social Context*, ed. B. Hoffmaster, 199–221. Philadelphia: Temple University Press.

Botkin, J. R. 2005. "Research for Newborn Screening: Developing a National Framework." *Pediatrics* 116:862–871.

———. 2009. "Parental Permission for Research in Newborn Screening." In *Ethics and Newborn Genetic Screening: New Technologies, New Challenges*, ed. M. A. Baily and T. H. Murray, 255–273. Baltimore: Johns Hopkins University Press.

Botkin, J. R., E. W. Clayton, N. Fost, W. Burke, T. Murray, M. A. Baily, B. Wilfond, A. Berg, and L. F. Ross. 2006. "Newborn Screening Technology: Proceed with Caution." *Pediatrics* 117:1793–1799.

Boulton, M., and R. Williamson. 1995. "General Practice and New Genetics: What Do General Practitioners Know about Community Carrier Screening for Cystic Fibrosis?" *Public Understanding of Science* 4:255–267.

Bronfenbrenner, U. 1979. *The Ecology of Human Development: Experiments by Nature and Design.* Cambridge, Mass.: Harvard University Press.

Brosco, J. P., L. M. Sanders, R. Dharia, G. Guez, and C. Feudtner. 2010. "The Lure of Treatment: Expanded Newborn Screening and the Curious Case of Histidinemia." *Pediatrics* 125:417–419.

Brosco, J., M. Seider, and A. Dunn. 2006. "Early History of Universal Screening for PKU and Galactosemia in the U.S." Mailman Center for Child Development, Department of Pediatrics, University of Miami, Quarterly Narrative Report, January–March.

Brown, P., S. McCormick, B. Mayer, S. Zavestoski, R. Morello-Frosch, G. Altman, and L. Senier. 2006. "'A Lab of Our Own': Environmental Causation of Breast Cancer and Challenges to the Dominant Epidemiological Paradigm." *Science, Technology, and Human Values* 31:499–536.

Calonge, N., N. S. Green, P. Rinaldo, M. Lloyd-Puryear, D. Dougherty, C. Boyle, M. Watson, T. Trotter, S. F. Terry, and R. R. Howell. 2010. "Committee Report: Method for Evaluating Conditions Nominated for Population-Based Screening of Newborns and Children." *Genetics in Medicine* 12:153–159.

Campbell, E., and L. F. Ross. 2003. "Parental Attitudes Regarding Newborn Screening of PKU and DMD." *American Journal of Medical Genetics* Part A. 120:209–214.

Centers for Disease Control and Prevention [CDC]. 1997. "Newborn Screening for Cystic Fibrosis: A Paradigm for Public Health Genetics Policy Development." http://www.cdc.gov/mmwr/PDF/RR/RR4616.pdf.

———. 2004. "Cystic Fibrosis Meeting—Criteria for Newborn Screening." *Morbidity and Mortality Weekly Report* 53(RR-13):1–35.

———. 2008. "Impact of Expanded Newborn Screening—United States, 2006." *Morbidity and Mortality Weekly Report* 57(37):1012–1015:

Church, J., D. Saunders, M. Wanke, R. Pong, C. Spooner, and M. Dorgan. 2002. "Citizen Participation in Health Decision-Making: Past Experience, Future Prospects." *Journal of Public Health Policy* 23:12–32.

Clayton, E. W. 1992a. "Issues in State Newborn Screening Programs." *Pediatrics* 90:641–646.

———. 1992b. "Symposium: Legal and Ethical Issues Raised by Human Genome Project, Screening and Treatment of Newborns." *Houston Law Review* 29:85–148.

———. 1995. "Removing the Shadow of the Law from the Debate about Genetic Testing of Children." *American Journal of Medical Genetics* 57:630–634.

———. 2005. "Talking with Parents before Newborn Screening." *Journal of Pediatrics* 147:S26–S29.

———. 2009a. "Lessons to Be Learned from the Move toward Expanded Newborn Screening." In *Ethics and Newborn Genetic Screening: New Technologies, New Challenges*, ed. M. A. Baily and T. H. Murray, 125–135. Baltimore: Johns Hopkins University Press.

———. 2009b. "Ten Fingers, Ten Toes: Newborn Screening for Untreatable Disorders." *Health Matrix Cleveland* 19:199–203.

Cleary, M., G. E. Hunt, and J. Horsfall. 2009. "Delivering Difficult News in Psychiatric Settings." *Harvard Review of Psychiatry* 17:315–321.

Collins F. S., E. D. Green, A. E. Guttmacher, and M. S. Guyer. 2003. "A Vision for the Future of Genomics Research: A Blueprint for the Genomics Era." *Nature* 422:835–847.

Collins, H., and T. Pinch. 2005. "Vaccination and Parents' Rights." In *Dr. Golem: How to Think about Medicine*, ed. H. Collins and T. Pinch, 180–205. Chicago: University of Chicago Press.

Collins, V., J. Halliday, S. Kahler, and R. Williamson. 2001. "Parents' Experiences with Genetic Counseling after the Birth of a Baby with a Genetic Disorder: An Exploratory Study." *Journal of Genetic Counseling* 10:53–72.

Condit, C. M. 1999. *The Meanings of the Gene: Public Debates about Human Heredity.* Madison: University of Wisconsin Press.

Conrad, P. 1997. "Public Eyes and Private Genes: Historical Frames, New Constructions, and Social Problems." *Social Problems* 44:139–154.

———. 2001. "Media Images, Genetics, and Culture." In *Bioethics in Social Context*, ed. B. Hoffmaster, 90–111. Philadelphia: Temple University Press.

Conrad, P., and J. Schneider, eds. 1992. *Deviance and Medicalization: From Badness to Sickness.* Philadelphia: Temple University Press.

Corbin, J., and A. Strauss. 1990. "Grounded Theory Research: Procedures, Canons, and Evaluative Criteria." *Qualitative Sociology* 13:3–21.

Crane, B. 2000. "Roots and Branches of Family Support—Building a Theory of Change and a Logic Model for an Empowerment-Based Family Support Training and Credentialing Program." Typescript. Author files.

Cunningham, G. 2002. "The Science and Politics of Screening Newborns." *New England Journal of Medicine* 346:1084–1085.

Cunningham-Burley, S., and M. Bouton. 2000. "The Social Context of the New Genetics." In *Handbook of Social Studies in Health and Medicine*, ed. G. L. Albrecht, R. Fitzpatrick, and S. C. Scrimshaw, 173–188. London: Sage Publications.

De Mars Cody, J. 2009. "An Advocate's Perspective on Newborn Screening Policy." In *Ethics and Newborn Genetic Screening: New Technologies, New Challenges*, ed. M. A. Baily and T. H. Murray, 89–105. Baltimore: Johns Hopkins University Press.

DeVries, J., and A. Waller. 1997. "Parent Advocacy in FAS Public Policy Change." In *Challenge of Fetal Alcohol Syndrome: Overcoming Secondary Disabilities*, ed. A. Steissguth and J. Kanter, 171–180. Seattle: University of Washington Press.

Dickie, M., and V. L. Messman. 2004. "Parental Altruism and the Value of Avoiding Acute Illness: Are Kids Worth More Than Parents?" *Journal of Environmental Economics and Management* 48:1146–1174.

Donzelot, J. 1997. *The Policing of Families.* Baltimore: John Hopkins University Press.

Dostoevsky, F. [1880] 1957. *The Brothers Karamazov.* New York: Penguin Classics.

Dougherty, D. E. 2000. "Testing of Newborns Can Be a Lifesaver." Letter to the editor. *Boston Globe.* March 4.

Dougherty, M. 2010. "The Genetics of Complex Traits: What Are the Implications of Education?" Paper presented at Sarah Lawrence College, Public Health Genetics/ Genomics Certificate Program, June 7.

Downie, J., and S. Wildeman. 2001. "Genetic and Metabolic Screening of Newborns: Must Health Care Providers Seek Explicit Parental Consent?" *Health Law Journal* 9:61–100.

Downs, A. 1972. "Up and Down with Ecology: The 'Issue Attention' Cycle." *Public Interest* 28:38–50.

Dreifus, C. 2005. "A Sociologist Confronts 'the Messy Stuff.'" *New York Times.* October 18.

Dresser, R. 1999. "Public Advocacy and Allocation of Federal Funds for Biomedical Research." *Milbank Quarterly* 77:257–274.

Duff, A., and K. Brownlee. 2008. "Psychosocial Aspects of Newborn Screening Programs for Cystic Fibrosis." *Children's Health Care* 37:21–37.

Dupuis, A., D. Hamilton, D. E. Cole, and M. Corey. 2005. "Cystic Fibrosis Birth Rates in Canada: A Decreasing Trend since the Onset of Genetic Testing." *Journal of Pediatrics* 147:312–315.

Duster, T. 2003. *Backdoor to Eugenics*. 2d ed. New York: Routledge.

Eckholm, E. 2007. "In Turnabout, Infant Deaths Climb in South." *New York Times*. April 22.

Edelson, E. 2003. "More Newborn Screening Urged." *HealthDay*. www.healthday.com. Accessed October 2004.

Ehrenreich. B., and D. English. 1978. *For Her Own Good: 150 Years of the Experts' Advice to Women*. Garden City, N.Y.: Anchor Press.

Elborn, J. S., M. Hodson, and C. Bertram. 2009. "Implementation of European Standards of Care for Cystic Fibrosis—Control and Treatment of Infection." *Journal of Cystic Fibrosis* 8:211–217.

Epstein, S. 1995. "The Construction of Lay Expertise: AIDS Activism and the Forging of Credibility in the Reform of Clinical Trials." *Science, Technology, and Human Values* 20:408–437.

Farrell, M. H., and P. M. Farrell. 2003. "Newborn Screening for Cystic Fibrosis: Ensuring More Good than Harm." *Journal of Pediatrics* 143:707–712.

Farrell, P. M., M. R. Kosorok, M. J. Rock, A. Laxova, L. Zeng, H. Lai, G. Hoffman, R. H. Laessig, M. L. Splaingard, and the Wisconsin Cystic Fibrosis Neonatal Screening Study Group. 2001. "Early Diagnosis of Cystic Fibrosis through Neonatal Screening Prevents Severe Malnutrition and Improves Long-Term Growth." *Pediatrics* 107:1–13.

Faulkner, L. A., L. B. Feuchtbaum, S. Graham, J. P. Bolstad, and G. C. Cunningham. 2006. "The Newborn Screening Educational Gap: What Prenatal Care Providers Do Compared with What Is Expected." *American Journal of Obstetrics and Gynecology* 194:131–137.

Feldman, R., and A. I. Eidelman. 2007. "Maternal Postpartum Behavior and the Emergence of Infant-Mother and Infant-Father Synchrony in Preterm and Full-Term Infants: The Role of Neonatal Vagal Tone." *Developmental Psychobiology* 49:290–302.

Fisher, S. 1986. *In the Patient's Best Interest: Women and the Politics of Medical Decisions*. New Brunswick, N.J.: Rutgers University Press.

Fox, M. 2009. "Comment to the Meeting of the Advisory Committee on Heritable Disorders in Newborns and Children." September 25. http://www.hrsa.gov/ heritabledisorderscommittee/presentations/sep09.

Fox, Renee C. 2000. "Medical Uncertainty Revisited." In *The Handbook of Social Studies in Health and Medicine*, ed. G. Albrecht, R. Fitzpatrick, and S. Scrimshaw. Thousand Oaks, Calif.: Sage Publications.

Frank, A. 1995. *The Wounded Storyteller*. Chicago: University of Chicago Press.

———. 2006a. "At the Margins of Health: Qualitative Methods and Practice." *Qualitative Sociology* 29:241–251.

———. 2006b. "Health Stories and Connectors and Subjectifiers." *Health: An Interdisciplinary Journal for the Social Study of Health, Illness, and Medicine* 10:421–440.

Freudenberg, N., and M. Golub. 1987. "Health Education, Public Policy, and Disease Prevention: A Case History of the New York City Coalition to End Lead Poisoning." *Health Education Quarterly* 14:387–401.

Fyro, K., and G. Bodegard. 1987. "Four-Year Follow-Up of Psychological Reactions to False Positive Screening Tests for Congenital Hypothyroidism." *Acta Paediatrica Scandinavica* 76:107–114.

Genzyme Genetics. "Cystic Fibrosis Mutation Analysis." http://www.genzymegenetics
.com/pdf/cf_physician_brochure.pdf. Accessed November 8, 2005.

Gill, T. 2007. *No Fear: Growing Up in a Risk Averse Society*. London: Calouste
Gulbenkian Foundation.

Goldberg, C. 2000. "Big Gap in Screening U.S. Infants for Hereditary Ills." *New York
Times*. February 26.

Goodwin, G., M. Msall, B. Vohr, L. Rubin, and J. Padbury. 2002. "Newborn Screening:
An Overview with an Update on Recent Advances." *Current Problems in Pediatric and
Adolescent Health Care* 32:144–172.

Götz, I., and M. Götz. 2006. "How and Why Parents Change Their Attitudes to Prenatal
Diagnosis." *Clinical Child Psychology and Psychiatry* 11:293–300.

Green, M., and A. J. Solnit. 1964. "Reactions to the Threatened Loss of a Child:
A Vulnerable Child Syndrome: Pediatric Management of the Dying Child, Part III."
Pediatrics 34:58–66.

Green, M. J., and J. R. Botkin. 2003. "'Genetic Exceptionalism' in Medicine: Clarifying
the Differences between Genetic and Nongenetic Tests." *Annals of Internal Medicine*
138:571–575.

Greendale, K., and R. E. Pyeritz. 2001. "Empowering Primary Care Health Professionals
in Medical Genetics: How Soon? How Fast? How Far?" *American Journal of Medical
Genetics* 106:223–232.

Grob, R. 2008. "Is My Sick Child Healthy? Is My Healthy Child Sick? Changing Parental
Experiences of Cystic Fibrosis in the Age of Expanded Newborn Screening." *Social
Science and Medicine* 67:1056–1064.

———. Forthcoming. "A House on Fire: Newborn Screening, Parents' Advocacy, and the
Discourse of Urgency." In *Patients as Policy Actors*, ed. B. Hoffman, N. Tomes,
R. Grob, and M. Schlesinger. New Brunswick, N.J.: Rutgers University Press.

Grob, R., and M. Schlesinger. 2008. "Astigmatism in the Public Eye: An Analysis of
Gaps in the Media Coverage of the Ethical and Social Issues Regarding Newborn
Genetic Screening." Paper presented at Translating ELSI: Ethical, Legal, and Social
Implications of Genomics Conference, Cleveland, May 2.

———. Forthcoming. Epilogue to *Patients as Policy Actors*, ed. B. Hoffman, N. Tomes,
R. Grob, and M. Schlesinger. New Brunswick: Rutgers University Press.

Groopman, J. 2003. "Annals of Medicine, the Reeve Effect." *New Yorker*. November 10,
80–93.

Grosse, S., and M. Gwinn. 2001. "Assisting States in Assessing Newborn Screening
Options." *Public Health Reports* 116:169–172.

Grosse, S. D., C. A. Boyle, A. Kenneson, M. J. Khoury, and B. S. Wilfond. 2006. "From
Public Health Emergency to Public Health Service: The Implications of Evolving
Criteria for Newborn Screening Panels." *Pediatrics* 117:923–929.

Gurian, E. A., D. D. Kinnamon, J. J. Henry, and S. E. Waisbren. 2006. "Expanded Newborn
Screening for Biochemical Disorders: The Effect of a False-Positive Result." *Pediatrics*
117:1915–1921.

Guthrie, P. 2005. "Georgia Is Behind on Newborn Tests." *Atlanta Journal-Constitution*.
July 12.

Guthrie, R. 1996. "The Introduction of Newborn Screening for Phenylketonuria: A
Personal History." *European Journal of Pediatrics* 155, Suppl. 1:S4–S5.

Hackett, M. 2007. "Unsettled Sleep: The Construction and Consequences of a Public
Health Media Campaign." Ph.D. diss., City University of New York Graduate Center.

Hale, J., R. Parad, and A. Corneau. 2008. "Newborn Screening Showing Decreasing
Incidence of Cystic Fibrosis." *New England Journal of Medicine* 358:973–974.

Hallowell, N., C. Foster, R. Eeles, A. Arden-Jones, V. Murday, and M. Watson. 2003. "Balancing Autonomy and Responsibility: The Ethics of Generating and Disclosing Genetic Information." *Journal of Medical Ethics* 29:74–110.

Hampton, M. L., J. Anderson, B. S. Lavizzo, and A. B. Bergman. 1974. "Sickle Cell 'Nondisease': A Potentially Serious Public Health Problem." *American Journal of Diseases of Children* 128:58–61.

Hays, S. 1997. *The Cultural Contradictions of Motherhood*. New Haven: Yale University Press.

Heath, D., R. Rapp, and K. S. Taussig. 2004. "Genetic Citizenship." In *A Companion to the Anthropology of Politics*, ed. J. Vincent, 152–167. Malden, Mass.: Blackwell.

Hedgecoe, A. M. 1993. "Expansion and Uncertainty: Cystic Fibrosis, Classification, and Genetics." *Sociology of Health and Illness* 25:50–70.

Hehmeyer, C. P. 2001. "The Case for Universal Newborn Screening." *Exceptional Parent Magazine*. August, 88.

Helft, P. R. 2005. "Necessary Collusion: Prognostic Communication with Advanced Cancer Patients." *Journal of Clinical Oncology* 23:3146–3150.

Helft, P. R., and S. Petronio. 2007. "Communication Pitfalls with Cancer Patients: 'Hit-and-Run' Deliveries of Bad News." *Journal of the American College of Surgeons* 205:807–811.

Henderson, M. 2009. "Genetic Mapping of Babies by 2019 Will Transform Preventive Medicine." *The Times/Sunday Times*. February 9. http://www.timesonline.co.uk/tol/news/science/article5689052.ece.

Hewlett, J., and S. E. Waisbren. 2006. "A Review of the Psychosocial Effects of False-Positive Results on Parents and Current Communication Practices in Newborn Screening." *Journal of Inherited Metabolic Disease* 29:677–682.

Hill, S. A. 1994. *Managing Sickle Cell Disease in Low-Income Families*. Philadelphia: Temple University Press.

Hiller, E., G. Landenburger, and M. R. Natowicz. 1997. "Public Participation in Medical Policy-Making and the Status of Consumer Autonomy: The Example of Newborn-Screening Programs in the United States." *American Journal of Public Health* 87:1280–1289.

Hochschild, A. 1997. *Time Bind: When Work Becomes Home and Home Becomes Work*. New York: Metropolitan Books.

Hoff, T., and A. Hoyt. 2006. "Practices and Perceptions of Long-Term Follow-Up across State Newborn Screening Programs." *Pediatrics* 117:1922–1929.

Hoffman, B. 2006. "Bringing the Patient Back In: Health Policy History from the Bottom Up." Typescript. Author files.

Hoffman, B., N. Tomes, R. Grob, and M. Schlesinger, eds. Forthcoming. *Patients as Policy Makers*. New Brunswick, N.J.: Rutgers University Press.

Holtzman, N. A. 1991. "What Drives Neonatal Screening Programs?" *New England Journal of Medicine* 325:802–804.

Howell, R. R. 2006a. "Advisory Committee on Heritable Disorders and Genetic Diseases in Newborns and Children." *Mental Retardation and Developmental Disabilities Research Reviews* 12:313–315.

———. 2006b. "We Need Expanded Newborn Screening." *Pediatrics* 117:1800–1805.

Howse, J. L., M. Weiss, and N. S. Green. 2006. "Critical Role of the March of Dimes in the Expansion of Newborn Screening." *Mental Retardation and Developmental Disabilities Research Reviews* 12:280–287.

Hubbard, R. 1982. "Legal and Policy Implications of Recent Advances in Prenatal Diagnosis and Fetal Therapy." *Women's Rights Law Reporter* 7:210–218.

Hubbard, R., and R. C. Lewontin. 1996. "Sounding Board: Pitfalls of Genetic Testing." *New England Journal of Medicine* 334:1192–1194.

Hubbard, R., and E. Wald. 1999. *Exploding the Myth: How Genetic Information Is Produced and Manipulated by Scientists, Physicians, Employers, Insurance Companies, Educators, and Law Enforcers.* Boston: Beacon Press.

Hulbert, A. 2003. *Raising America: Experts, Parents, and a Century of Advice about Children.* New York: Knopf.

Janson, A. D. 2007. "Newborn Screening for Cystic Fibrosis: Variation in Priorities Guiding Laboratory Decision-Making in North America." Master's thesis, Sarah Lawrence College.

Jasanoff, S. 2005. *Designs on Nature.* Princeton: Princeton University Press.

Jennings, B. 2003. "The Liberalism of Life: Bioethics in the Face of Biopower." *Raritan* 22:132–139.

Jennings, B., and A. Bonnicksen. 2009. "Ethics and Newborn Genetic Screening: New Technologies, New Challenges." In *Ethics and Newborn Genetic Screening: New Technologies, New Challenges,* ed. M. A. Baily and T. H. Murray, 136–159. Baltimore: Johns Hopkins University Press.

Jewkes, R., and A. Murcott. 1998. "Community Representatives: Representing the Community?" *Social Science and Medicine* 46:843–858.

Katz, M. 1986. *In the Shadow of the Poor House.* New York: Basic Books.

Kaye, C., and the Committee on Genetics. 2006. "Newborn Screening Fact Sheets." *Pediatrics* 118:e934–e963.

Kemper, A. R., C. A. Boyle, J. Aceves, D. Dougherty, J. Figge, J. L. Fisch, A. R. Hinman, C. L. Greene, C. A. Kus, and J. Miller. 2008. "Long-Term Follow-Up after Diagnosis Resulting from Newborn Screening: Statement of the US Secretary of Health and Human Services' Advisory Committee on Heritable Disorders and Genetic Diseases in Newborns and Children." *Genetics in Medicine* 10:259–261.

Kemper, A. R., R. L. Uren, K. L. Moseley, and S. J. Clark. 2006. "Primary Care Physicians' Attitudes Regarding Follow-Up Care for Children with Positive Newborn Screening Results." *Pediatrics* 118:1836–1841.

Kerr, A., and T. Shakespeare. 2002. *Genetic Politics: From Eugenics to Genome.* Cheltenham, U.K.: New Clarion Press.

Kessler, S., T. Field, L. Worth, and H. Mosbarger. 1987. "Attitudes of Persons at Risk for Huntington Disease toward Predictive Testing." *American Journal of Medical Genetics* 26:259–270.

Kevles, D. J. 1985. *In the Name of Eugenics: Genetics and the Uses of Human Heredity.* New York: Knopf.

Khoury, M., M. Gwinn, P. W. Yoon, N. Dowling, C. A. Moore, and L. Bradley. 2007. "The Continuum of Translation Research in Genomic Medicine: How Can We Accelerate the Appropriate Integration of Human Genome Discoveries into Health Care and Disease Prevention?" *Genetics in Medicine* 9:665–674.

Kleinman, A. 1988. *The Illness Narratives.* New York: Basic Books.

Kleinman, A., and D. Seeman. 2000. "Personal Experience of Illness." In *The Handbook of Social Studies in Health and Medicine,* ed. G. C. Albrecht, R. Fitzpatrick, and S. C. Scrimshaw, 230–242. London: Sage Publications.

Knapp, A. A., A. R. Kemper, and J. M. Perrin. 2009. *Evidence Review: Krabbe Disease.* Boston: Massachusetts General Hospital.

Kolata, G. 1987. "Panel Urges Newborn Sickle Cell Screening." *Science* 236:259–260.

———. 2005. "Panel to Advise Tests on Babies for 29 Diseases." *New York Times*. February 21.

Leiberman, A., and S. Chaiken. 1992. "Defensive Processing of Personally Relevant Health Messages." *Personality and Social Psychology Bulletin* 18:669–679.

Lerner, B. 2006. *When Illness Goes Public: Celebrity Patients and How We Look at Medicine*. Baltimore: Johns Hopkins University Press.

Lipstein, E. A., J. M. Perrin, S. E. Waisbren, and L. A. Prosser. 2009. "Impact of False-Positive Newborn Metabolic Screening Results on Early Health Care Utilization." *Genetics in Medicine* 11:716–721.

Litt, J. 2000. *Medicalized Motherhood*. New Brunswick, N.J.: Rutgers University Press.

Lloyd-Puryear, M. A., and I. Forsman. 2002. "Newborn Screening and Genetic Testing." *Journal of Obstetric, Gynecologic, and Neonatal Issues* 31:200–207.

Lomas, J. 1997. "Reluctant Rationers: Public Input to Health Care Priorities." *Journal of Health Services Research and Policy* 2:103–111.

Lupton, D. 1995. *The Imperative of Health: Public Health and the Regulated Body*. London: Sage Publications.

———. 1999. *Risk*. London: Routledge.

———, ed. 2000. *The Social Construction of Medicine and the Body*. San Francisco: Sage.

———. 2001. "Risk as Moral Danger: The Social and Political Functions of Risk Discourse in Public Health." In *The Sociology of Health and Illness: Critical Perspectives*, ed. P. Conrad, 394–401. New York: Worth Publishers.

Macintyre, S. 1995. "The Public Understanding of Science or the Scientific Understanding of the Public? A Review of the Social Context of the 'New Genetics.'" *Public Understanding of Science* 4:223–232.

Makoul, G. 2001. "Essential Elements of Communication in Medical Encounters: The Kalamazoo Consensus Statement." *Academic Medicine: Journal of the Association of American Medical Colleges* 76:390–393.

Marano, H. E. 2008. *A Nation of Wimps: The High Cost of Invasive Parenting*. New York: Broadway Books.

Marcus, A. D. Forthcoming. "The Power of Us: A New Approach to Advocacy for Breast Cancer." In *Patients as Policy Makers*, ed. B. Hoffman, N. Tomes, R. Grob, and M. Schlesinger. New Brunswick, N.J.: Rutgers University Press.

Marshall, E. 2001. "Fast Technology Drives New World of Newborn Screening." *Science* 294:2272–2274.

Marteau, T., and M. Richards. 1996. *The Troubled Helix: Social and Psychological Implications of the New Human Genetics*. Cambridge: Cambridge University Press.

Marteau, T. M., M. van Duijn, and I. Ellis. 1992. "Effects of Genetic Screening on Perception of Health: A Pilot Study." *Journal of Medical Genetics* 29:24–26.

Martin, J. A., B. E. Hamilton, P. D. Sutton, S. J. Ventura, F. Menacker, S. Kirmeyer, and T. J. Mathews. 2009. "Births: Final Data for 2006." *National Vital Statistics Reports* 57, no 7. Hyattsville, Md.: National Center for Health Statistics.

Massie, J., L. Curnow, L. Gaffney, J. Carlin, and I. Francis. 2010. "Declining Prevalence of Cystic Fibrosis since the Introduction of Newborn Screening." *Archives of Disease in Childhood* 95:531–533.

Maternal and Child Health Bureau, Health Resources and Services Administration, U.S. Department of Health and Human Services [MCHB]. "Newborn Screening: Toward a Uniform Screening Panel and System." http://www.mchb.hrsa.gov/screening/summary.htm.

Maynard, D. 1996. "On 'Realization' in Everyday Life: The Forecasting of Bad News as a Social Relation." *American Sociological Review* 61:109–131.

McDonough, J. E. 2001. "Using and Misusing Anecdote in Policy Making." *Health Affairs* 20:207–212.

Mehlman, M., and J. Botkin. 1998. *Access to the Genome: The Challenge to Equality.* Washington, D.C.: Georgetown University Press.

Meilaender, G. C. 2008. "Personal Statement." In *The Changing Moral Focus of Newborn Screening: An Ethical Analysis by the President's Council on Bioethics*, 117–120. Washington, D.C.: President's Council on Bioethics.

Mérelle, M. E., J. Huisman, A. Alderden-van der Vecht, F. Taat, D. Bezemer, R. W. Griffioen, G. Brinkhorst, and J. E. Dankert-Roelse. 2003. "Early versus Late Diagnosis: Psychological Impact on Parents of Children with Cystic Fibrosis." *Pediatrics* 111:346–350.

Miller A., and P. Guthrie. 2003. "Newborns at Risk: How Georgia's Health Screening Practices Can Put Newborns at Risk; Limited Testing, Poor Follow-up Allow Disorders to Go Untreated." *Atlanta Journal-Constitution.* February 2.

Miller, F. A., C. Ahern, J. Ogilvie, M. Giacomini, and L. Schwartz. 2005. "Ruling In and Ruling Out: Implications of Molecular Genetic Diagnoses for Disease Classification." *Social Science and Medicine* 61:2536–2545.

Miller, F. A., M. Paynter, R. Z. Hayeems, J. Little, J. C. Carroll, B. Wilson, J. Allanson, J. P. Bytautas, and P. Chakraborty. 2010. "Understanding Sickle Cell Carrier Status Identified through Newborn Screening: A Qualitative Study." *European Journal of Human Genetics* 18:303–308.

Miller, F. A., J. S. Robert, and R. Z. Hayeems. 2009. "Questioning the Consensus: Managing Carrier Status Results Generated by Newborn Screening." *American Journal of Public Health* 99:210–215.

Minkler, M., A. G. Blackwell, M. Thompson, and H. Tami. 2003. "Community-Based Participatory Research: Implications for Public Health Funding." *American Journal of Public Health* 93:1210–1213.

Minkler, M., and N. Wallerstein, eds. 2008. *Community-Based Participatory Research for Health.* 2d ed. San Francisco: Jossey-Bass.

Minnesota Lawyer Staff. 2009. "Hennepin County District Court Rules MDH Not in Violation of Privacy Laws." *Minnesota Lawyer.* December 7.

Mischler, E., B. S. Wilfond, N. Fost, and A. Laxova. 1998. "Cystic Fibrosis Newborn Screening: Impact on Reproductive Behavior and Implications for Genetic Counseling." *Pediatrics* 102:44–53.

Morgan, J., D. Robinson, and J. Aldridge. 2002. "Parenting Stress and Externalizing Child Behavior." *Child and Family Social Work* 7:219–225.

Morone, J. A. 1990. *The Democratic Wish: Popular Participation and the Limits of American Government.* New York: Basic Books.

Moskowitz, S., J. Chmiel, D. Sterner, E. Cheng, and G. Cutting. 2005. "CFTR-Related Disorders." *Gene Reviews.* http://www.ncbi.nlm.nih.gov/books/NBK/250/.

Moyer, V., N. Calonge, S. Teutsch, and J. Botkin, on Behalf of the U.S. Preventive Services Task Force. 2008. "Expanding Newborn Screening: Process, Policy, and Priorities." *Hastings Center Report* 38:32–39.

Mulick, J. A., and E. M. Butter. 2002. "Educational Advocacy for Children with Autism." *Behavioral Interventions* 17:57–74.

Murphy, E., and R. Dingwall. 2003. *Qualitative Methods and Health Policy Research.* New York: Aldine de Gruyter.

Neergaard, L. 2010. "Hunting Newborn Tests for Super-Rare Gene Diseases." Associated Press. January 5.

Nelkin, D. 1995. *Selling Science: How the Press Covers Science and Technology*. New York: W. H. Freeman.

———. 1996. "The Social Dynamics of Genetic Testing: The Case of Fragile-X." *Medical Anthropology Quarterly* 10:537–550.

Nelkin, D., and L. Tancredi. 1994. *Dangerous Diagnostics: The Social Power of Biological Information*. New York: Basic Books.

Nelson, R. M., J. R. Botkin, E. D. Kadish, M. Levetown, J. T. Truman, B. S. Wilfond, C. E. Harrison, A. Kazura, E. Krug III, P. A. Schwartz et al. 2001. "Ethical Issues with Genetic Testing in Pediatrics." *Pediatrics* 107:1451–1455.

Newborn Screening [NBS] Task Force. 2000. "Serving the Family from Birth to the Medical Home. Newborn Screening: A Blueprint for the Future. A Call for a National Agenda on State Newborn Screening Programs." *Pediatrics* 106:386–427.

Oliver, L. 2002. "Newborn Genetic Screening." *Genetics Brief* 10, National Conference of State Legislatures. June.

Parsons, E., and D. M. Bradley. 2003. "Psychosocial Issues in Newborn Screening for Cystic Fibrosis." *Pediatric Respiratory Reviews* 4:285–292.

Parton, N. 1994. "'Problematics of Government,' (Post) Modernity, and Social Work." *British Journal of Social Work* 24:9–32.

Paul, D. 1997. "The History of Newborn Phenylketonuria Screening in the U.S." In *Promoting Safe and Effective Genetic Testing in the United States: Final Report of the Task Force on Genetic Testing*, ed. N. A. Holtzman and M. S. Watson, 137–160. Bethesda, Md.: National Institutes of Health.

———. 1998. *The Politics of Heredity: Essays on Eugenics, Biomedicine, and the Nature-Nurture Debate*. New York: State University of New York Press.

———. 1999. "Contesting Consent: The Challenge to Compulsory Neonatal Screening for PKU." *Perspectives in Biology and Medicine* 42:207–219.

———. 2000. "A Double-Edged Sword." *Nature* 405:515.

———. 2008. "Patient Advocacy in Newborn Screening: Continuities and Discontinuities." *American Journal of Medical Genetics*. Part C, *Seminars in Medical Genetics* 148C:8–14.

Paul, D., and P. J. Edelson. 1998. "The Struggle over Metabolic Screening." In *Molecularising Biology and Medicine: New Practices and Alliances, 1930s–1970s*, ed. S. de Chadarevian and H. Kamminga, 203–220. Reading, U.K.: Harwood Academic Publishers.

Penticuff, J. H. 1996. "Ethical Dimensions in Genetic Screening: A Look into the Future." *Journal of Obstetric, Gynecologic, and Neonatal Nursing* 14:785–789.

Peters, B. G., and B. W. Hogwood. 1985. "In Search of the Issue-Attention Cycle." *Journal of Politics* 47:238–253.

Petersen, A., and R. Bunton. 2002. *The New Genetics and the Public's Health*. London: Routledge.

Petersen, A., and D. Lupton. 1996. *The New Public Health: Health and Self in the Age of Risk*. London: Sage Publications.

Pollack, A. 2008. "Redefining Disease, Genes and All." *New York Times*. May 6.

Popenoe, D. 1988. *Disturbing the Nest: Family Change and Decline in Modern Societies*. New York: Aldine de Gruyter.

Poppelaars, F.A.M., L. Henneman, H. J. Adèr, M. C. Cornel, R.P.M.G. Hermens, G. Van Der Wal, and L. P. Ten Kate. 2004. "Preconceptional Cystic Fibrosis Carrier Screening: Attitudes and Intentions of the Target Population." *Genetic Testing* 8:80–89.

Potter, B. K., D. Avard, and B. J. Wilson. 2008. "Newborn Blood Spot Screening in Four Countries: Stakeholder Involvement." *Journal of Public Health Policy* 29:121–142.

PR Newswire. 2004. "March of Dimes Statement on Newborn Screening Report." September 22. www.LexisNexis.com/hottopics/lnacademic.

———. 2008. "Pro Football Hall of Fame Member Jim Kelly Urges Congress to Approve the Newborn Screening Saves Lives Act; Legislation to Improve Screening of Newborns Vulnerable for Rare Metabolic Conditions." April 8. Press release available from March of Dimes, http://www.marchofdimes.com/.

———. 2009. "States Expand Newborn Screening for Life-Threatening Disorders; New March of Dimes Report Finds State-by-State Gaps Nearly Eliminated." February 18. www.LexisNexis.com/hottopics/lnacademic.

Prasad, A., E. Main, and M. E. Dodd. 2008. "Findings Consensus on the Physiotherapy Management of Asymptomatic Infants with Cystic Fibrosis." *Pediatric Pulmonology* 43:236–244.

President's Council on Bioethics. 2008. *The Changing Moral Focus of Newborn Screening: An Ethical Analysis by the President's Council on Bioethics.* Washington, D.C.: President's Council on Bioethics.

Prosser, L. A., J. A. Ladapo, D. Rusinak, and S. E. Waisbren. 2008. "Parental Tolerance of False-Positive Newborn Screening Results." *Archives of Pediatric and Adolescent Medicine* 162:870–876.

Putnam, R. 2001. *Bowling Alone: The Collapse and Revival of American Community.* New York: Simon and Schuster.

Quittner, A. L., D. L. Espelage, L. C. Opipari, B. Carter, N. Eid, and H. Eigen. 1998. "Role Strain in Couples with and without a Child with Chronic Illness: Associations with Marital Satisfaction, Intimacy, and Daily Mood." *American Psychological Association* 17:112–124.

Rapp, R. 2000. *Testing Women, Testing the Fetus: The Social Impact of Amniocentesis in America.* New York: Routledge.

Reventlow, S., A. C. Hvas, and K. Malterud. 2006. "Making the Invisible Body Visible: Bone Scans, Osteoporosis, and Women's Bodily Experiences." *Social Science and Medicine* 62:2720–2731.

Richards, M.P.M. 1993. "The New Genetics: Some Issues for Social Scientists." *Sociology of Health and Illness* 15:567–586.

Rieff, P. 1966. *The Triumph of the Therapeutic: Uses of Faith after Freud.* New York: Harper and Row.

Riessman, C. 1990. "Strategic Uses of *Narrative in the Presentation of Self and Illness.*" *Social Science and Medicine* 30(11):1195–1200.

Rose, N. 1989. *Governing the Soul: The Shaping of the Private Self.* 2d ed. London: Routledge.

Roser, M. A. 2009. "Blood Storage Changes Sought." *Austin American-Statesman.* March 6.

Rosner, J. 2004. "Lullabies for Sophia." *Hastings Center Report* 34(6):20–21.

Ross, L. F. 2003. "Minimizing Risks: The Ethics of Predictive Diabetes Mellitus Screening Research in Newborns." *Archives of Pediatrics and Adolescent Medicine* 157:89–95.

Rothenberg, L. 2003. *Breathing for a Living: A Memoir.* New York: Hyperion.

Rothman, B. K. 1986. *The Tentative Pregnancy.* New York: Viking.

———. 1989. *Recreating Motherhood.* New York: Norton.

———. 1993. *Encyclopedia of Childbearing.* New York: Henry Holt.

———. 1998. *Genetic Maps and Human Imaginations.* New York: Norton.

————. 2000. *Spoiling the Pregnancy: The Introduction of Prenatal Diagnosis to the Netherlands*. Bilthoven, Netherlands: Catharina Schrader Stichting of the Dutch Organization of Midwives.

Rubin, R. 2006. "Saved by a Drop of Blood; States Expand Routine Testing of Newborns." *USA Today*. July, 9D.

Ryan, C. 1991. *Prime Time Activism: Media Strategies for Grassroots Organizing*. Boston: South End Press.

Salander, P. 2002. "Bad News from the Patient's Perspective: An Analysis of the Written Narratives of Newly Diagnosed Cancer Patients." *Social Science and Medicine* 55:721–732.

Sandel, M. J. 2004. "The Case against Perfection." *The Atlantic*. April, 51–62.

Sawyer, S. M., B. Cerritelli, L. C. Carter, M. Cooke, J. A. Glazner, and J. Massie. 2006. "Changing Their Minds with Time: A Comparison of Hypothetical and Actual Reproductive Behaviors in Parents of Children with Cystic Fibrosis." *Pediatrics* 118:e649–e656.

Schild, S. 1979. "Psychological Issues in Genetic Counseling of Phenylketonuria." In *Genetic Counseling: Psychological Dimensions*, ed. S. Kessler. New York: Academic Press.

Schlesinger, M. Forthcoming. "The Canary in the Gemeinschaft: The Public Voice of Patients as a Means of Enhancing Health System Performance." In *Patients as Policy Actors*, ed. B. Hoffman, N. Tomes, R. Grob, and M. Schlesinger. New Brunswick, N.J.: Rutgers University Press.

Schneider, C. E. 2008. "Personal Statement." In *The Changing Moral Focus of Newborn Screening: An Ethical Analysis by the President's Council on Bioethics*, 121–124. Washington, D.C.: President's Council on Bioethics.

Schubert, D., and M. Murphy. 2005. "The Struggle to Breathe: Living the Life of Expectancy with Cystic Fibrosis." *Oral History Review* 32:35–55.

Scotet, V., M. De Braekeleer, G. Rault, P. Parent, M. Dagome, H. Journel, A. Lemoigne, J.-P. Codet, M. Catheline, V. David et al. 2000. "Neonatal Screening for Cystic Fibrosis in Brittany, France: Assessment of 10 Years' Experience and Impact on Prenatal Diagnosis." *Lancet* 356:789–794.

Shamoo, A. E., and F. A. Kihn-Maung-Gyi. 2002. *Ethics of the Use of Human Subjects in Research*. London: Garland Science Publishing.

Sims, E. J., A. Clark, J. McCormick, G. Mehta, G. Connett, and A. Mehta. 2007. "Cystic Fibrosis Diagnosed after 2 Months of Age Leads to Worse Outcomes and Requires More Therapy." *Pediatrics* 119:19–28.

Skinner, D., K. Sparkman, and D. Bailey. 2003. "Screening for Fragile X Syndrome: Parent Attitudes and Perspectives." *Genetics in Medicine* 55:378–384.

Smith, K. C., D. Twum, and A. C. Gielen. 2009. "Media Coverage of Celebrity DUIs: Teachable Moments or Problematic Social Modeling?" *Alcohol and Alcoholism* 44:256–260.

Somerson, M. D. 2000. "State Urged to Test Babies for More Disorders." *Columbus Dispatch* (Ohio). February 14.

Southern, K. W. 2004. "Newborn Screening for Cystic Fibrosis: The Practical Implications." *Journal of the Royal Society of Medicine* 97, Suppl. 44:57–59.

Stacey, M. 1994. "The Power of Lay Knowledge." In *Researching the People's Health*, ed. J. Popay and G. Williams, 85–98. London: Routledge.

States News Service. 2008a. "Dodd, Hatch Laud House Passage of Their Bill to Improve Health Screenings for Newborn Children." April 8. http://www.marchofdimes.com/.

———. 2008b. "Congresswoman Lucille Roybal-Allard Newborn Screening Saves Lives Act Wins Final Passage in Congress." April 8. www.LexisNexis.com/hottopics/lnacademic.

Stearns, P. 2003. *Anxious Parents: A History of Modern Childrearing in America.* New York: New York University Press.

Stein, R. 2009. "Some Samples Are Stored and Used for Research without Parents' Consent." *Washington Post.* June 30.

Strauss, A. L., and J. M. Corbin. 1990. *Basics for Qualitative Research: Grounded Theory Procedures and Techniques.* Newbury Park, Calif.: Sage Publications.

Sweetman, L., D. S. Millington, B. L. Therrell, W. Hannon, B. Popovich, M. S. Watson, M. Y. Mann, M. A. Lloyd-Puryear, and P. C. van Dyck. 2006. "Naming and Counting Disorders (Conditions) Included in Newborn Screening Panels." *Pediatrics* 117:S308–S314.

Szasz, T. 1961. *The Myth of Mental Illness.* New York: Harper and Row.

Taner-Leff, P., and E. H. Walizer. 1992. *Building the Healing Partnership: Parents, Professionals, and Children with Chronic Illnesses and Disabilities.* Brookline, Mass.: Brookline Books.

Tarini, B. A., W. Burke, C. R. Scott, and B. S. Wilfond. 2008. "Waiving Informed Consent in Newborn Screening Research: Balancing Social Value and Respect." *American Journal of Medical Genetics.* Part C, *Seminars in Medical Genetics* 148C:23–30.

Tarini, B. A., D. A. Christakis, and H. G. Welch. 2006. "State Newborn Screening in the Tandem Mass Spectrometry Era: More Tests, More False-Positive Results." *Pediatrics* 118:448–456.

Tarini, B. A., D. Singer, S. Clark, and M. Davis. 2009. "Parents' Interest in Predictive Genetic Testing for Their Children When a Disease Has No Treatment." *Pediatrics* 124:e432–e438.

Tassicker, R. J., B. Teltscher, M. K. Trembath, V. Collins, L. J. Sheffield, E. Chiu, L. Gurrin, and M. B. Delatycki. 2009. "Problems Assessing Uptake of Huntington Disease Predictive Testing and a Proposed Solution." *European Journal of Human Genetics* 1:66–70.

Taylor, B. 2009. "Missouri Family Seeks More Newborn Testing." Associated Press state and local wire. April 9.

Themba, M. 1999. *Making Policy/Making Change: How Communities Are Taking Law into Their Own Hands.* Berkeley, Calif.: Chardon Press.

Therrell, B. 2001. "U.S. Newborn Screening Policy Dilemmas for the Twenty-first Century." *Molecular Genetics and Metabolism* 74:64–74.

Tibbena, A. 2007. "Predictive Testing for Huntington's Disease." *Brain Research Bulletin* 72:165–171.

Tluczek, A., R. L. Koscik, P. M. Farrell, and M. J. Rock. 2005. "Psychosocial Risk Associated with Newborn Screening for Cystic Fibrosis: Parents' Experience While Awaiting the Sweat-Test Appointment." *Pediatrics* 115:1692–1703.

Tomes, N. 2006. "Patient as a Policy Factor: A Historical Case Study of the Patient/Survivor Movement in Mental Health." *Health Affairs* 25:720–729.

———. 2007. "Patient Empowerment and the Dilemmas of Late-Modern Medicalisation." *Lancet* 369:698–700.

Urban, P. 2007. "Newborn Test Program Boosted." *Connecticut Post Online.* December 14. www.LexisNexis.com/hottopics/lnacademic.

U.S. General Accounting Office [U.S. GAO]. 2003. *Newborn Screening: Characteristics of State Programs.* GAO-03-449.

Wailoo, K., and S. Pemberton. 2006. *Troubled Dream of Genetic Medicine: Ethnicity and Innovation in Tay-Sachs, Cystic Fibrosis, and Sickle Cell Disease.* Baltimore: Johns Hopkins University Press.

Waisbren, S. E., S. Albers, S. Amato, M. Ampola, T. G. Brewster, L. Demmer, R. B. Eaton, R. Greenstein, M. Korson, and C. Larson. 2003. "Effect of Expanded Newborn Screening for Biochemical Genetic Disorders on Child Outcomes and Parental Stress." *JAMA* 290:2564–2574.

Wald, N. 2007. "Neonatal Screening: Old Dogma or Sound Principle?" *Pediatrics* 119:406–407.

Waldholz, M. 2004. "Parents Prod States to Boost Newborn Testing." *Wall Street Journal.* July 30.

Wallack, L., L. Dorfman, D. Jernigan, and M. Themba-Nixon. 1993. "Thinking Media Advocacy." In *Media Advocacy and Public Health*, ed. L. Wallack, L. Dorfman, D. Jenigan, and M. Themba-Nixon, 86–120. Newbury Park, Calif.: Sage Publications.

Warren, N. S., T. P. Carter, J. R. Humbert, and P. T. Rowley. 1982. "Newborn Screening for Hemoglobinopathies in New York State: Experience of Physicians and Parents of Affected Children." *Journal of Pediatrics* 100:373–377.

Watson, M. S. 2006. "Current Status of Newborn Screening: Decision-Making about the Conditions to Include in Screening Programs." *Mental Retardation and Developmental Disabilities Research Reviews* 12:230–235.

Watson, M. S., M. Y. Mann, M. A. Lloyd-Puryear, P. Rinaldo, R. R. Howell, and American College of Medical Genetics Newborn Screening Expert Group. 2006. "Newborn Screening: Toward a Uniform Screening Panel and System—Executive Summary." *Pediatrics* 117:S296–S307.

Wertz, D. C., and J. C. Fletcher. 2004. *Genetics and Ethics in Global Perspective.* Dordrecht, Netherlands: Kluwer Academic.

White, D. 2000. "Consumer and Community Participation: A Reassessment of Process, Impact, and Value." In *The Handbook of Social Studies in Health and Medicine*, ed. G. Albrecht, R. Fitzpatrick, and S. Scrimshaw. Thousand Oaks, Calif.: Sage Publications.

Whitehead, N. S., D. S. Brown, and C. M. Layton. 2010. *Developing a Conjoint Analysis Survey of Parental Attitudes Regarding Voluntary Newborn Screening.* RTI Press Publication MR-0014–1002. Research Triangle Park, N.C.: RTI International.

Wieser, B. 2010. "Public Accountability of Newborn Screening: Collective Knowing and Deciding." *Social Science and Medicine* 70:926–933.

Wilcken, B. 2003. "Ethical Issues in Newborn Screening and the Impact of New Technologies." *European Journal of Pediatrics* 162:S62–S66.

Wilcken, B., V. Wiley, J. Hammond, and K. Carpenter. 2003. "Screening Newborns for Inborn Errors of Metabolism by Tandem Mass Spectrometry." *New England Journal of Medicine* 348:2304–2312.

Wilcox, S. 2010. "Lay Knowledge: the Missing Middle of the Expertise Debates." In *Configuring Health Consumers: Health Work and the Imperative of Personal Responsibility*, ed. R. Harris, N. Wathen, and S. Wyatt, 45–64. Hampshire, U.K.: Palgrave Macmillan.

Wilfond, B. S. 1995. "Screening Policy for Cystic Fibrosis: The Role of Evidence." *Hastings Center Report* 25:S21–S24.

Wilfond, B. S., R. B. Parad, and N. Fost. 2005. "Balancing Benefits and Risks for Cystic Fibrosis Newborn Screening: Implications for Policy Decisions." *Journal of Pediatrics* 147, 3 Suppl.:S109–S113.

Wilson, J.M.G., and G. Jungner. 1968. *Principles and Practice of Screening for Disease.* Geneva: World Health Organization.

World Health Organization [WHO]. 2000. *Classification of Cystic Fibrosis and Related Disorders.* Report of a joint WHO/ICF(M)A/ECFS/ECFTN Meeting. June, Stockholm, Sweden.

Wright, L., A. Brown, and A. Davidson-Mundt. 1992. "Newborn Screening: The Miracle and the Challenge." *Journal of Pediatric Nursing* 7:26–42.

Wrigley, J. 1989. "Do Young Children Need Intellectual Stimulation? Experts' Advice to Parents, 1900–1985." *History of Education Quarterly* 29:41–75.

Wynne, S. K. 2006. "A Fighting Chance." *St. Petersburg Times* (Florida). April 25.

Zelkowitz, P., A. Papageorgiou, C. Bardin, and T. Wang. 2009. "Persistent Maternal Anxiety Affects the Interaction between Mothers and Their Very Low Birthweight Children at 24 Months." *Early Human Development* 85:51–58.

Index

abnormal screen results: with inconclusive follow-up, 217; increasing number of, 207; and parental support, 224; parents' reaction to, 21, 42; recipients of, 161. *See also* positive screening results

Accurso, Frank J., 31

ACMG. *See* American College of Medical Genetics

administrators, NBS, 199, 200; concerns of, 138–139; interviews with, 160, 240n. 2. *See also* directors

advisory boards, 180

Advisory Committee on Heritable Disorders in Newborns and Children, HHS, 191, 229

advisory committees, 181, 241n. 20; Canadian, 242n. 23; and issues of representation, 179–180; membership of, 177; parents on, 176, 179–180; recruitment for, 241n. 21; tension on, 178–179

advocacy: diverse strategies for, 181–182; in history of NBS, 227; and media coverage, 182–184; process of, 184

advocacy, ad hoc, 167–171, 168; and new NBS, 180; recruitment of, 176–177, 241n. 21

advocacy, parental: in media, 184; motivation for, 147; population-based focus for, 164

advocacy groups/organizations: formal, 172–173; impact on NBS expansion of, 174–175; and new NBS, 180; recruitment of, 176–177, 241n. 21; work of, 173

advocates: for NBS expansion, 161–162; parents as, 142–151. *See also* parent advocates

African Americans, cystic fibrosis among, 30

Alexander, Duane, 11, 188, 189, 191

alternative or complementary health care, 239n. 1

American Academy of Pediatrics, 6

American College of Medical Genetics (ACMG), 21, 64; on conditions for NBS, 13; recommendations of, 10–11, 235n. 7; 2005 report of, 15, 99, 173, 174, 175, 180, 182, 185, 186, 198, 229, 235n. 6, 241n. 13, 242n. 29

American College of Obstetricians and Gynecologists (ACOG), 53

American Society of Human Genetics, 21

amniocentesis, impact of, 232

antibiotics, 101

anxiety, of parents, 86–88

Aronowitz, Robert, 211

Asian Americans, cystic fibrosis among, 30

Association for Retarded Citizens, 5

asymptomatic children, 211; and discourse of danger, 244n. 4; families of, 157–158; parenthood and, 219; parents of, 93–94, 95, 157–159; in risk discourse, 212; and risk of doubt, 219

Austria, knowledge and collective choice in, 228–229

autism, and public policy, 163

Baily, MaryAnn, 20, 196

Baio, Renee, 171

Baio, Scott, 171

benefits of NBS, 184; "being prepared," 214; in cystic fibrosis, 33; identification of affected children, 186. *See also* "diagnostic odyssey"

Bioethics, President's Council on, 188, 189

birth: beginning preventive care at, 107; parents of children diagnosed at, 202; saving lives by preventing, 200–206; testing at, 23

blood spot, heel: concerns about storage and use of, 242n. 24; and MS/MS, 164. *See also* heel stick

Bluebond-Langner, Myra, 110

Boland, Carol, 95

experts, role of, 231–232. *See also*
    professionals, health care

false-positive results, 18–19; avoidance of,
    62; in CF screening, 19; family reaction
    to, 20, 22
families: with asymptomatic children,
    157–158, 158–159; consequences of NBS
    for, 4; impact of false-positive screening
    results on, 22; impact of professional
    expectations on, 154; new CF diagnosis
    in, 73–74, 238n. 18; reaction to
    false positives of, 20; support and
    services for, 224
family history: and CF diagnosis, 51; and
    follow-up tests, 62
family planning, NBS's impact on, 201–203,
    243n. 44
Family Support Group for Fatty Oxidation
    Disorders, 173
fathers, interviews with, 35–36
fetal alcohol syndrome, and parent
    advocates, 163
"fighter moms," 163
follow-up, 139; access to, 17; for
    asymptomatic babies, 239n. 3; parent
    reliance on, 125
follow-up testing: and family history, 62;
    overseeing of, 157
fostering dependency scale, 95
Fox, Michelle, 192
Fox, Renee, 136
fragile X syndrome, 212
Frank, Arthur, 24, 117
Freidson, Eliot, 112
future: planning for, 118; providers'
    circumspection about, 140

GA1 disorder, 171
galactosemia, 19, 171
gene therapy, 110
Genetic Alliance, 172, 185, 208
"genetic citizenship," 207
genetic counseling, 23, 224
genetic counselors, and efficacy of NBS, 192
genetic diagnosis: devastation of, 38;
    effect of, 2; parents' experience with,
    38; and phenotypic expression, 13;
    presymptomatic, 12; and uncertainty, 12

genetic disorders, 116, 172, 207; clinical
    manifestations of, 40; diagnosis of,
    39–46; and "geneticization" of patient,
    210; newborns with, 55; parental
    response to, 34; and politics of
    nomenclature, 199; risk for, 163–164;
    separated from identity, 233; testing for,
    190–191; threat of, 195–197; treatability
    of, 165, 166
genetic information: importance of, 8;
    inadequate protection of, 18; value of, 10.
    See also information
Genetic Information Nondiscrimination Act
    (2008), 225
genetic profiling, 208; newborn, 213;
    vs. health promotion, 228
genetics, media coverage of, 16–17
genetic testing, in U.S., 5–6, 235n. 2.
    See also newborn screening
genetic traits, in newborn screening, 1
genomic revolution, 15
Georgia, 196
germs, parental concern about, 87–88
Giordano, Jessica, 3
grandparents, and CF diagnosis, 75
Green, Michael, 8
Green, Morris, 21
grief, parental, 35
Grosse, Scott, 13
grounded theory, 25, 28
Guthrie, Robert, 5

Hatch, Sen. Orrin, 231
health: defining, 23; social determinants of,
    195–196
health care providers, 120; caution of, 141;
    "cookie-cutter approaches" of, 128, 135;
    information withheld by, 129–131; and
    medical uncertainty, 224; number and
    diversity of, 142, 239n. 5; parent reliance
    on, 124–128, 125–126; paternalism of,
    130–131; in postdiagnosis period, 133;
    reliance on, 143–144; unpreparedness
    of, 137. *See also* professionals, health
    care
health care system, transforming policy in,
    225–226
health information: life-altering, 50; for new
    parents, 44–45; parents' access to, 58–59;

About the Author

Rachel Grob, M.A., Ph.D., is Scholar in Residence and Director of National Initiatives at the Center for Patient Partnerships, University of Wisconsin–Madison. She is also a faculty member in the Health Advocacy Program and consultant to the Child Development Institute at Sarah Lawrence College. Grob holds a B.A. from Wesleyan University, an M.A. in health advocacy from Sarah Lawrence College, and a Ph.D. in sociology from the City University of New York Graduate Center.

Leo B. Slater, *War and Disease: Biomedical Research on Malaria in the Twentieth Century*

Matthew Smith, *An Alternative History of Hyperactivity: Food Additives and the Feingold Diet*

Rosemary A. Stevens, Charles E. Rosenberg, and Lawton R. Burns, eds., *History and Health Policy in the United States: Putting the Past Back In*

Barbra Mann Wall, *American Catholic Hospitals: A Century of Changing Markets and Missions*